WOOD
IN AUSTRALIA
Types, properties and uses

SECOND EDITION

T0357942

WOOD
IN AUSTRALIA
Types, properties and uses

SECOND EDITION

KEITH R. BOOTLE

The *McGraw·Hill* Companies

Sydney New York San Francisco Auckland
Bangkok Bogotá Caracas Hong Kong
Kuala Lumpur Lisbon London Madrid
Mexico City Milan New Delhi San Juan
Seoul Singapore Taipei Toronto

National Library of Australia Cataloguing-in-Publication data:

Bootle, K.R. (Keith R.).
Wood in Australia.

    2nd ed.
    Includes index.
    ISBN 10: 0071014012
    ISBN 13: 9780071014014

    1. Wood—Australia—Handbooks, manuals, etc. 2. Timber—Australia—
    Handbooks, manuals, etc. I. Title.

674.10994

Published in Australia by
McGraw-Hill Australia Pty Ltd
Level 2, 82 Waterloo Road, North Ryde NSW 2113
Acquisitions editor: Meiling Voon
Cover and internal design: Jan Schmoeger, Designpoint
Cover image: Forests NSW
Production editor: Sybil Kesteven
Copy editor: Carolyn Pike
Illustrator: Dimitrios Prokopis, Provisuals Visuals & Design
Proofreader: Tim Learner
Indexer: Max McMaster
Typeset in 9/10 Trump Mediaeval by Jan Schmoeger, Designpoint
Printed in Australia by SOS Print + Media

Contents

About the author

Keith Bootle was educated at Dubbo High School and Sydney University before joining what was then the Forestry Commission of New South Wales in 1949 as a research officer in the Division of Wood Technology. In 1953 he became officer-in-charge of the Commission's wood utilisation activities. He retired from the Commission in 1983 and died in 1992.

His first book, *Commercial Timbers of New South Wales and Their Use,* was published in 1971.

The first edition of *Wood in Australia* received the National Book Award of the Building Science Forum of Australia in 1985.

This second edition was prepared as a collaboration between Forests NSW, the Timber Development Association of NSW and the Forest and Wood Products Research and Development Corporation. Through their guidance this book has been updated so that it remains the industry's premier text.

Individuals and organisations with the relevant experience in the field of expertise required for each chapter were used as reviewers, making changes or additions as necessary. Every effort has been made to maintain the original character and style of the book so it remains the work of Keith Bootle. Corrections, additions and amendments have been undertaken to reflect the changes in the industry or in timber supply that have occurred since this book was first written.

Introduction

While there are many publications available on the scientific studies of the use of forest products in Australia, especially from the CSIRO and the State Forestry Departments, in the early 1980s a need had existed for some time for a book that provided a brief summary of the main aspects of wood utilisation—not only for the timber producer and user but also for the general reader.

In earlier years, such publications as E. H. F. Swain's *Timbers and Forest Products of Queensland* (1928), I. H. Boas's *Commercial Timbers of Australia* (1947), N. K. Wallis's *Australian Timber Handbook* (1956), and K. R. Bootle's *Commercial Timbers of New South Wales and Their Use* (1971) served this purpose in varying degrees, but these sources of information had become out of date.

The nature of the timber resource was changing significantly. The virgin forests of large-diameter trees had been largely cut over, not only in this country but in most parts of the world's readily accessible forests. The main supplies of timber for general construction purposes were destined to come from intensively managed plantation stands, harvested at a relatively early age because of the effect of compound interest charges on the cost of production.

Such artificial forests were predicted to yield wood products that may be somewhat different from those of the past. Changes in strength, shrinkage and durability would need to be determined and there would be a greater recourse to reconstituted products, such as particleboard, hardboard and fibreboard, to achieve full utilisation of the thinnings from such forests. However, one must bear in mind that there is a very considerable energy saving in utilising such trees, whenever possible, in the form of sawn timber rather than as reconstituted board material. The increasing use of wood residue for fuel and for composting was also predicted to create competition for the raw material of reconstituted products.

Sawmilling practices were also undergoing change. The thick, large-diameter saws that were used to convert the huge trees of the past into usable timber were obviously inappropriate for cutting small plantation logs. The young, rapidly grown plantation tree was (and still is) subject to considerable growth stress, especially the hardwood species, and this characteristic complicated the task of designing the most appropriate sawmilling and drying equipment.

The rapid decline in availability of the rainforest species of fine appearance and medium density was a worldwide phenomenon. In Australia it led to greater consideration for decorative use of many of our eucalypt hardwoods, of rich colour and beautiful figure, but which could present production difficulties because of their high density. However, these difficulties had not been insurmountable, as was already indicated by the increasing use of a number of hardwoods as furniture, polished flooring and decorative panelling.

Because of space it had not been possible in the book to deal in depth with the various topics, so further sources of information were suggested at appropriate points. The species whose general properties were described were limited to those that were subjectively selected as being of general interest or commercial importance. However, the number of other species of local and overseas origin deserving of mention was such as would occupy another book. The further reading list on page 363 provides a source of information on many such species.

Keith Bootle's working life was associated with the Forestry Commission of New South Wales (now called Forests NSW) in the field of wood utilisation and the text inevitably concentrated, to some extent, on eastern Australian species but every effort was made to incorporate the main species of all the other states in addition to those species of other countries that received some mention in Australia.

Some 22 years have passed since this book was first published in 1983. Obviously, there have been a number of significant changes in sections of the production processes of timber and timber products and, indeed, in the utilisation of timber and timber products since then.

Accordingly, it was considered that it was now an appropriate time to review this book so that it might reflect the changes in knowledge, practices and methods of production and utilisation.

The changes in some instances have been rather subtle; in some instances, a little more dramatic. Such changes include:

- some of the species harvested in 1983, such as brushwoods and rainforest species, are no longer harvested
- the timber resource available for harvesting has decreased considerably with the increase in National Parks
- there is greater use of manufactured timber, called engineered wood products, in ever-growing volumes
- drying techniques have been refined and species not considered suitable for drying in the past are now regularly dried for decorative products, such as flooring and furniture
- some of the chemicals used to preservative treat timbers in the early 1980s have been replaced with new chemicals that have new methods of treatment—a number of the chemicals are still used but the retention and penetration requirements have changed
- there is a greater consideration of how timber will perform in fires, which is reflected in a new chapter that has been added
- multi-storey residential construction using timber as the framework is now commonplace
- requirements today for thermal efficiency and sound insulation for single- and multi-residential buildings have become much more

'demanding' on the materials used for construction compared with the requirements of the early 1980s—timber has a part to play here

- the new Australian Standard for durability gives appropriate durability ratings for timber that is used externally but not in ground contact—in the 1980s we just had to assume that the timber that was used in such a situation would perform at least as well as its in-ground rating predicted; because of the ratings for external above-ground use, many timbers can now be used even though Standards prevented their use in the 1980s—this Standard for durability has made an impact on Part 2 of the book
- with all the progress in the timber and associated industries, many Australian Standards have been updated to accommodate the advancements—there are some new Standards and some have been withdrawn so that the review of this book brings all the references to appropriate Standards up to date.

Acknowledgments

Keith Bootle acknowledged the invaluable help received over many years from other workers in wood science and technology in Australia and overseas and, in particular, from his colleagues in the Wood Technology and Forest Research Division of the Forestry Commission of New South Wales.

A number of organisations and individuals assisted with this review. Their contribution is gratefully acknowledged. Contributors to the review included:

- Charlie Herbert of Forests NSW and Andrew Dunn of the Timber Development Association (TDA) of NSW—Chapters 1, 11, 12, 13, 18, 20 and 22 and Part 2 Timber Properties
- Barry La Fontaine—Chapter 11
- Bruce Stevenson of the Wood Panel Association of Australia—Chapter 10
- Simon Dorries of the Plywood Association of Australasia—Chapter 9
- Harry Greaves—Chapters 15, 16 and 19
- Colin Mackenzie and Dave Haywood of Timber Queensland—Chapters 5, 6, 7, 14 and 17
- Boris Iskra of the Timber Promotion Council—Chapters 2 and 4
- Geoff Boughton of TimberEd—Chapters 3 and 8
- Andrew Dunn of TDA NSW—new chapter 21
- Dave Barnes of NSW Department of Primary Industries—most of the photographs

Part 1

Wood: characteristics and applications

Chapter 1

The nature of wood

All plant material consists of cells of various shapes and arrangements. The presence of the very complex organic substance known as *lignin* is an essential feature of those plants described as being 'woody'. It bonds the various types of cell together, producing the degree of rigidity that is associated with wood, and enables woody plants to attain their large size.

Structural components

All wood cells are formed in the very narrow *cambium layer*, which separates bark and wood. On its inner side new cells are continuously added to the *xylem* (woody tissue transporting mineral nutrients and water upward), while on its outer side new cells are added to the *phloem* (bark-like tissue that transports food material downward).

The cell wall is made up of a network of *microfibrils*, which are complex chains of cellulose molecules. Aggregations of microfibrils are sometimes called *micelles*. As the cell matures, further layers of microfibrils are formed at angles to each other. These layers are often referred to as the S1, S2 and S3 layers and compose the secondary wall. The membrane at the outside of these layers, which separates the cells from each other, is called the *middle lamella*. The term *micellar angle* often appears in discussions about longitudinal shrinkage. It is a measurable attribute of the tree that can be useful in tree breeding work, and is measured in the S2 layer, which is much wider than the other layers. The smaller the micellar angle to the longitudinal axis, the greater the tensile strength of the fibre and the smaller its shrinkage.

In some regions of the cell wall the secondary wall does not develop; these regions are called *pits* and they permit liquids to flow from one cell to another. The pits vary in shape and size and may have a flexible membrane, which can close (aspirate) if air enters the adjacent cell or if heartwood is formed. Aspiration is a feature of earlywood pits; latewood pits do not close.

When the formation of the cell wall is complete, impregnation with lignin begins in the middle lamella and gradually extends throughout the cell wall. The many capillaries present between the microfibrils become filled with polyphenols and other extractives when sapwood changes into heartwood.

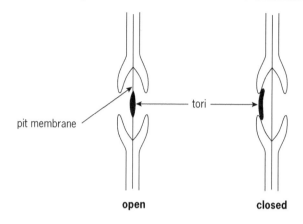

Fig. 1.1 Diagram of pits between cells. Magnification × 2000. The pit membrane has a thickened centre (the torus) supported by a flexible cellulose web, which allows it to move across and block the opening of the pit

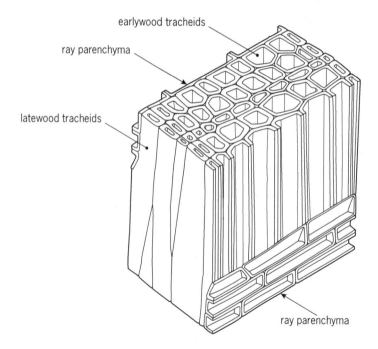

Fig. 1.2 Diagram of a cube of softwood. Magnification × 250. The pits in the cell walls have been omitted

The newly formed cell on the inner side of the cambium may become one of four types of wood tissue: *parenchyma cell, fibre, tracheid* and *vessel*. Each type of tissue serves one or more special functions: the parenchyma cells conduct and store food materials and water; the fibre's main role is to provide mechanical support; and tracheids and vessels conduct water and dissolved mineral salts from the roots to the leaves to provide basic materials for photosynthesis, as well as providing mechanical support. The term 'fibre' is loosely applied in general use, embracing the tracheid as well. Vessels (also called 'pores') occur only in hardwoods and are their main distinguishing feature. Softwoods are much less complex in structure than hardwoods and their cells are of simpler form.

Parenchyma cells are brick-shaped, with thin walls and simple pits. Tracheids are elongated cells with rounded ends and walls that have characteristic pits. Fibres are long, pointed cells with very small pits. Tracheids, which are not common in hardwoods, are longer (3–8 mm) than fibres (0.7–2 mm). Vessels are formed from a vertical row of cells whose end walls disappear to produce a long pipe.

On the outer side of the cambium a new layer of bark is formed continuously to protect the new tissue on the inner side against water loss and fungal invasion. The bark has to suffer splitting to accommodate

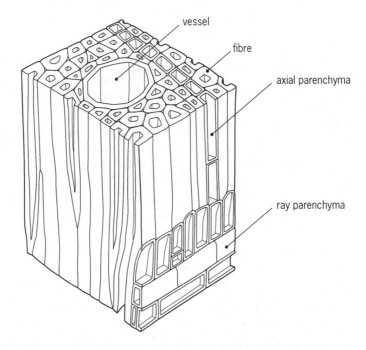

Fig. 1.3 Diagram of a cube of hardwood. Magnification × 250. The pits in the cell walls have been omitted

the increase in girth and thus produces the fissured surface common on those trees that do not lose their outer bark annually.

Another type of wood tissue, the *ray*, links all the above-mentioned types. It extends from the inner bark right across to the pith at the centre of the tree. The rays consist mainly of parenchyma cells (Plate 1) and enable liquids to move between the various types of tissue; they function as the conveyor and storer of plant food. The parenchyma cells lose this ability with the transition from sapwood to heartwood.

Sapwood and heartwood

Heartwood (sometimes given the name 'truewood') appears to provide only structural support for the plant; its cells become blocked with deposits that contribute considerably to the colour of the wood and are mainly responsible for the enhanced durability of heartwood.

At the time of heartwood formation, balloon-shaped intrusions called *tyloses* extend from the parenchyma into the vessels of hardwoods and sometimes into the resin canals of pines, and they also contribute to the clogging of the tissue. The combination of deposits and tyloses make heartwood difficult to penetrate with preservatives. Closing of the pits between some cells at heartwood formation also adds to the difficulty of penetration.

The amount of sapwood present on a tree stem is a genetic characteristic of a species and varies from a narrow band of perhaps 10 mm to instances where the whole cross-section of a large tree is sapwood.

There are numerous theories seeking to explain why sapwood is converted to heartwood but it seems clear that as a tree gets bigger there is usually no need for the whole cross-section to be involved in the conduction of sap and the storing of food reserves. A balance is reached: the redundant sapwood is converted into physiologically inert heartwood and the valuable minerals previously held in these cells are used to promote the production of more wood. Thus, the tree makes full use of the minerals within reach of its root system. In some species (e.g. spotted gum), there can be a transition zone between sapwood and heartwood but usually there is a sharp line of demarcation indicated by a distinctive change in the colour of the wood, provided that it is not a pale-coloured species.

Although the moisture content of the sapwood in green timber is usually considerably higher than that of the heartwood, there are numerous exceptions to this. However, the greater absorbency of the sapwood can often be used as a means of its visual separation from heartwood when colour differences do not apply. Even a short period of dipping of the end grain in water or in a dye solution (such as a 0.5 per cent solution of safranin in alcohol) may show up the intersection line on the end grain of a log section.

Starch is used by plants as a reserve stock of food for growth and is frequently found in the living parenchyma cells. The presence of starch indicates sapwood but its absence does not necessarily indicate heartwood. Starch gives a blue-black colour in the presence of iodine, so the use of an aqueous iodine solution is a common method of detecting sapwood. The method of preparation of the solution is referenced on page 189.

Bamber (1979) describes a number of chemicals that give colour changes indicative of sapwood.

The presence of starches and sugars in the sapwood makes it considerably more susceptible than heartwood to fungal and insect attack, while the materials deposited in heartwood in the changeover from sapwood often contain chemicals that repel such destructive agencies. The strength of the sapwood is much the same as that of the adjacent heartwood when considered at the same moisture content. Since its cells are still capable of rapid conduction of liquid plant food, sapwood is generally easy to impregnate with preservatives, but for the same reason it is unsuitable for the construction of liquid storage containers, such as vats and barrels, which would be likely to leak.

Earlywood and latewood

The wood produced in the flush of growth in springtime is called *earlywood* (or 'springwood') and it produces fibres that are larger in diameter, shorter in length and with thinner walls than those produced later in the growing season in the *latewood* (or 'summerwood'). The distinctive characteristics of these differing responses vary with species and climatic conditions. In the pines, there is an abrupt transition that shows up as easily countable growth rings, whereas in other species the transition is often undetectable by the unaided eye. In species with a pronounced difference, the tensile strength and modulus of elasticity are greater in the latewood, whose fibres are longer.

Softwoods and hardwoods

The trees that produce the wood that is sawn into the *timber* (or 'lumber', as it is called in North America) of commercial value belong to the divisions of the plant world known as *gymnosperms* and *angiosperms*.

Gymnosperms, the more ancient in evolutionary development, produce uncovered seeds, usually in cone-like structures, and hence the application of the term 'conifers' to a major portion of the trees classified as gymnosperms and described as *softwoods* by botanists. However, this term has no relation at all to the softness of the wood, and confusion often results because carpenters and timber merchants frequently use the term to describe timbers that are easy to work but which are not necessarily softwoods in the botanical sense.

Angiosperms are flowering plants whose seeds are formed inside a ripening fruit. They are subdivided into monocotyledons, which include the palms and bamboos, and dicotyledons, to which the term *hardwood* is applied.

The conifers are most commonly found in temperate and cool climates and the world contains about 600 different species. The hardwoods, of more recent evolution and more complex structure, are widespread in all climatic zones capable of sustaining trees and there are many thousands of species.

The essential structural distinction between the wood types is that hardwoods have vessels and softwoods do not. As the vessels are usually much larger in cross-section than the other wood tissue, an examination of the end grain of the wood with a low power (×10 or ×20) hand lens following a clean cut with a sharp razor blade will easily resolve the question. Vessels are also called pores and the terms 'pored' and 'non-pored' woods are often applied to hardwoods and softwoods, respectively.

The vessels are arranged in a pattern that is characteristic of each group of species but the main visual elements of softwoods, the tracheids, are rather uniform in appearance. Accurate identification of hardwoods is generally much easier, therefore. The softwood may have to be sectioned very carefully and examined with a powerful microscope and even then the exact species may not be ascertained with certainty. The resin canals of some softwoods might, at first glance, be confused with vessels.

In softwoods, fibres (including tracheids) represent at least 90 per cent of the wood volume, the remainder being mainly ray parenchyma and resin canals. Hardwoods usually have significantly less fibres; between 10 per cent and 20 per cent is represented by vessels. The rays, consisting of parenchyma cells, are usually much larger in hardwoods than in softwoods.

The actual wood substance of the cell wall has a density of about 1500 kg/m³ but as a lot of space in the timber is taken up by the cell cavity (and the pores, in hardwoods) the density of the timber of the various species is considerably less than this, even of the densest hardwoods. Density is the most important single characteristic of a species and is generally indicative of its strength.

Organic components

Apart from extractives, described more fully below, the three major chemical components of wood are cellulose, hemicelluloses and lignin. *Cellulose* consists of thousands of glucose molecular units joined end to end in long chains. It is made up of 44.4 per cent carbon, 6.2 per cent hydrogen and 49.4 per cent oxygen and is relatively unaffected by alkalis and dilute acids. It represents between 40 and 45 per cent of wood. *Hemicelluloses* act as a matrix for the cellulose microfibrils, are of relatively low molecular weight and of a rather gelatinous nature, soluble in alkalis and converted by acids into carbohydrates. They represent between 15 and 30 per cent of hardwoods and about 20 per cent of softwoods. The hemicelluloses of softwoods differ somewhat from those in hardwoods. *Lignin*, which constitutes between 22 and 30 per cent of wood, occurs in the form of very complex chain polymers of high molecular weight, consisting of about 65 per cent carbon, 6 per cent hydrogen and 29 per cent oxygen and is virtually impossible to dissolve without being broken down into simpler substances. The lignin in softwood is a little different from that in hardwoods and represents a higher percentage of the wood. A simple method of detecting lignin is to smear the clean wood surface with a 2 per cent solution of phloroglucinol in alcohol, followed by a drop of concentrated hydrochloric acid. The presence of lignin will cause the formation of a bright red colour.

All these components are formed from the sugars produced in the leaves by *photosynthesis*. The water obtained from the roots is combined with carbon dioxide from the atmosphere, by complex biochemical processes dependent on *chlorophyll*, which is able to absorb from sunlight the energy needed, to form simple sugars. When these sugars are conveyed from the leaves to the wood cells, they are changed into the much more complex cellulose, hemicelluloses and lignin.

Extractives

In addition to cellulose, hemicelluloses and lignin, wood also contains a wide variety of compounds that can be extracted by solvents. These have been termed 'extractives'.

Although not part of the essential wood structure, extractives are of major importance to wood properties. They contribute to colour, taste, odour, density, durability, flammability and hygroscopicity (moisture absorbency), and can be polyphenols, oils, fats, gums, resins, waxes or starches. In many species the sapwood is low in extractives; the greatest concentration is in the outer heartwood, and there is a progressive diminution towards the centre of the tree. Such diminution is probably the reason for the lower durability of the inner heart of many species and is often manifested in the form of a hollow pipe, or material that is weak (brittleheart) and subject to decay.

Extractives may represent from 5 per cent to as high as 30 per cent of the dry wood mass, varying with species, sapwood or heartwood, rate of growth and season. They can be removed from the wood by extraction with a variety of inert solvents, such as water, ethyl alcohol, acetone, benzene and ether.

Main types of extractives

Carbohydrates

Small amounts of soluble carbohydrates are present in the sap stream as simple sugars, such as sucrose, glucose and fructose, while starch is present in the form of grains in the food storage tissue of the parenchyma and rays. The sapwood of some species can contain up to 5 per cent of starch.

Exudates

Injury to the cambium provokes a protective response in the form of exudates; some species, particularly pines, produce a flow of resin that seems to occur without apparent external response, although its abundance is increased by such factors.

The pale brown *resins* produced by conifers are soluble in turpentine but not in aqueous or alcoholic solvents, whereas the *gums* produced by hardwoods are of a carbohydrate nature and are relatively insoluble in organic solvents but can be dissolved by alcohol or water. The dark reddish-coloured exudate from the eucalypts is called *kino* and is soluble in dilute alkali and in alcohol. The abundance of resins in some pines can lead to erroneous results when the moisture content of the timber is determined by oven-drying methods.

The southern pines, of which slash pine and loblolly pine are the main species that have been planted in Australia, have an especially abundant flow of resin. Distillation of the resin yields wood turpentine and rosin.

This pine resin was an important source of raw material for the coatings and pharmaceutical industries in past years, especially in the United States, where the large-scale extraction of resin was referred to as the 'naval stores' industry; this name arose from the large-scale use of rosin (resin from which the wood turpentine fraction has been distilled) in earlier times for the caulking of the seams of wooden ships. The naval stores industry declined because of competition from petroleum products but the decline in oil resources could prompt a renewal of interest in the resin yield of pines.

The process of regular tree wounding in the cambial region and collection of the ensuing flow of resin is akin to that used in the collection of latex from the rubber tree (*Hevea brasiliensis*). The flow is increased greatly by spraying the fresh wound with sulfuric acid or organic chemicals, such as paraquat.

Phenolic compounds

Phenolic compounds are more prevalent in heartwood and are responsible for some of its darker colour and greater durability. Flavones, stilbenes, quinones, lignins and tannins are the main types of phenolic compounds present in wood; because of their chemical structure the term 'polyphenols' is often applied to these types of extractives. The tannins precipitate proteins from solution and are used for the conversion of animal hides into leather. There are two main groups of tannins: the hydrolytic tannins, which are esters of a sugar (usually glucose) with one or more polyhydric alcohols (usually gallic or ellagic acid); and the condensed tannins, of greater complexity and based on catechin. The condensed tannins are converted by acids into insoluble red-coloured phlobaphenes.

In addition to their use in the production of leather, tannin extracts are used to control the viscosity of oil-well drilling muds, for ore flotation in mining, and for the production of tannin–formaldehyde adhesives.

Tannins are much more common in the wood of hardwoods than that of softwoods, although softwood bark (e.g. that of radiata pine) can have a high tannin content. Bark is a richer source of tannins than is wood.

Nitrogen compounds

Nitrogen compounds generally represent less than 0.2 per cent by weight of wood and are mainly proteins and amino acids present in the living cells of the sapwood. The amount of nitrogen is considerably greater in species producing alkaloids, which contain nitrogen in their chemical structure. The nitrogen in sapwood plays an important part in assisting the development of organisms that are responsible for decay and borer damage.

Minerals

Minerals absorbed by the roots from the soil play an essential role in the process of wood formation. Wood from temperate climatic zones generally has an ash content well below 1 per cent but tropical woods may sometimes contain as much as 5 per cent. The main elements are calcium, potassium, magnesium, sulfur and iron, plus small amounts of aluminium, sodium, manganese, phosphorus and zinc, although the relative abundance varies considerably between species, between wood and bark, and between sapwood and heartwood. The ash content of the bark can be very much higher than that of the wood, while the sapwood usually contains a higher percentage than the heartwood.

As well as varying with species, the ash content varies with position in the tree, the age of the tree and the season. The relative abundance of potassium in wood ash makes it a useful soil supplement.

Silica

Since silica is not dissolved by the usual solvents it cannot really be considered an extractive but it is convenient to consider it here alongside other mineral constituents of wood.

Silica is generally observed, with the aid of a microscope, as small grains that are most frequently found in the rays. There is a very considerable within-species variation in the amount of silica present in species known to contain it.

Timber with more than 0.3 per cent silica is likely to cause rapid blunting of saws, but it has the advantage of enhanced resistance to marine borers and termites, evidently due to the abrasive action of the silica on these creatures' cutting equipment.

Apart from the kauris, in which silica may be present but not to a significant extent, softwoods are virtually free of silica but many hardwoods contain enough to make them difficult to work, especially when seasoned. Mention is made in the descriptions of the individual species of those that are likely to have a significant amount of silica.

Influence of extractives on wood properties

Colour

The basic structural components of wood (cellulose, lignin and hemicelluloses) do not give it any colour. The colours that give species their individual aesthetic appeal are complex organic compounds, such as flavones and quinones, which are more concentrated in the heartwood than the sapwood, and hence the common colour distinction between them. When subject to long-term exposure to sunlight, these compounds undergo chemical change: blond woods acquire a yellowish tint and red woods become brownish. Such changes are limited to the surface layers of wood and the original colour can be regained by sanding or planing the surface.

Staining

The colouring matter is often partly soluble in water and this is a common cause of difficulty, for when the surface of the wood is wetted there is a chance that colour will migrate and cause water marks when the wood redries. The run-off of rain from freshly installed wood is also likely to stain surfaces on which it impinges: the tannins, in particular, are likely to react with alkaline surfaces, such as concrete paths, to form a brown stain. The eucalypts are particularly prone to cause such staining. The bleaching effect of sunlight and rain will eventually remove such stains if they are not continually reinforced by further leaching from the wood. If they are so unsightly as to require urgent action, they can generally be removed (so long as they are of recent origin) by washing down the affected surface with dilute acids (citric or hydrochloric acid can be used). Appropriate design detailing or careful choice of species should obviate this problem.

As alkaline solutions can cause the formation of a brownish stain on wood, adhesives of an alkaline nature, such as casein, can cause difficulties when bonding thin veneers through which the adhesive may penetrate and from which it will be difficult to sand off the stain. Strongly acidic adhesives may cause pink colours to form with some species (e.g. imported sapele and sycamore).

Wood that has a relatively high tannin content is liable to be discoloured with black stains when it comes into contact with iron compounds while in the unseasoned condition, as inevitably occurs during the sawing of logs. Such timber when seasoned is not usually affected but, if it becomes temporarily wetted in service or during installation, then any ferrous fixings are liable to cause staining. All external fixings, unless they can be protected by a waterproof coating system, should be of heavily galvanised steel or of non-ferrous metals.

Durability

The great difference between the durability of the sapwood and heartwood of many species is essentially due to the concentration of toxic compounds of phenolic type in the heartwood.

The presence in some softwoods of high concentrations of resins, although not of much inherent toxicity, can be of some value in promoting durability because they restrict the uptake of moisture.

Allergic reactions

The processing of wood products creates a lot of fine particles, which can affect the worker's skin and mucous membranes. The provision of efficient dust-extracting equipment, good ventilation and extra attention to personal hygiene by the worker, especially in hot weather, will solve most problems, but there are some species whose dust is more than usually irritant to some people, who can develop an allergy to it. Species requiring extra care in this regard include Crow's ash, black bean, silky beech, blackwood, western red cedar, miva mahogany, silky oak, cypress, teak and guarea. This subject is discussed further on page 206.

Effect on finishes

Oleoresins, which flow under the influence of hot sunlight and which are present in many pines and Douglas fir, may exude through coatings and form sticky globules on the surface. Such globules are best removed with a sharp knife-edge, resulting in minimum disturbance to the coating and obviating the need for any touch-up of the surface. Kiln drying of such species is recommended, for the heat involved in the process drives off the more volatile constituents and so the resins are less liable to flow during exposure to warm conditions. Resins are soluble in mineral turpentine but not in alcohol; the reverse applies to gums. Rose mahogany and northern silky oak sometimes exude gums that can have a harmful effect on finishes. If only small amounts are present, the surface should be washed with alcohol (methylated spirits) to dissolve the gum before applying finishes. Badly affected wood should be excluded from uses involving surface finishes.

Extractives can affect the drying rate of finishes; those in teak, Brazilian rosewood and Parana pine are examples of this.

Effect on curing of cement

When wood fibres are used in combination with cement for building boards, the presence of sugars and tannins can severely weaken the bond with the cement; it appears that they may form a skin around the cement particles and inhibit hydration. The addition of a small amount of calcium chloride is beneficial, although it may not completely solve the problem.

Atypical wood

Reaction wood

The wood of greatest commercial value generally comes from the straight main stem of the tree. Wood from the branches, apart from not being sufficiently straight to provide reasonable lengths of timber, has considerable growth stresses in it owing to the formation of what is known as 'reaction wood'.

Reaction wood is formed by the tree when it is subject to prolonged structural stress, such as can occur with leaning trunks, or if it is continually exposed to strong winds, and is inevitably present in branches. The formation of reaction wood is usually associated with eccentric growth of wood, with more tissue being formed on the upper side of the leaning stem or branch of hardwoods, and on the lower side of softwoods. Thus, the reaction wood of hardwoods is called 'tension wood' and of softwoods 'compression wood'.

Compression wood is harder, denser and more brittle than normal wood; the tracheids are shorter and thicker (Plate 2). It is darker in colour, the latewood is wider than normal and the lignin content is higher. Although denser, its strength properties are usually below those of normal wood. It has less lateral shrinkage but longitudinal movement is increased considerably. When a piece of timber is part normal wood and part compression wood, very considerable warping can occur during drying.

Tension wood is not as easily identified as compression wood. It may be darker but this colour change does not always occur and indeed it can sometimes be paler. The best indicator is the woolliness of the freshly sawn surface of green timber and it can also be observed on freshly peeled veneer. Longitudinal shrinkage is high but not as abnormal as that in compression wood. Radial shrinkage is normal but that in the tangential direction is increased. Non-recoverable collapse occurs during drying.

The fibres have rather gelatinous inner walls, which are low in lignification. Compression strength parallel to the grain is reduced considerably.

Knots

Knots, the tissue of the branches, are usually considerably harder and, in softwoods, darker in colour and more resinous than the wood enclosing them. Because of the presence of reaction wood they are likely to suffer increased shrinkage and stress; those in softwoods are likely to contain a considerably greater amount of resin than the enclosing wood.

Visual characteristics

Those features of wood that play an important part in determining the wood's suitability for decorative use include texture, grain and figure.

Texture

This is described as being fine or coarse, even or uneven. It is determined by the size and arrangement of the cells, and by variations in density, such as result from earlywood and latewood.

Grain

This refers to the general direction of growth of the woody tissue, and is indicated by the way it tends to separate when the piece of timber is split. It can be straight, spiral, sloping, interlocked, curly, wavy or rippled. Plates 3–5 show different types of grain

Spiral grain

The helical orientation of grain can be caused by environmental factors, such as persistent strong wind, but it is more often a genetic feature that deserves attention when selecting elite trees for seed and for tree breeding. Impact resistance and bending strength can be severely affected. *Interlocked grain* is virtually a double spiral effect in which the alternate bands of growth have their fibres oriented in opposite directions. The effect on strength is unlikely to be as great as pronounced spiral grain but the wood is difficult to split and also difficult to dress, with the likelihood of tearing out small pieces of the wood. Interlocked grain produces a fiddleback appearance (see Plate 6).

Figure

This describes the ornamental markings seen on the dressed surface and produced by the arrangement of the various wood tissues and variations in colour. There are numerous descriptions of figure, such as fiddleback, ribbon, striped, silver, burl and bird's eye.

Tree growth

The main trunk of the tree is a very elongated cone rather than a cylinder. The amount of taper can vary considerably but a rough guide for mature trees would be about 10 mm of diameter change per metre length of trunk.

The increase in height of the trunk, or the length of the branch, is due to the activity of special cells at the extreme tip, whose elongation is the only lengthwise growth that occurs in the tree; these special cells are thin walled and do not produce woody tissue. A short distance away from the tip the outside cells change to form the cambium, while the inner cells break down and become the *pith*, which in pines is often brown in colour and soft and spongy.

In cool climates growth has a seasonal pattern, often reflected in the formation of *growth rings*, which are very obvious when the wood is viewed on end section. In warm and tropical climates growth rings are less common. Softwood tracheids in the later period of annual growth have thicker walls and, often, smaller overall dimensions; in hardwoods the vessels formed early in the growing season may be larger and more numerous than the later ones, while fibres in the later wood may be thicker walled and perhaps smaller.

Identification of species

Density, odour and the colour of the heartwood are valuable aids in identification but the botanist relies basically on the microscopic examination of very thin cross-sections of the wood, which are compared with those of known species. Even this may be insufficient to distinguish between closely related species and it will then be necessary to obtain the leaves, fruit and bark of the tree for examination. Thus, it is always desirable to provide a range of botanical material when an identification is sought, particularly in those instances when great similarities exist (e.g. the pines and the stringybarks).

People with no botanical training but with long experience in timber production and distribution often acquire the ability to identify very accurately those species met in day-to-day contact. However, it is not a subject that can be mastered without a lot of practical experience and because of this no attempt is made in this book to provide guidelines for wood identification.

Wood and the energy crisis

The small amount of solar energy that is absorbed by plant life undergoing photosynthesis maintains all living matter. Only about 25 per cent of the sunlight reaching the earth's surface is of a wavelength such as to promote photosynthesis and only a fraction of this is actually used; factors limiting the productivity of photosynthesis in a particular location include the amount of sunlight actually received by the plant, the temperature, and the availability of carbon dioxide, water, nitrogen, phosphorus and trace amounts of a number of other elements.

Photosynthesis combines molecules of carbon dioxide and water to produce carbohydrates and oxygen. The atmosphere contains about 0.032 per cent of carbon dioxide but the current rate of burning of fossil fuels (coal, oil) is increasing this amount. While increased levels of carbon dioxide are a favourable stimulus to plant growth, there is also a negative aspect since the carbon dioxide in the atmosphere captures some of the infra-red energy radiated from the earth's surface and an increase in its concentration will have a warming effect on the planet. It has been suggested that this could eventually melt much more of the polar ice caps and thus raise the level of the oceans. This is known as the greenhouse effect.

The ultraviolet portion of the sun's radiation has the power to break chemical bonds, which explains its destructive effect on many materials (e.g. surface coatings, fabrics) and on human skin.

Decomposition of oxygen in the stratosphere by ultraviolet radiation results in the formation of ozone, which is an absorber of such radiation and acts as a filter, reducing the amount of potential damage to objects on the earth's surface. Some recent products as a result of technological developments (e.g. pressure pack propellants, jet engine exhaust gases) are alleged to have the potential to affect the stability of that protective ozone layer.

It seems, then, that the relative availabilities of carbon dioxide and oxygen have a very significant effect on life on earth and this is the basis of the concern felt about the rapid increase in atmospheric pollution caused by the scale of current industrial activity.

Wood, as a major product of photosynthesis, is a continually renewable resource that has obvious advantages in the light of this environmental concern. In the construction industry, for example, materials based on non-renewable resources usually need a considerably greater amount of energy for their fabrication than does timber.

A study in the United States (Boyd et al., 1977) produced a number of interesting comparisons of energy requirements. For example, to make the equivalent of the corresponding timber product, steel floor joists require about 50 times as much energy, aluminium framing for external walls 20 times, steel framing for external walls 13 times, aluminium cladding 4 times and brick veneering 25 times.

There are other factors that could modify these claims, such as a consideration of the relative rates of deterioration or the relative costs of material in a particular locality, but the figures do illustrate the important role of wood in a world where energy consumption is a critical factor in social progress.

It is important to bear in mind that these comparisons of energy requirement are related essentially to sawn timber. When the wood raw material is reconstituted as hardboard, fibreboard or particleboard, the advantage is much less pronounced.

FURTHER READING

Bamber, R. K. (1976). Heartwood, its function and formation.
Wood Sci and Tech 10: 1–8.

Bamber, R. K. (1979). Sapwood and heartwood. Tech. pubn. no. 2 (revised).
Sydney: Forestry Commission of NSW.

Boyd, C. W. et al. (1977). Wood for structural and architectural purposes.
For Prod J 27(2): 10–20.

Core, H. A., Cote, W. A., Day, A. C. (1979). *Wood structure and identification.*
2nd edn. New York: Syracuse University Press.

Gates, D. M. (1971). The flow of energy in the biosphere. *Sci Am* 224(3):
89–100.

Glasser, W. G. (1981). Potential role of lignin in tomorrow's wood utilisation
technologies. *For Prod J* 31(3): 24–9.

Goldstein, I. S. (1981). Chemicals from biomass: present status. *For Prod J*
1(10): 63–8.

Lambert, M. J. (1981). Inorganic constituents in wood and bark of New South
Wales forest tree species. Research note 45. Sydney: Forestry Commission
of NSW.

Lanyon, J. W. (1981). Card key for the identification of the commercial timbers
used in New South Wales. Research note 40. 2nd edn. Sydney: Forestry
Commission of NSW.

Panshin, A. J. and de Zeeuw, C. (1970). *Textbook of wood technology.* Vol. 1.
3rd edn. New York: McGraw-Hill.

Richards, P. W. (1973). The tropical rainforest. *Sci Am* 229(6): 58–67.

Chapter 2

Colour changes in wood

Much of the visual appeal of wood can be attributed to its colour. Because it comes from a naturally grown resource (trees), within-species variation in colour can be considerable. This variability is a valued characteristic and prevents the monotony that is usually found in products that try to imitate wood's appearance. The colour depends mainly on the presence of polyphenolic compounds and quinones. The former can be colourless but are easily oxidised to quinones, which are usually coloured.

Sapwood is generally of a distinctively lighter colour than heartwood, except in pale species. The colour of freshly cut wood often changes with exposure to the air and ultraviolet light. The change in colour with heartwood is partly due to the oxidation of phenolic substances. Freshly cut sapwood can often acquire a surface browning somewhat similar to that which occurs when an apple is peeled, and both are caused by an oxidation process.

It is not practicable to maintain the colour exactly as it appears on the freshly dressed wood surface. Sunlight, even when not impinging directly on it, will have a gradual bleaching effect on dark colours and a yellowing effect on blond colours. Even very clear finishes will change the colour considerably because they fill the air spaces among the wood fibres and, as they have a higher refractive index than air, the result is a darkening of the colour. The amount of air that is replaced varies with the type of wood tissue, the angle of the grain and other factors that affect absorption. Because of this differential absorption, special features are made more visible and generally the final effect will be more striking than the uncoated surface; although not necessarily as beautiful. To obtain an indication of the effect of a clear finish on the colour of the wood, wetting a small area with water will give speedy guidance.

Quick-drying finishes forming only a surface film give a paler initial colour than those that soak into the wood; although if they are prone to yellowing this initial advantage may not be maintained for long. Most finishes tend to oxidise gradually and acquire a yellowish colour, which can detract from the appearance of the pale-coloured timbers. Eventually, it may be necessary to strip off the old coating and sand down to a bright new wood surface before applying a new coating.

Weathering

When wood is exposed externally to sunlight, rain and dew, initially dark colours become paler through leaching and bleaching and pale colours darken because of oxidation, but in time all surfaces exposed to the elements become silver-grey. This colour change is confined to the surface layers, which eventually are composed mainly of cellulose. The lignin that cements the wood cells together is degraded by long exposure to weather and is washed away, together with sugars, starches and extractives.

The silver-grey colouring that results may be dirty and blotchy in situations favouring fungal organisms. In a dry climate, or in coastal locations where salt spray inhibits fungal invasion, the silvery grey colour that develops may be considered attractive.

Stains due to natural causes

Wood can be stained in many ways. In the living tree, damage to the bark may permit many types of organism to enter (Plate 7). The extractives present in the wood may also behave erratically at times. During the drying process, invasion of the sapwood by bluestain fungi is a common hazard, especially for pale-coloured species, while during the wood's service life there is the possibility of stains arising from leaching or decay. These aspects are now discussed in more detail.

Stains arising from damage to the living tree

The rupturing of the protective bark permits the entry of oxygen and a wide variety of organisms to the living wood tissue, which reacts and forms protective materials, which are mostly phenolic compounds in hardwoods and terpenes in softwoods. The pioneering invaders can be bacteria, decay fungi or other kinds of fungi, and the wood, in the area of invasion, is often discoloured.

The nature of the invaders and the rate at which discolouration occurs is influenced by the season of the year when attack occurs and the severity of the wound.

One example of this type of stain is the black 'pencil streak' often found in the pale-coloured, cooler climate eucalypts of south-eastern Australia (Plate 8) and occasionally in jarrah and tallowwood. It arises from fungal penetration of the cells of the rays and may affect considerable lengths of the rays; dark-coloured polyphenolic materials indicate the tree's protective response. Such 'pencil streaks' are not necessarily an indication of the presence of decay but could suggest that such wood is at greater risk than unaffected material. Invasion by the pin-hole borer is a common source of the initial infection.

Chemical changes in wood extractives

During the wood's growth, pigments differing from those usually produced may show up as streaks and blotches and may enhance its decorative value. After it is processed, colour changes can also occur because of the oxidation of extractives, which is accentuated by exposure to light. The extractives can cause some staining problems when timber is exposed to the leaching effect of weather. Racking (spacer) sticks of eucalypt hardwood, which are used to separate the layers of boards during drying, have been known to cause discolouration of the boards if the stack was unprotected from rain. The discolouration results in imprints of the racking sticks appearing on the surface of the boards. In some instances these marks go right through the boards and sanding does not remove them. In the grading rules they are referred to as 'sticker marks'.

Stains due to leaching

Intermittent wetting of the surface of an uncoated piece of timber can cause migration of colouring materials, which results in a stained and blotchy appearance on the dried timber surface, particularly if the species has a lot of extractives.

This same migration of water-soluble extractives can lead to the deposition of brown stains on adjacent painted woodwork, on brick walls and on concrete paths, the problem being exacerbated in the latter two because of their alkaline nature and their potential iron content. The bleaching effect of sunlight and rain will gradually remove the stain if it is not further added to. Alternatively, commercial cleaners are available for cleaning affected areas.

Superficial stains from moulds

During the early stages of drying, when the sawn timber has a moisture content considerably above 20 per cent, superficial moulds of black or a dirty green colour feed on carbohydrates in the wood cells on the surface but do not destroy the wood tissue. Such stains are limited to the surface and are removed in the dressing of the timber.

Sapstain or bluestain

Bluestain fungi may invade the sapwood and outer heartwood of felled logs and sawn timber of both softwoods and hardwoods. The speed of attack can be very rapid in the warmer months and it is important that there be a minimum of delay between the felling of the tree and its seasoning if it is of a species that is susceptible to infection. The plantation pines, with their large amount of sapwood, are particularly prone to such staining.

The bluestain fungi live on the contents of the cells of freshly felled timber but do not attack the cell walls, so the effect on strength is small. However, the timber can become streaked and unsightly as a result of the fungal invasion and, hence, its acceptability to buyers is considerably impaired. The stain arises from the presence of fine dark threads of fungal hyphae in the cells, especially in the ray cells. The spores of the fungus responsible are present everywhere, so if conditions are favourable attack is very likely.

Rapid conversion of sawn timber after felling and speedy drying of the sawn material will practically eliminate staining. If susceptible timber is to be dried it is generally advisable to dip it in a fungicide as it comes from the saw. A commonly used formulation is 4 per cent weight–weight of sodium pentachlorphenate and 12 per cent weight–weight of borax dissolved in water. Once the timber has dried to a moisture content of 20 per cent, the danger of bluestain is past but covering of the stack is needed to prevent leaching of the protective chemicals. The same formulation is effective in protecting timber against the mould growth that may occur in the early stages of drying.

Stains due to decay

The presence of decay is often indicated by pronounced colour changes in the wood. There may be streaks or patches of reddish-brown or whitish wood depending on the type of fungal organisms involved. If attack is well advanced, such wood may be considerably softer than surrounding tissue and will generally give a brittle fracture when an attempt is made to lever out a splinter with a sharp knife. This decay is rendered inactive by seasoning the timber and maintaining it in the seasoned condition.

Stains caused by chemical reaction

Many species have a high tannin content, which reacts with iron to form black and insoluble iron tannates if the wood is in a wet condition. Thus, one often sees a dark colouration on sawn timber as a result of contact with the steel saw. Such a stain is limited to the surface. Seasoned timber is unaffected so there is no danger of such stains arising when dressing or resawing the dried boards. Ordinary mild steel nails have the same effect, and hence the necessity to punch them below the surface and give them some protective cover when they are used for fixing timber exposed to the weather. Spotty iron tannate staining may result from atmospheric fallout of particles produced in tool sharpening, the use of an angle grinder, and so on.

Copper nails tend to cause a slight reddish brown colour on some timbers when used externally. Aluminium, monel metal, stainless steel and high-quality galvanised steel do not cause staining but in the latter case it is important that the galvanising remains undamaged during the driving of the nail; hence, hot-dipped galvanised fixings are typically specified for use in external environments.

Colour changes in veneers

The top veneer in plywood, or laid on other bases, may sometimes suffer from undesirable colour changes. This can arise from the effect of strongly acid adhesives on the natural extractives in the wood, or from the reaction between extractives and strong alkalis.

The presence of veneer jointing tape can be 'telegraphed' through by colour changes. Glue viscosity and veneer porosity can affect the light refraction of the veneer surface, especially if the veneer is very thin.

Stains on hands

Handlers of green eucalypt hardwood timber soon find that their hands are stained a dark bluish colour because of the extractives in the wood. The problem seldom arises with seasoned material, except perhaps in very hot humid weather, when the sweat on the hands may attract some of the extractives. If normal washing of the hands is followed by rubbing with a cut lemon, most of the staining should be removed.

Chapter 3

Mechanical properties of timber

Species vary considerably in their mechanical properties and the figures given in most tabulations (e.g. in Appendix 3) represent averages from which considerable variation can occur. The age of the tree, climatic, environmental and genetic factors, even the position in the tree from which the small clear test sample was taken, all have a significant effect on the results obtained. Because of this, small differences in the figures obtained from various species should not be regarded seriously; this is one reason for classifying species into strength groups within which all are assumed to have the same essential characteristics.

There is also considerable variability of growth characteristics between species. However, grading of timber to relevant Australian Standards ensures that commercial timber has appropriate properties.

A distinction should be clearly made between the properties of 'small clear' wood specimens and those of commercial timber. The terms *wood* and *timber* are often confused in the same way as are *concrete* and *cement*. Essentially, *wood* refers to the material in the tree trunk (made up of wood fibre) and to the material in a piece of timber (the wood fibre). *Timber* refers to a commercial product that has been cut from the wood of a tree, such as veneers, beams, poles, scantling and so on. *Small clears* are samples obtained by carefully cutting them so that they contain no knots or other strength-reducing characteristics, such as gum veins, splits or checks. These samples contain only wood fibre that is aligned with the long axis of the sample (no sloping grain) and can be used to determine the upper boundary of timber properties for that species. Clear wood is very strong in tension and when subjected to bending tends to fail in the compression zone. Clear wood bending failures are generally ductile.

Commercial timber contains some clear wood but knots and other characteristics are also present. The mechanical properties of timber are therefore less than that of clear wood of the same species. The failure of commercial timber under bending or tension is often initiated on the tension edge in the vicinity of knots, other growth characteristics or steep localised slope of grain. All of these can interrupt the continuity of the wood fibres and induce tension perpendicular to the grain. Commercial timber must have all of the properties expected for its use; these include strength and stiffness (mechanical properties), straightness and dimensional stability (utility) or appearance. The mechanical properties and utility of commercial timber are discussed in later sections of this chapter.

Factors affecting properties of small clear specimens of wood

The main factors affecting the mechanical properties of wood that are significant in studying the results of tests on small clear specimens are listed below.

Density

In general, the denser the species, the greater the mechanical properties of its clear material. However, young trees may often have a significant amount of wood in their central core, which is much lower in density than normal for the species.

Some reference books quote specific gravity figures instead of densities. Specific gravity is defined as the ratio of the density of wood to the density of water at 4°C. In practice, the specific gravity of wood is usually the oven-dry weight of the wood divided by its volume at a specified moisture content.

If the species' specific gravity figures at 12 per cent moisture content are given, the respective densities (in kg/m³) at 12 per cent for a limited range of figures can be interpolated from Table 3.1.

Table 3.1 Relationship between density and specific gravity

Specific gravity	Density (kg/m³)	Specific gravity	Density (kg/m³)
0.30	336	0.52	581
0.32	359	0.54	604
0.34	381	0.56	626
0.36	404	0.58	649
0.38	426	0.60	671
0.40	448	0.62	694
0.42	471	0.64	716
0.44	493	0.66	738
0.46	516	0.68	761
0.48	537	0.70	783
0.50	559		

Rate of growth

In many species, particularly hardwoods with an absence of visible growth rings, it is difficult to assess the rate of growth. Timber of a medium rate of growth is likely to have some superiority over timber of a very fast or very slow rate of growth within the same species.

Climatic factors can have an effect on density and strength. Generally, the warmer the climate, the stronger the wood. For example, timber from some species from northern New South Wales are stronger than timber from the same species from more southern areas.

Percentage of latewood

Some species of pronounced seasonal growth habits have thicker-walled cells in the wood formed late in the growing season and such wood is denser and stronger than that formed at the beginning of the season.

Position in tree

Wood from butt logs may be expected to be slightly denser and stronger, as may wood from the outer heartwood.

Moisture content

The moisture content of wood has a significant effect on its strength, stiffness and stability. Clear wood usually increases in strength as it dries, although this effect does not begin until the water within the cell has dried out and it is starting to be lost from the cell walls (i.e. at a wood moisture content in the vicinity of 25–30 per cent). At 12 per cent moisture content the modulus of rupture and compression strength parallel to the grain of small clears may have improved by 75–100 per cent; its stiffness, as indicated by its modulus of elasticity, will be less affected but it may have increased by up to 30 per cent. Not every strength property improves with a decrease in moisture content; impact resistance may, in fact, decrease due to the fact that dry wood will not deform as far as unseasoned (green) wood before failure, although it will usually carry a greater load.

The mechanical properties given in reference books may be quoted for a variety of moisture contents so it may be helpful to note the adjustment factors (Table 3.2) that enable an approximate comparison to be made for properties of small clears.

Table 3.2 Adjustment factors for mechanical properties of small clears

Small clear properties	Percentage change per 1 per cent property change in moisture content
Modulus of rupture	4
Modulus of elasticity	2
Tension perpendicular to grain	1.5
Compression parallel to grain	6
Compression perpendicular to grain	5.5
Shear parallel to grain	3
Impact (falling weight test)	0.5
Hardness (end)	4
Hardness (side)	2.5

The increase in strength obtained by drying is usually greater for small sections than for large ones because seasoning defects tend to have more influence on the latter. The magnitude of the increase varies considerably between species.

Temperature

Above-normal temperatures tend to lower the strength properties of wood, and lower temperatures tend to raise them. The magnitude of the effect will be related to the moisture content of the wood and the period of exposure to the abnormal conditions. After return to normal conditions, most of the original strength is recovered, provided the abnormality is not severe.

Prolonged exposure to temperature in excess of about 90°C will make the strength loss irreversible but dry wood can be exposed to temperatures up to 65°C for as long as a year without much permanent loss of strength. The amount of strength loss due to elevated temperature depends on the temperature reached, the moisture content of the wood, the time period, the species and the size of the member.

The temperature change may alter the relative humidity of the air, which will affect the moisture content of the wood, which will in turn affect the mechanical properties. If increased temperature is accompanied by a lower relative humidity, the weakening effect from temperature will tend to be counterbalanced by an increase in strength due to drying.

Factors affecting properties of commercial timber

The properties of commercial timber are affected by all of the factors that determine the fibre properties, as discussed in the section on the strength of small clear pieces of timber. However, the presence of growth characteristics that are specifically excluded from small clears has a significant influence on the properties of the timber that will be used in construction.

Density

Species of high density are slow to dry so are often used structurally in the unseasoned condition. However, provision should be made for the gradual but small reduction in cross-section as the timber seasons. Milled products such as floorboards are used in the seasoned condition to avoid as much dimensional change as possible in the fitted product. Species of high density generally have high ratings for hardness and abrasion resistance.

Density has some correlation with many structural properties, but is particularly important in hardness and connection capacities. Abnormally low-density wood should be rejected from highly stressed structural applications for this reason.

Brittleheart

Wood near the heart may have suffered high compressive stress in the early stages of growth of the tree and may be abnormally low in impact or shock resistance and liable to abrupt failure at comparatively small deflections. It fractures cleanly in the same way as a snapped carrot with little or no splintering, which enables it to be identified when a small splinter is prised out of the suspect member with a pocket knife.

Grading rules for structural hardwood timber usually either reject heart or, in large sections, require it to be enclosed fully by timber of normal strength (boxed heart). Grading rules for structural softwood timber usually make provision for heart material.

Knots

Knots are specifically excluded from small clears, so the considerable effect of knots on properties is only seen when testing commercial timber.

Knots are the remnants of branches that have been captured by the growing trunk. Timber cut at the junction of the main trunk and side branch will contain a knot. On the tangential, or 'back-cut', surface of the board the knot will be round or oval but if the radial, or quarter-cut, surface of the timber cuts through the knot it will appear in section and is elongate or a longitudinal section through the branch.

If the branch was still living when it was captured by the trunk, the knot will be fully or partially intergrown with the wood which encloses it (Plate 9); but if the branch died many years before but was not shed by the tree, it will be encased (Plate 10), often with its bark still present, so it is then much more likely to be dislodged from the sawn timber and may be considered equivalent to a knot hole.

Knots can have a major effect on mechanical properties since they interrupt the continuity and change the direction of the wood fibres. The extent of their influence depends on their size, shape and location in the piece of timber, and the type of stress to which they are subjected.

Knots contribute no strength to a member in tension and can be considered equivalent to a hole. Knots increase hardness and strength in compression perpendicular to the grain. They appear to have a much smaller effect on stiffness than on strength, although they can have a serious effect on the stiffness of columns. They have no adverse effect on shear strength.

Knots are a major cause of deviations in grain direction. (The effect of sloping grain is described below.) Intergrown knots can cause the grain to change direction and run into the branch (almost at right angles to the grain in the trunk). They may cause considerable deviation of grain and can therefore significantly reduce timber properties. Encased knots may be loose or even drop out so are less acceptable in decorative products. Clusters of knots have a much greater effect than the sum of their diameters might suggest because the grain will be distorted around the whole area.

The location of knots is also important. For example, in bending members, they are much more harmful on the tension side of a beam than on the compression side, while their location in the outer third of the width of a member is more serious in effect than if located more centrally.

Both intergrown and encased knots in round timber have much less effect than in sawn timber because nature provides a collar of sound wood to give additional strength. Because of this it is unwise to trim bumps off poles and piles and thereby thwart nature.

Grain distortion

Small clears, by definition, have straight grain, so there is no effect on properties as a result of any grain distortion. However, commercial timber often includes deviation of grain, which can have a significant effect on its behaviour.

Slope of grain is introduced by irregularities in the growth of the tree, or by knots and other growth characteristics. Local grain distortion is caused by the presence of knots as discussed above, but more general sloping grain can arise in the sawing of a misshapen log, or when the saw is not cutting parallel to the outside edge of the log. General grain distortion can be described as spiral grain, diagonal grain, interlocked grain and curly grain.

Spiral grain, caused by the wood fibres growing in a spiral rather than a vertical fashion, is especially common in the case of small-diameter radiata pine logs. While in the tree, the grain completes a spiral shape from top to bottom; in any one piece of sawn timber, the grain will appear as a general slope throughout the piece. In addition to its effect on strength, it makes timber containing it subject to twisting as it dries.

Diagonal grain is produced when the saw cut is made parallel to the central axis rather than parallel to the line of the growth rings. It is of common occurrence when processing logs that are crooked, or subject to swellings, or if they have a pronounced taper. In this case, the sloping grain may not be uniformly distributed through the piece. One end can have parallel grain and the other can have sloping grain.

Interlocked grain is a form of grain structure in which the angle of the wood fibres changes or reverses periodically in successive layers. *Wavy* and *curly grain* are akin to interlocked grain. Such localised changes in grain direction have little effect on the strength of large sections.

The weakening effect of sloping grain arises from the fact that the timber may be 20 to 40 times stronger parallel to the grain than perpendicular to it, so any considerable slope of grain away from the axis of the piece will be significant, particularly in regard to resistance to impact loads. Stiffness of timber is also affected by sloping grain, as the stiffness parallel to grain is around 30 to 50 times the stiffness perpendicular to grain. Since shrinkage across the grain is very much greater than along the grain, a considerable slope of grain, especially in unseasoned material, will have a noticeable effect on length stability (important in applications such as tiling battens or barge boards for roofs), and it will also increase the likelihood of twist.

Sloping grain can be a serious strength-reducing defect in sawn timber but is seldom of consequence in round timbers, such as poles and piles. In theory, the strength of sawn beams can be reduced approximately 20 per cent by a grain slope of 1 in 16, 30 per cent by 1 in 12 and 50 per cent by 1 in 8. In practice, the interaction of knots and other defects with general and local sloping grain can produce a wide range of strengths of commercial timber.

Observation of a surface gives one component of the sloping grain. When both radial and tangential surfaces have sloping grain, the true slope may be greater than that showing on these surfaces and can be calculated by taking the square root of the sum of the squares of the slopes of grain observed on the radial and tangential faces, or the face and edge of the piece (see AS/NZS 1080.2.1–2.4:1998 *Timber—Methods of Test—Slope of Grain*). The design values for commercial timber are much less than those of the clear wood strengths principally to take this effect into account.

Gum veins and gum pockets

Gum veins and gum pockets are common features of most eucalypt hardwoods but can be present in other species as well. The gum is formed as a protective response to some injury to the tree, such as from insect attack, fire or mechanical damage.

Gum pockets (see Plate 11) and resin pockets are cavities in the wood containing gum (if hardwood) or resin (if softwood). The gum of eucalypts is more accurately called *kino*. Large pockets that extend through the piece can have an effect on strength properties.

Gum veins (see Plate 12) are not as wide as gum pockets and often appear as dark streaks parallel to the growth rings. If the gum vein is bridged at close intervals by woody tissue, it is called a *tight gum vein*. If there is little or no bridging, the vein will tend to open after seasoning so it is called a *loose gum vein*. Tight gum veins do not significantly affect strength or stiffness, but loose gum veins can reduce shear and connection strength because of the discontinuity across the grain of the wood.

Shakes, splits and checks

These defects all cause separations of the wood fibre parallel to the grain.

A *check* is often the smallest of the three but there can be quite a number of them in seasoned timber. It is a separation that extends along the grain and results from stresses developed as the surface layers of wood lose moisture and shrink while the main body of material underneath is fully distended. A check does not extend from one surface of the piece to another. Checks do not cause reductions in properties, but if they are too wide, they can affect nail-holding power.

A *split* is a grain separation that extends from one surface to another. It opens a gap between the fibres that can cause a reduction in shear and connection strength. As splits are more common near the end of the timber (where there are usually connections), particular care is needed in identifying and limiting *end splits*.

A *shake* is a complete or partial separation due to causes other than shrinkage (Plates 13, 14). It may be a felling shake caused by the severe stress when the falling tree hits the ground, or a heart shake, which can develop in the central region of the tree as a result of growth stresses or wind stresses. Some shakes follow the growth rings of the tree and are difficult to identify from the outside of a piece.

These forms of fibre separation reduce resistance to shear stress so they should not be present in quantity at joints.

Wane and Want

These features are both used to describe pieces of timber missing from the cross-section.

Wane occurs when a corner is missing from a piece of timber that has been cut too close to the outside of the log. It may have some bark still attached.

Want refers to timber that is missing from a piece due to mechanical damage during processing. Want can occur on any piece of timber and is not limited, as wane is, to pieces cut from the outside of the log.

Both can reduce the bending and tensile strength of commercial timber as they reduce the cross-section, but they are more important to bearing strength as they have the potential to lead to a significant reduction in bearing area.

Moisture content

Properties of commercial timber have different relationships with moisture compared to small clear specimens.

The strength of commercial timber tends to be limited more by the presence of growth characteristics, such as knots, sloping grain or overgrowth of injury. Moisture content has very little effect on the strength of those characteristics, although as discussed previously, it has a significant effect on the strength of clear wood.

On the other hand, the stiffness of timber is affected by all of the wood fibre in the cross-section (features and clear wood alike), so the stiffness of commercial timber tends to show similar relationships with moisture content to those discussed previously for clear wood.

The moisture content of timber will adjust to be in equilibrium with the moisture in the environment. This is explored further in Chapter 7. However, timber is most effective when specified at a moisture content that is close to the equilibrium moisture content of its service environment.

The structural grading rules classify timber into different stress grades depending on its moisture content. Typically, seasoned products will be one stress grade higher than the same quality and species of timber in the unseasoned condition. Particularly in the higher grades of commercial timber, the properties of the unseasoned product improve as it dries in service in a dry environment. After some years, this initially unseasoned product has properties closer to that of the seasoned product.

Some species of high-density hardwoods are slow to dry so are often used structurally in the unseasoned condition, with provision being made for the gradual but small reduction in cross-section as the timber seasons.

Temperature

For covered structures the temperature effect can usually be ignored, except when high humidity and high temperature occur together, as in tropical areas, or in those industrial situations in which these conditions are created by manufacturing processes. High-temperature seasoning can cause some loss in strength, particularly in impact resistance.

Duration of load

Commercial timber responds to long-term loads differently from the way it responds to short-term loads.

The strength of wood is affected by the length of time and the magnitude of the load to which it is subjected. A member loaded continuously for 10 years could carry only about 60 per cent of what it would easily sustain for a few minutes. A much greater load could be borne if the loading rate was very rapid and applied for a very short time. However, repeated applications tend to be cumulative in effect.

This occurs because the fibres in the wood stretch and move relative to each other under long-term stresses. The movement of fibres can cause damage on a microscopic scale. Over very long periods of loading, this can lead to loss of strength, increase in deformation (creep) and fatigue. The timber engineering standard AS 1720.1-1997 *Timber Structures—Design Methods* provides factors to take account of the duration of the load.

Timber, being of a non-crystalline nature, is less subject to *fatigue* failure than metals, but it is not immune. For example, in tests on small clears, a cycle of stresses repeated 10 million times may lead to a modulus of rupture that is only 25 per cent of that of the initial figure. Fatigue strength may be reduced by the presence of knots.

Some limited tests on larger sections have confirmed that these duration of load models for strength are valid.

Initial moisture content and the prevailing temperature will have a considerable effect on the amount and rate of creep that occurs. A beam of unseasoned (green) timber may have a deflection, after several years, of three to six times its initial deflection, whereas the same beam, if seasoned prior to installation, may have deflected only twice the initial amount. If the moisture content of the beam were to vary cyclically, the deflection would be greater still. Green timber drying under full load has the largest deformation; most deformation occurs in the first few years of service.

Compression failures

Compression failures are localised creases in the wood arising from severe stress in the tree due to high winds, or the felling operations. On dressed surfaces an irregular line of buckled cells may be visible, as shown in Plate 15.

They can cause a serious reduction of tensile strength and impact resistance, leading to a brittle fracture. However, they can be difficult to detect visually or by machine grading of the sawn timber. Fortunately, they are relatively rare.

Decay

Some decay fungi consume wood fibre. When they have become well established the affected wood has little strength, particularly in regard to impact resistance.

Chapter 15 gives more information on biological hazards that may damage wood, and Chapter 16 outlines some methods of improving durability of timber.

If timber is suspected of having decay, its use should be avoided in structural members. The heart rot sometimes found in the conversion of durable eucalypts is less of a problem in this regard.

Factors affecting the utility of commercial timber

Some factors (other than those that are strength reducing) limit the usefulness of commercial timber in its intended application. These utility considerations include distortion of the cross-sectional shape or changes in the cross-sectional dimensions. In some applications, the appearance of the timber may affect the way in which it can be used.

Bow, spring and twist

These terms are applied to deviations from straightness due either to growth stresses present in the tree or to those that develop during the seasoning process. They are illustrated in Figure 3.1, and limits are included in each of the graded product standards.

- *Cup* is a curvature across the width of the cross-section. (Edges move upwards.)
- *Bow* is a deviation from the plane of the width of the piece. (The ends move upwards.)
- *Spring* is a deviation from the plane of the edge of the piece. (The ends move sideways.)
- *Twist* is a turning of the plane of the piece along its length. It may be due to spiral grain (a common occurrence in *radiata pine*), or to sloping grain, or to stresses caused by uneven stacking for the drying process.

Cup produces little structural effect and is relatively easy to accommodate in most structural applications. If the timber is visible in a structure, a badly cupped member may be rejected for aesthetic reasons.

In framing applications, bow and twist can often be removed using noggings or blocking pieces. These can apply minor axis bending or torsion to straighten the member.

Spring is much more difficult to correct as the cross-section is very stiff in this direction. Excessive spring in flooring boards can make it difficult to bring boards into close contact when laying, unless the boards are cut into shorter lengths.

Most sawmilling operations use cutting patterns that minimise residual stresses in sawn timber products and hence reduce the number of pieces affected by these deformations.

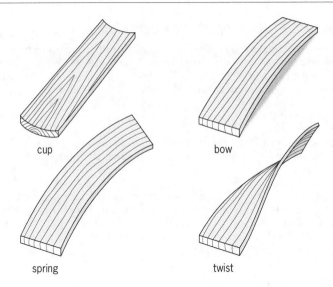

cup

bow

spring

twist

Fig. 3.1 Types of warping

Bow and spring are more of a problem in longer pieces. The amount of deviation at one end of the curved piece from the imaginary tangent to the curve at the other end increases by the square of the length of the piece. Thus, a piece twice as long would have four times as much deviation for the same shape of curve.

Bluestain

The sapwood of some species can be discoloured by bluestain fungi, particularly when milled in warm, humid weather. (In some softwood species, the heartwood can also be affected.) These fungi feed mainly on the contents of the wood cells, not on the cell wall, so they do not have much effect on mechanical properties.

While it has no consequences for most structural timber, the blue colouration caused by bluestain can be a problem for timber with appearance uses.

Pin-hole borer damage

The ambrosia or pin-hole borer can cause a serious weakening in strength if there is a large concentration of holes. Species most affected are the less dense eucalypts of south-eastern New South Wales and north-eastern Victoria.

Compliance with the restrictions imposed by the relevant Australian Standards on the number of allowable holes usually provides an adequate safeguard.

Growth features in appearance products

Some products (including joinery, mouldings, furniture and lining materials) that have minimal structural requirements are selected because of their visual impact or aesthetic appeal. The distribution and extent of growth features becomes important in the grading of the product:

- Select appearance grades have few visually discernable growth characteristics.
- Feature grades have many more growth characteristics and it is recognised by customers that they enhance the appearance of the product.

Most gum pockets or resin pockets are unwelcome in appearance grades and any later migration of gum or resin can affect the performance of coating systems. Gum veins, on the other hand, are often considered to enhance the character and appeal of the product and there is little or no likelihood of gum migration.

Moisture content

Drying (whether in the mill or in service after construction) can cause utility issues for timber including:

- checks, splits and honeycombing—these may originate during seasoning and reduce the utility of the timber product
- warping—(including development of cup, bow, spring or twist) discussed above
- shrinkage—this is a reduction in cross-sectional dimension and is discussed in Chapter 7; the increase in strength and stiffness on drying more than compensate for the reduction in section size that accompanies drying, provided the drying process has not caused a lot of degrade.

Changes in moisture content while the timber is in service can be in either direction, and seasoned timber that is used in a humid environment may swell. This can lead to jamming or the development of unintended load paths if inadequate clearance is allowed.

Development of design properties

The mechanical properties necessary for the designer when timber is required for structural members include:

1. the basic properties of the individual species, which lead to bearing capacities and joint strength properties
2. the modulus of elasticity (MoE) and strengths of the graded products, which are a function of the stress grade awarded
3. factors that take account of special loading requirements and the environmental conditions of the site.

Characteristic properties

Because of the way in which it is formed, wood has different properties in the longitudinal, tangential and radial axes. The most commonly measured properties are its modulus of rupture in bending; tension and compression strength, both perpendicular and parallel to the grain; shear strength parallel to the grain; impact bending strength; and hardness. Some of these properties for the more common species are summarised in Appendix 3. Forces tending to pull a material apart are called *tensile* forces, those that tend to crush it are *compression* forces, while the force tending to make one layer of material slide over that which is adjacent is called *shear*. When members are loaded they *deflect*; the measure of resistance to deflection is called the *modulus of elasticity (MoE)* or *stiffness* of the material. A piece of timber might be sufficiently strong to carry a certain load but if it deflects excessively under that load it might cause lining material to crack or might set up vibrations in the structure when subject to transient loads.

The following are different measures of the properties of timber:

1. *Modulus of rupture* (bending strength) can be considered as a measure of the ultimate short-term load-carrying capacity of a beam when the load is applied slowly. The major critical use of timber in structures is as beams, so this value is of great importance in assessing the structural suitability of a species. (Species- and grade-dependent property.)
2. *Tensile strength parallel to the grain* is the ultimate strength attained under a stretching load slowly applied parallel to the grain, and indicates the relative suitability of species for tension members (such as truss bottom chords). (Species- and grade-dependent property.)
3. *Tensile strength perpendicular to the grain* is the ultimate strength attainable when a force acts uniformly on an area across the grain in a manner tending to cause the member to separate transversely (This is a rare problem but can exist at complex connections.) (Species-dependent property only.)
4. *Compression strength parallel to the grain* is the ultimate strength attained under a compressing load slowly applied parallel to the grain, and indicates the relative suitability of a species for short columns. (Species- and grade-dependent property.)
5. *Compression strength perpendicular to the grain* is the maximum across-the-grain stress of a few minutes duration that can be applied through a plate covering only a portion of the timber surface without causing injury to the timber. It is an important property for the design of bearings under beams. (Species-dependent property only.)
6. *Shear strength parallel to the grain* is the ultimate strength attained when the applied force causes the member to fail by the sliding of one part upon another along the grain. (Species- and grade-dependent property.)
7. *Cleavage strength* is the ultimate resistance to a force acting across the grain and tending to split the member. It is an indicator of nail-holding ability. (Species-dependent property only.)
8. *Impact strength* is a measure of the energy needed to break a standard-sized specimen. (Generally taken as species-dependent property only.)

There are three common test methods:

(a) The Izod impact test. In this test (the one most commonly used in Australia) a notched specimen is broken at the notch by a falling pendulum and the energy absorbed in breaking the specimen is read directly from a dial.

(b) The Dension toughness test. In this test a small beam is broken in the centre by a stirrup attached to a chain pulled by a falling pendulum.

(c) The falling weight test. A standard weight is dropped from gradually increasing heights until the specimen is broken, the result being expressed as the height of the drop.

9. The *hardness* of timber, representing its resistance to wear and marking, is usually determined by the test called the Janka indentation test, which measures the force required to embed in the wood a steel ball of 11.18 mm diameter to half that diameter. (Species-dependent property only.)

10. The *modulus of elasticity* (MoE) of a material is a measure of its dimensional response under stress and for most materials is measured under tensile or compressive actions. For timber, the MoE is calculated from bending tests and incorporates some shear deformation. This makes it a useful property for the determination of the deflection of beams. (Species- and grade-dependent property.)

Establishing properties that are species-dependent only

Rather than providing tables of bearing, tension perpendicular to grain and joint strength properties for each individual species, which would be cumbersome and needlessly confusing, it has been customary to allocate species to a limited number of strength groupings.

Each species has been allocated a strength group, with an 'S' prefix for unseasoned (green) material and an 'SD' prefix for seasoned material, using the figures relevant to 12 per cent moisture content. The allocation is on the basis of the minimum species mean test values, which are obtained from small clear samples, on both unseasoned and seasoned (12 per cent moisture content) products. Minimum values are given in Tables 3.3 and 3.4. The density can also be used to assist in the allocation of strength group and joint group, as shown in Tables 3.5 and 3.6, respectively. AS/NZS 2878:2000 *Timber—Classification into Strength Groups* gives the required values and analysis methods to allocate a strength group to a species. It also contains rules for fitting species into the strength groups where all of the test data does not match exactly with one or other of the groups.

Species have been given either a positive or provisional strength grouping, depending on the amount of test data available, and either classification may be subject to change if further testing indicates significant differences, but in the meantime the classifications given by AS/NZS 2878:2000 *Timber—Classification into Strength Groups* are to be used in association with AS 1720.1-1997 *Timber Structures—Design Methods*, AS 1684:1999 *Residential Timber-Framed Construction* and the various other standards for structural timber.

Table 3.3 Minimum values for strength groups for unseasoned (green) timber (MPa)

Property	S1	S2	S3	S4	S5	S6	S7
Modulus of rupture	103	86	73	62	52	43	36
Modulus of elasticity	16 300	14 200	12 400	10 700	9100	7900	6900
Maximum crushing strength	52	43	36	31	26	22	18

Table 3.4 Minimum values for strength groups for seasoned timber (MPa)

Property	SD1	SD2	SD3	SD4	SD5	SD6	SD7	SD8
Modulus of rupture	150	130	110	94	78	65	55	45
Modulus of elasticity	21 500	18 500	16 000	14 000	12 500	10 500	9100	7900
Maximum crushing strength	80	70	61	54	47	41	36	30

In determining the classifications the following rules are used:

1. *For positive strength grouping*
   The species mean values for modulus of rupture, modulus of elasticity and maximum crushing strength in compression parallel to the grain are obtained from standard tests on small clear specimens of at least five trees representative of the species population.

2. *For provisional strength grouping*
   Where insufficient data are available to enable positive grouping, provisional classifications are made in the light of the information that is available.
   If there is sufficient information on only the seasoned material, then the unseasoned material is rated one step lower (i.e. confirmed SD5 would have a provisional S6 and, conversely, if the unseasoned material is definitely S6, then the dry material would be provisionally SD5). When provisional strength groupings are given for both unseasoned and seasoned material, the classifications should not vary by more than one strength group, with any adjustment required being on the conservative side.

When only density values are available, the provisional classification is based on the figures shown in Table 3.5. In AS 2858:2004 *Timber— Softwood—Visually Graded for Structural Purposes*, provisional classifications are indicated by enclosing the rating in brackets.

Appendix 3 gives some mechanical properties of small clear specimens from Australian species, and these can be used with AS/NZS 2878:2000 *Timber—Classification into Strength Groups* to check on the provisional strength and joint grouping. When there is a difference between the groupings from this data and those given in current Australian Standards, then the groupings in the Standards take precedence. In view of the changing pattern of timber production, with its accent on improved seed selection, plantation environment and early felling, there will be inevitable changes in strength properties from those of the mature natural growth that has been the basis for most of the earlier work, so there is a need for occasional reassessment of the classifications of the species involved.

The species density is the main parameter in allocating a joint group. These are different from the strength groups and have a 'J' prefix for unseasoned (green) material and a 'JD' prefix for seasoned material. The densities used to allocate joint group are shown in Table 3.6. Different values are used for provisional allocation of strength group (Table 3.5) compared with the joint group (Table 3.6). There is not necessarily a correlation between strength group and joint group for each species.

Table 3.5 Provisional classifications into strength groups based on density values

Strength group	Minimum density at 12 per cent moisture content (kg/m³)	Strength group	Minimum density at 12 per cent moisture content (kg/m³)
S1	1180	SD1	1200
S2	1030	SD2	1080
S3	900	SD3	960
S4	800	SD4	840
S5	700	SD5	730
S6	600	SD6	620
S7	500	SD7	520
		SD8	420

Table 3.6 Classifications into joint groups based on density values

Strength group	Basic density (kg/m³)	Strength group	Minimum density at 12 per cent moisture content (kg/m³)
J1	750	JD1	940
J2	600	JD2	750
J3	480	JD3	600
J4	380	JD4	480
J5	300	JD5	380
J6	240	JD6	300

For structural designers, the strength group of a species of timber can be found in AS 1720.1-1997 *Timber Structures—Design Methods* and AS 1720.2-1990 *Timber Structures—Timber Properties* or AS/NZS

2878:2000 *Timber—Classification into Strength Groups*. It is then used to determine the bearing strength of the species and the shear strength at joints, by consulting Table 2.3 in AS 1720.1-1997 *Timber Structures—Design Methods*.

Establishing properties that are species- and grade-dependent

During production, different pieces of timber from a single species can be sorted into a number of stress grades, each of which contains timber with similar structural properties.

Australian Standards provide the requirements of graded structural timber products. Producers mark the products with the stress grade. The stress grades are the link to many of the structural properties for the products. In order to determine the full suite of properties for structural timber, it is necessary not only to know the species or species group to which the timber belongs but also to know to which stress grade it has been allocated.

Australia now has a number of different stress grades used for structural timber products:

- F grades have been used for most visually graded hardwood and softwoods, and for some mechanically graded hardwood and softwoods. The properties are given in Table 3.7.
- MGP grades are used for machine stress-graded softwoods and have the properties given in Table 3.8.
- GL grades are used for the range of manufactured structural glued laminated (glulam) products, and have the properties given in Table 3.9.
- The A17 grade is used for visually stress-graded seasoned ash eucalypts and has the properties given in Table 3.10.
- Other manufactured structural products, such as plywood, laminated veneer lumber (LVL), I-beams, oriented strand board (OSB), parallel strand lumber (PSL) and laminated strand lumber (LSL), each have properties published by the manufacturer directly.

In each case, the stress grade is usually designated as some letters followed by a number, in a form such as F14, MGP10, A17 and so on.

Stress-graded timber products are produced using a number of different standards, including:

- visual stress-grading standards for hardwood or softwood
- machine stress grading
- manufacturing processes, such as those in glulam, LVL or plywood production.

The process of stress grading is detailed later in this chapter.

F-grade products can be graded by almost any method but are frequently visually stress-graded. They can be sourced from Australian hardwoods or softwoods and may be either seasoned or unseasoned. Some imported products are visually graded to the F grades. The properties of the F grades are presented in Table 3.7.

Table 3.7 Structural design properties for F grades (from AS 1720.1-1997 *Timber Structures—Design Methods*)

		Characteristic strength (MPa)				
Stress grade	Bending (f'_b)	Tension parallel to grain (f'_t)		Shear in beams (f'_s)	Compression parallel to grain (f'_c)	Modulus of elasticity (E)
		H'wood	S'wood			
F34	100	60	50	7.2	75	21 500
F27	80	50	40	6.1	60	18 500
F22	65	40	35	5.0	50	16 000
F17	50	30	26	4.3	40	14 000
F14	40	25	21	3.7	30	12 000
F11	35	20	17	3.1	25	10 500
F8	25	15	13	2.5	20	9 100
F7	20	12	10	2.1	15	7 900
F5	16	9.7	8.2	1.8	12	6 900
F4	13	7.7	6.5	1.5	9.7	6 100

MGP grades are specifically used for seasoned softwoods that are machine stress-graded. The MGP grades originated with in-grade tested Australian-grown pine, and the production must still be accompanied by a testing and monitoring program. In-grade testing is described later in this chapter. Mostly they are sourced from within Australia, but there is imported machine-graded softwood products in the local market marked as MGP timber from New Zealand, Chile or Scandinavia. The design values for the MGP grades are presented in Table 3.8.

Table 3.8 Structural design properties for MGP grades (from AS 1720.1-1997 *Timber Structures—Design Methods*)

		Characteristic strength (MPa)			
Stress grade	Bending (f'_b)	Tension parallel to grain (f'_t)	Shear in beams (f'_s)	Compression parallel to grain (f'_c)	Modulus of elasticity (E)
MGP15	41	23	9.1	35	15 200
MGP12	28	15	6.5	29	12 700
MGP10	16	8.0	5.0	24	10 000

Glulam timber is a manufactured wood product, which is sold as stress-graded timber. While its production differs significantly from the milling of sawn timber (see Chapter 8), the stress grades make it as easy to specify as sawn timber. The stress grades for glulam products (hardwood or softwood) are presented in Table 3.9.

Table 3.9 Structural design properties for GL grades for Glulam timber (from AS 1720.1:1997 *Timber Structures—Design Methods*)

Stress grade	Characteristic strength (MPa)				
	Bending (f'_b)	Tension parallel to grain (f'_t)	Shear in beams (f'_s)	Compression parallel to grain (f'_c)	Modulus of elasticity (E)
GL18	50	25	5.0	50	18 500
GL17	42	21	3.7	35	16 700
GL13	33	16	3.7	33	13 300
GL12	25	12	3.7	29	11 500
GL10	22	11	3.7	26	10 000
GL8	19	10	3.7	24	8 000

The A17 grade has also come about because of in-grade testing. It is sourced from mixed mountain and alpine ash (principally from Victoria), which has been visually graded to rules that target it specifically. In-grade testing was used to define the grade properties and it is periodically used to check the performance of the graded material. The A17 properties are presented in Table 3.10.

Table 3.10 Structural design properties for A17 grade (from AS 1720.1-1997 *Timber Structures—Design Methods*)

Stress grade	Characteristic strength (MPa)				
	Bending (f'_b)	Tension parallel to grain (f'_t)	Shear in beams (f'_s)	Compression parallel to grain (f'_c)	Modulus of elasticity (E)
A17	50	30	5.8	45	16 000

Use of timber grades in design

Designers make use of Australian Standards to model the behaviour of timber in the anticipated service conditions.

- Engineers designing timber elements to AS 1720.1-1997 *Timber Structures—Design Methods* must identify the specific service conditions for the timber being designed, so the appropriate modification factors can be applied.

Members for use in domestic structures can be sized using the span tables in AS 1684: 1999 *Residential Timber-Framed Construction*. The modification factors used by AS 1720.1-1997 *Timber Structures—Design Methods* are embedded in the tables.

Choosing timber for structural purposes

Other considerations as well as strength or stiffness are taken into account when deciding which species to use.

- Species vary in stability—some have a high shrinkage, or they may be subject to the excessive distortion known as 'collapse'. When varying moisture contents are anticipated in service, these dimensional stability issues may be seen as important.
- Species also vary in natural durability. Species of adequate durability for the conditions of use should be considered. If none of these are available locally, then perhaps a treated timber (see Chapter 16) should be considered.

Rather than specify a particular species, it is often more appropriate to specify only the stress grade of the required timber, and if it is for external use, its durability classification.

When the species name is specified, to avoid misunderstanding, standard trade names, as provided by Australian Standard AS/NZS 1148:2001 *Timber—Nomenclature—Australian, New Zealand and Imported Species*, should be used since many species have a variety of local names, which is likely to cause confusion.

Specification of timber should include the following details:

- size—width (depth) × thickness (breadth) (in mm)
- stress grade—this includes the stress grade designation (e.g. F8, MGP12, etc.) and the grading method, which is usually specified by referring to the Australian Standard that describes the graded timber product (these are listed below)
- moisture content—usually as 'seasoned' or 'unseasoned', but for particular applications, the moisture content can be specified at a percentage range
- species or durability information—either the species of timber or the natural durability class; if necessary, a preservative treatment can be specified.

Grading methods

Grading is simply sorting timber so that the timber in each grade has similar properties. There are different methods of sorting that are detailed in appropriate Australian or industry standards that specify the way in which timber is graded and marked for commercial use, either for appearance or structural applications.

Timber that will be used for appearance purposes, such as joinery, cabinetry, flooring, lining boards and furniture, is always visually graded by trained graders, as the presence or absence of characteristics or features such as knots, gum veins and so on is critical for such applications. There are specific appearance grading rules for these products.

However, for structural purposes, where the strength and stiffness of the material is of importance, producers can use a number of methods to sort the timber into groups with similar structural properties. These methods include:

- visual stress grading
- machine stress grading
- proof-grading.

Whichever method of grading is used, the outcome of the sorting process must produce results that are both consistent and repeatable. To achieve this level of reliability, rules for acceptable stress-graded products have been developed and are detailed in relevant Australian Standards, including:

- AS/NZS 1748:1997 *Timber—Stress-Graded—Product Requirements for Mechanically Stress-Graded Timber*
- AS 2082:2000 *Timber—Hardwood—Visually Stress-Graded for Structural Purposes*
- AS 2858:2004 *Timber—Softwood—Visually Graded for Structural Purposes*
- AS 3519:1993 *Timber—Machine Proof-Grading.*

Visual grading

Visual grading of structural timber relies on a correlation between the size of growth characteristics, as observed on the surface of the piece, and its effect on strength and stiffness. The grading rules in Australian Standards list the various growth characteristics (i.e. features likely to have some effect on the usefulness of the piece in which they occur). Each characteristic has limitations on its size and frequency of occurrence for each grade. Limits are also placed on cutting tolerances, machining defects and the degree of distortion resulting from bow, spring or twist. The acceptable moisture content range for seasoned timber is also stated (generally not more than 15 per cent).

In the Australian Standards pertaining to the visual grading of structural timber, tables are provided that establish the relationship between strength groups and stress grades for both seasoned and unseasoned timber. For example, in AS 2082:2000 *Hardwood—Visually Stress-Graded for Structural Purposes*, the following relationship is given between the various quality grades (described as no. 1 structural through to no. 4 structural), the strength group for the species and the stress grade in terms of F. For both seasoned and unseasoned timber the relationship is set out as shown in Table 3.11 on page 44.

These four grades are based on the allowance of characteristics to the extent that the strength of the material will be theoretically 75 per cent, 60 per cent, 47.5 per cent and 38 per cent, respectively, of that of small clear samples.

In the softwood visual grading standard, as a reflection of the weaker timber, strength groups S7, SD7 and SD8 appear. In the Australian Standards relevant to the particular softwood under consideration there is a table showing the relationship between the name of the grade, the F rating and the strength group of the species. The species-specific information takes precedence over the more general information provided in Table 3.11.

In Table 3.11 seasoned timber has its strength group as one of the SD1 to SD8 series. Unseasoned timber strength groups are in the S1 to S7 series.

Table 3.11 Stress grades of visually graded hardwood timber (from AS 2082:2000 *Timber—Hardwood—Visually Stress-Graded for Structural Purposes*, Appendix B)

Strength group (species property)		Stress grade (assigned to each piece of timber from VSG)			
		Structural grade no. 1	Structural grade no. 2	Structural grade no. 3	Structural grade no. 4
–	SD1	–	F34	F27	F22
–	SD2	F34	F27	F22	F17
S1	SD3	F27	F22	F17	F14
S2	SD4	F22	F17	F14	F11
S3	SD5	F17	F14	F11	F8
S4	SD6	F14	F11	F8	F7
S5	SD7	F11	F8	F7	F5
S6	SD8	F8	F7	F5	F4
S7	–	F7	F5	F4	–

VSG = visual stress grade.

The process of grading a particular species or group of species requires trained visual stress graders to examine each piece of timber and classify it according to the growth characteristics in it. The grading rules need to be relatively simple, fast and easy to apply, because the speed with which the timber passes along a sawmill production line is such that split-second decisions have to be made and there is no opportunity for careful measurement and calculations.

The grader must examine each board on all surfaces before placing it in a stack corresponding to structural grade 1 (highest strength properties) through to structural grade 4 or 5 (lowest strength properties). Timber with large knots and other strength-reducing characteristics are assigned a lower structural grade than is timber that possesses smaller knots and more clear wood. The appropriate stress grade as given in the grading standard is then marked on each piece.

Knots

All trees have branches and hence sawn timber will have knots. However, trees grown deep within forests have few branches low in the trunk as the lack of light means that those branches die early as the lower branches are shaded by the higher ones. For those trees, the outer wood in the mature trunk is essentially free of knots. This is the case for many hardwood species drawn from managed native forests.

Plantation-grown trees sustain their lower branches because the trees are all much the same height, allowing more light to reach branches that are relatively low in the tree. Hence, the timber from pine-type softwoods contains a larger number of knots.

Knots in softwoods are generally darker in colour and contrast well with the light-coloured wood and are therefore quite obvious. Knots in hardwoods are generally similar in colour to the surrounding wood but are readily distinguishable.

Plate 9 shows a photograph of an *encased knot* with the sapwood and bark on the branch quite visible. When branches are pruned and dead, new wood can grow over the end of the pruned branch as the trunk continues to become wider. This feature is known as an *occluded branch stub* and a section through one is shown in Plate 10. While the effects of the knot are still clearly present, depending on how the piece is milled, the grader may not be able to see the extent of the pruned branch.

The visual grading standards define a number of different types of knots. The Australian Standard's visual grading rules for structural softwoods differentiate knots on size using a measurement of Knot Area Ratio (KAR). This is the percentage of the cross-section that is occupied by the knot or knot group. Illustrations of how KAR is used in measuring knots are shown in Appendix B of AS 2858-2004 *Timber—Softwood—Visually Graded for Structural Purposes*.

The Australian Standard's visual grading rules for structural hardwoods differentiate knots on size using a measurement of the knot as it appears in relation to the timber surface.

The visual grading rules for both hardwood and softwood milled products measure the knot as it appears in relation to the timber surface.

Sloping grain

There is no doubt that slope of grain is one of the most important grading criteria, but it is also one of the hardest to detect at speed in a production environment. Here are some tips for assessment of slope of grain when there is the luxury of time.

A swivel-handled scribe (see Fig. 3.2) is very effective if the needle is pressed slightly into the surface and drawn steadily along in the apparent direction of the grain. If prominent growth rings are present, there is a tendency for the needle to be trapped in the earlywood between the bands of denser latewood, so it is important in such cases to repeat the operation a number of times to obtain consistency of results. A suitable scribe can be made by using the hub of the front wheel of a bicycle as the swivelling handle and fitting a bent steel rod to it. The arm of the rod should be about 170 mm long and have a replaceable needle, held in place by a small screw, near the end. It is important that the needle moves independently of any influence from the operator's hand, so the handle should be fitted with ball bearings for freedom of movement.

Another method is to probe the surface of the timber with a sharp blade (e.g. that of a pocket knife) and prise up as long a splinter as possible. The direction of the splinter should give an indication of the slope of grain but it will be appreciated that the shortness of the measured slope obtained in this way will not give a very accurate assessment.

A third method, appropriate for sawn timber that has undergone some drying, is to examine the slope of grain revealed by surface checking, such as is common in the denser hardwoods.

A fourth method, of only limited applicability because of its destructive nature, is to split a portion of the timber in question and observe the natural separation lines in the wood.

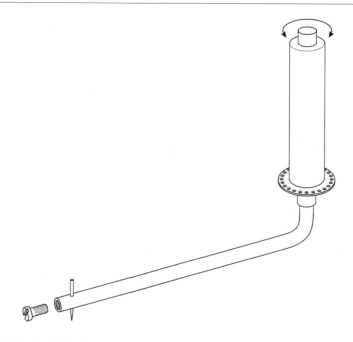

Fig. 3.2 Scribe for detecting slope of grain

Gum pockets, resin pockets

The visual grading rules have limits on the size of gum pockets (Plate 11). Gum pockets are a significant problem if they pass right through the piece or are near the end of the piece (where connections are quite probable).

Gum veins

Tight gum veins do not cause serious structural problems for timber (Plate 12), so there are few limits on them in the visual grading standards.

However, loose gum veins can cause reduction in shear and connection strengths. The visual grading standards have limits on their size and whether or not they pass right through the piece.

Checks, splits and shakes

Checks have little effect on the structural response, so provided that they are truly checks and do not pass through the piece, the limits are quite generous.

However, there are limits on the size of all splits. Splitting within the body of the piece is not allowed in any grade. The only allowed splits occur at the ends and there are limits on the size of those splits.

Shakes, as illustrated in Plates 13–15, have size limits on them as well. Shakes that pass through the piece are not permitted. (The grading rules refer to wind shakes and felling shakes and the compression fracture shown as cross shakes, as they run across the grain.)

Pith and heart-in material

Pith is the first formed wood adjacent to the growing tip of the tree. It is different in structure from, and much weaker than, the wood that subsequently forms around it. In hardwoods it is usually so small as to be virtually unnoticed, but in pine-type softwoods it can be prominent as a brownish material 3–13 mm wide, as shown in Plate 16. Pith has poor resistance to wear and is an unsatisfactory basis for coatings.

Heart-in material is generally of low density and is the timber within 50 mm of the pith. Some of the softwood visual grades have restrictions on where heart-in material may occur.

Cone holes

Pine cones occasionally remain attached to the main stem for many years and the dead tissue that attaches them to the trunk does not become intergrown with the enclosing wood. When such logs are sawn, the cone stems fall out, leaving small holes, usually about 12 mm in diameter with a lining of bark. These are treated in the same way as knots in the visual grading standards.

Needle trace

In its early stage of growth, the stem of pine-type softwoods is liberally endowed with needles, such as one sees on the young branches. Sometimes, possibly due to a pathological condition, the tissue responsible for their production persists to some extent, leaving marks in the timber known as needle trace, as shown in Plate 17. Needle trace has no structural effect and is not included in the visual grading standards.

Wane and want

The cutting of rectangular shapes out of the circular log means that some pieces are going to have an edge showing some of the outer extremity of wood growth and will not have a continuously full cross-section of wood. This is called wane. Want refers to timber missing from a piece as a result of mechanical damage.

Want and wane are limited by grading rules depending on their size. There are limits on both the length of missing timber and the width.

Bow, spring and twist

These terms are applied to deviations from straightness due either to growth stresses that are present in the tree or to those that develop during the seasoning process.

The grading rules give dimensional limits for the out-of-straightness of graded timber, which depend on the length of the piece. The limits are presented in tables in the grading standards.

Primary rot

Decay present in the living tree is described as primary rot to distinguish it from fungal destruction arising in the converted material.

The hardwood visual grading standard provides limits on the size of any area of timber affected by primary rot.

Machine stress grading

Machine stress grading uses a machine (Plate 18) to bend each piece of timber about its minor axis to measure the minimum modulus of elasticity (*MoE*) of the piece. There are now many different configurations of machine stress grader, but all involve putting the timber under some bending stress and measuring both the load and its deflection. The dynamic *MoE* is calculated at regular intervals along the length as it passes quickly through the machine. The grade of a piece of timber can be marked on the piece in a number of ways, including:

- colour marks sprayed onto the timber
- laser-printed ink marks
- ink stamping
- indent branding
- printed labels either glued or stapled to the timber.

AS 1748:1997 *Timber—Stress-Graded—Product Requirements for Mechanically Stress-Graded Timber* is used for the mechanical grading of timber. The Standard requires calibrated test pieces to be passed through the machine at regular intervals to check the accuracy of its operation. Other continuously monitored data can warn if the machine drifts out of calibration during operation.

Each stress grade has a number of structural properties that must be achieved. The machine measures just one—stiffness—but there is a loose correlation between stiffness and strength, so pieces with high stiffness also tend to have a high enough strength to be included in a higher stress grade. Regular testing of graded products ensures that the properties are being achieved.

Machine stress-graded products must also achieve satisfactory utility, so the requirements for want and wane dimensional tolerances, as well as cup, bow, spring and twist, must also be applied by trained graders. These requirements are similar to those for visually graded products. Many machine-grading operations need to use visual stress grading to override the graded product. Typically, this may be an upper KAR limit. In each case, the very ends of the pieces are not fully evaluated by the machine, so a visual grade check is applied to the ends of the pieces.

Proof-grading

Proof-grading relies on the ability of the material to carry a predetermined load similar to that which it will be required to meet in service. Passage through the machine produces only a binary 'yes' or 'no' decision (i.e. does the timber pass or fail?). However, before the material is passed through the proof grader, it first must undergo preliminary sorting into structural grades. Each stress grade has its own proof stress, which is significantly higher than the stress at serviceability loads for that grade. The proof load is applied to each board in accordance with the guidelines in AS 3519-1993 *Timber—Machine Proof-Grading*, and those that do not break, deform excessively or survive without other signs of damage are deemed to qualify for the stress grade that corresponds to the applied proof stress.

Proof-grading is not as widely used as visual or machine stress-grading methods. However, it is used by a number of producers in limited applications for grading some hardwoods and cypress. It does offer some advantages to the producer, as weaker pieces that may have been assigned a grade by visual or machine grading processes will break in the proof grader, and so will not reach the marketplace and cause problems in service. Also, if more than the accepted 1–5 per cent of timber for a particular grade fails in the proof grader, the producer will know that the reliability of the preliminary grading method needs to be improved.

In-grade testing of structural timber

In-grade testing involves sampling of a particular species and grade of commercially available timber, and testing of a large number of full-sized lengths in a manner similar to the loading expected in service. For example, bending tests on the material use a third point load over a span 18 times the depth of the timber, and the bending moment diagram is similar in shape and scale to that produced by a uniformly distributed load, and the span to depth ratio is characteristic of bending members. The test results are reported in a way that accounts for sampling error, and are taken to represent the properties of the entire population of timber of that particular species, size and grade.

AS/NZS 4063:1992 *Timber—Stress-graded—In-Grade Strength and Stiffness Evaluation* specifies test and analysis methods for the in-grade testing of timber. Tests can be used for initial evaluation of timber properties for new products or grades, or can be applied to an existing product to confirm its properties. A number of the stress grades presented earlier in this chapter have been derived by in-grade testing commercial timber products (MGP grades and the A17 grade).

The properties derived from an in-grade testing program need to be continually checked by producers through continuous and periodic monitoring procedures to ensure that the material that they are marketing still meets the requirements of the specified grade.

FURTHER READING

American Society for Testing and Materials (2002). *Standard D245-Standard practice for establishing structural grades and related allowable properties for visually graded lumber.*

American Society for Testing and Materials (2003). *Standard D2915-Standard practice for evaluating allowable properties for grades of structural lumber.*

Anton, A. (1978). Mechanical stress grading of ladder stiles. Tech. paper 27. Sydney: Forestry Commission of NSW.

Forest Products Laboratory, US Dept of Agriculture (1999). *Wood handbook. Wood as an engineering material.* FPL-GTR-113. Washington, DC: Govt Printing Office.

Kloot, N. H. (1978). The strength group and stress grade systems. Newsletter no. 394. CSIRO Division of Forest Production.

Mack, J. J. (1979). Australian methods for mechanically testing small clear specimens of timber. Tech. Paper. (2nd series) 31. CSIRO Division of Building Research.

Madsen, B. (1978). In-grade testing—problem analysis. *For Prod J* 28(4): 42–50.

Madsen, B. (1992). *Structural behaviour of timber.* North Vancouver, Canada: Timber Engineering Ltd.

Pearson, R. G., Kloot, N. H., Boyd, J. D. (1962). *Timber engineering design handbook.* 2nd edn. Melbourne: Jacaranda Press.

Siemon, G. R. (1979). Bending strength of CCA-treated slash pine poles. Note 29. Qld Dept of Forestry Research.

Spaun, F. D. (1981). Reinforcement of wood with fibreglass. *For Prod J* 31(4): 26–33.

Standards Australia (1998). *Timber design handbook.* HB108. Sydney: Standards Australia.

Szymani, R. and McDonald, K. A. (1981). Defect detection in lumber: state of the art. *For Prod J* 31(11): 34–44.

Chapter 4

Other properties of timber

Acoustic properties

'Noise' is transmitted either as airborne sound, such as speech, or as impact sound, such as footsteps. Airborne sound is transmitted as pressure waves through the air and travels at a speed of 343 m/s at 20°C and increases with increasing air temperature. Impact sound travels at a speed that is dependent on the properties of the material that it is travelling through.

The acoustic properties of wood vary with its density and modulus of elasticity. The speed of sound decreases with increasing moisture content or temperature in proportion to their influence on these properties. Surface coatings will also alter the acoustic properties. The speed of sound wave dispersion in wood is approximately the same as that in most metals (except lead), but it is many times higher than that in air (see Table 4.1).

Table 4.1 Rate of sound wave dispersion

Material	Speed (m/s)
Dry air at 20°C	343
Cork	430–530
Lead	1300
Copper	3500
Wood (along the grain)	3700–4900
Iron	5000
Aluminium	5100

With airborne sound the distinct functions of sound absorption (the prevention of reflection) and sound insulation (the prevention of transmission) should not be confused. There is no direct relationship.

Sound absorption values vary with the porosity of the material, particularly its surface, and with the frequency of the sound. Porous materials absorb mainly the high frequencies and increased thicknesses are needed to absorb low and medium frequencies. Resonant materials absorb mainly the low frequencies.

The correct control of reverberations and reflected sound is of the utmost importance in places of public assembly, such as theatres and concert halls, and a knowledge of the sound-absorbing properties of all the contents, including the audience, is required. Even then the position may not be clear, for the absorption coefficients of the individual components may be inapplicable to the total assembly. The actual values will vary with the design of the structure and the stiffness and fit of the materials. Any gaps in or around an insulating panel, for example, will seriously reduce its performance.

In wood the speed of sound wave dispersion in longitudinal, radial and tangential directions is roughly in the ratio of 15:5:3.

Non-uniformity of structure, low density and coarse texture improve sound-proofing qualities. In the case of insulation boards, these factors are the basis of the use of the network of holes often seen, especially in the acoustic tiles used for ceilings and other areas not subject to mechanical damage. The holes or fissures trap the sound, so it is important that such crevices are never filled with paint. Because of this they are often sold prefinished.

Electrical resistance

When it is in a dry condition, wood has a high resistance to the passage of electric current. However, resistance falls off very considerably with an increasing percentage of moisture present and moisture meters based on this relationship are used for making instantaneous measurements of the moisture content of timber. For example, Douglas fir has a resistance along the grain of 22 400 MΩ at 7 per cent moisture content, 120 at 12 per cent and 0.46 at 25 per cent.

Resistance varies inversely with the density of the wood but any mineral constituents present will affect resistance; the variability due to species' differences is slight compared with that due to moisture content, but it is necessary to correct readings for species' differences when using moisture meters. Resistance across the grain is approximately twice that along the grain; it is slightly greater in the tangential than in the radial direction but the difference is so slight as to be negligible for practical purposes. Moisture content meter readings along the grain are likely to be about 1 per cent higher than the reading across the grain. When using a resistance-type moisture meter, care should be taken that the meter is used as the manufacturer intended (i.e. along the grain or across the grain).

Effect of temperature

The electrical resistance of wood decreases as temperature increases, approximately halving for each temperature increase of 10°C. The amount of voltage involved will have some effect on this figure.

Most moisture meters are likely to be calibrated at about 21°C, so if the temperature of the timber is substantially different, a correction figure, which could amount to several percentage points, must be applied (refer to temperature correction table for solid wood, AS/NZS 1080.1:1997

Timber—Methods of Test—Moisture Content). An approximate guideline, in the absence of the tables, is to subtract one percentage point from the meter reading for every 10°C that the temperature of the wood is above the calibration temperature, or vice versa for cold conditions.

Effect of additives

The presence of electrolytic substances, such as sea water or ionic preservatives, can cause a considerable decrease in resistance, especially when the true moisture content exceeds about 10 per cent. Consequently, moisture meter readings are likely to be too high. The amount of error increases greatly with rising moisture content and above 15 per cent it may be too large and variable for accurate estimations. Below this figure it may be up to 3 per cent too high.

Oil-borne organic preservatives, such as creosote and pentachlorophenol, usually have little effect; if anything, the reading is more likely to be slightly lower than the true figure.

Veneer immunised against lyctid borer attack by treatment with 3 per cent borax solution gives reasonably accurate readings when its moisture content is below 15 per cent.

The glue lines of plywood may cause inaccurate meter readings. If the meter reading increases sharply as the needle electrode contacts the first glue line, any results will be suspect and should be checked against results obtained by the oven-dry method of moisture content assessment.

The use of the oven-dry method (refer AS/NZS 1080.1:1997 *Timber—Methods of Test—Moisture Content*) is generally preferable for moisture content determination when wood preservatives and/or adhesives are present.

Thermal properties

The thermal properties of a material may be considered from four main aspects: thermal conductivity, specific heat, thermal diffusivity and the coefficient of thermal expansion.

Thermal conductivity is a measure of the rate of heat flow through the material when subjected to a temperature gradient. The thermal conductivity of wood is only a small fraction of that of most building materials.

For example, the conductivity of aluminium is about 1700 times as great, steel 400, concrete 10, brick and glass 6 times, but mineral wool has only about one-third of the conductivity of wood.

The rate of flow of heat along the grain is about 2.5 times that in the radial and tangential directions; it increases slightly with an increase in wood density, extractives content and moisture content.

The *specific heat* of a material is the ratio of its heat capacity to the heat capacity of water; heat capacity is the thermal energy required to produce unit change in temperature in unit mass of material.

The specific heat of wood increases with temperature and moisture content but is almost independent of density.

Thermal diffusivity is a measure of the speed with which a material absorbs heat from the surrounding environment. It is the ratio of thermal conductivity to the product of density and specific heat.

The thermal diffusivity of wood is only about 1.25 per cent of that of steel so it seldom feels very hot or very cold to the touch.

The coefficient of thermal expansion is a measure of the change in dimension caused by a change in temperature. For oven-dry wood, linear expansion parallel to the grain seems to be relatively independent of species and density and lies within the range 0.000 003 0–0.000 004 5 per degree Celsius. The expansion across the grain is related to density and can be five to ten times that parallel to the grain; the tangential expansion is greater than the radial expansion.

The position is much more complicated for wood containing moisture. Although a rise in temperature will tend to make the wood increase in size due to thermal expansion, it will also tend to shrink because of a consequent loss of moisture if the temperature rise is maintained for a significant period; unless the wood is very dry (say, below 4 per cent moisture content) the net result will be shrinkage, not expansion, although initially there may be a little expansion before the moisture loss is effected.

R values

The term 'R value' is commonly referred to in sales literature on insulation materials. It refers to the sum of the heat resistances of individual components plus a value applied to any air space between them and on exposed surfaces; it is equivalent to the reciprocal of the aggregate coefficient of heat transmission of the building's assemblage of components (U value).

Timber, being a natural insulating material, has good thermal properties compared with other construction materials. Its properties vary with species, moisture content and density. A 25-mm thick piece of timber with a density of 690 kg/m³ would achieve an R value of about R0.17, whereas with a density of 500 kg/m³ the R value would be about R0.25. Increasing or decreasing thickness will have a proportional effect on the R value.

For a fuller explanation and a table of figures applicable to a wide range of materials, the *Wood Handbook* should be consulted.

Resistance to wear

Species vary greatly in hardness and fineness of surface so it is important to give due consideration to those properties when selecting timbers for such purposes as factory flooring, decorative domestic flooring, wooden bearings and other uses involving frictional forces.

Friction characteristics of wood

Friction is the force that acts between two bodies at their surface of contact to resist their sliding on each other. The coefficient of friction is the ratio of the force required to slide a body along a horizontal plane to the mass of the body; it is related to the tangent of the angle of repose, which is the angle of inclination at which the body will just overcome its tendency to slide down a slope.

Species, such as tallowwood, with a relatively greasy surface, have somewhat lower than normal friction coefficients. Seasoned timber in contact with unpolished steel has a coefficient that decreases from a static value of about 0.65 to about 0.4 at 3.66 m/sec. The coefficient of friction between wood and wood is of a similar nature to that between wood and unpolished steel.

The most common application of the knowledge of wood's frictional behaviour is in the study of flooring and floor finishes. Slipperiness, in itself, is not necessarily dangerous. Everyone expects a dance floor to be slippery and makes due allowance when walking on it. It is the unexpected changes in slipperiness that cause accidents. The presence of dirt, wax, water or spilt food on a floor creates danger, while the nature of the material used for the sole of the shoe is as important as that of the floor surface in assessing slipperiness.

Safety at corners requires a friction coefficient above 0.3, although lower values are safe for straight, level floors. Staircases need a coefficient over 0.35.

Leather and steel tips have a lower friction coefficient on most surfaces than do rubber or synthetics, but the situation can be quickly reversed if the surface is wet or oily. The friction coefficient of most sole materials on clean, dry uncoated wood is above 0.35 and there is no problem. Friction coefficients on waxed floors depend on the thickness of the wax and coefficients as low as 0.15 have been reported between leather and smooth finished wood with a very thin coating of wax.

Heavily waxed floors can create dangers, not so much from the wax on the floor but because the excess wax accumulates on the footwear. This can lead to an unexpected reduction in friction when the walker moves to an adjacent surface.

The hard, clear synthetic floor finishes that are now used give lower friction coefficients than uncoated wood but the figures increase as the finish wears.

It is impossible to provide a satisfactory finish for the mutually contradictory requirements of some public halls, for example, when they are to be used for both dancing and gymnastics. Such multiple use should be disallowed in the interests of safety. Gymnasium floors should not be waxed.

Resistance to abrasion

A species' capacity to resist abrasion is often taken to be directly related to its hardness. However, it also depends on its uniformity of composition and the way it was cut; quarter-cut surfaces often wear better than those tangentially cut, especially in species with pronounced growth rings. Hardwoods with relatively high density, fine, even texture and small pores are the most suitable for industrial or heavy-duty floors. An exception to this would be the hardwood with relatively few widely dispersed pores but with a very high density to compensate for the possible weakness of large pores under abrasive action. The larger the pore, the greater the opportunity for small particles of grit to become embedded in the wood and hasten abrasion. The application of a sealer to fill the pores and form a thin surface coating can do a lot to increase floor life, provided it is maintained.

Hardness

Hardness is not directly related to workability but is a measure of the resistance of the wood to indentation. The hardness figures most commonly quoted are those obtained in the Janka hardness test, which involves the pressing of a steel ball into the test specimen until the ball has penetrated to half its diameter, forming a cavity with a projected area of 1 cm².

The wearing of stiletto heels causes a great deal of damage to all types of flooring, and hardness figures are sometimes used as a guide to species selection for flooring when they may be subject to such damage. Perhaps too much importance is attached to hardness as other factors, such as edge splintering and uneven wear, also have to be considered. Even though a timber floor may initially be somewhat blemished by slight indentations, after a few months the indentations can create such a uniform pattern that they are no longer visually irritating unless penetration is deep.

Janka hardness figures for many common species are listed among the mechanical properties given in Appendix 3. The figures given are for side grain and represent an average for tangential and radial surfaces. End-grain hardness is generally somewhat higher than side grain in softwoods but in the denser hardwoods there is little difference; in fact, the end-grain hardness of some species is less than that of the side grain. As some of the figures are based on only a small sampling, they are not appropriate for making fine distinctions between species.

Miscellaneous properties

Ageing

The mechanical properties of wood show little change with time when kept in relatively dry and moderate temperature conditions. Results of testing have indicated that significant losses in strength properties only occur after several centuries of 'normal' ageing conditions. The existence of centuries-old wooden structures is testament to this.

Effect of chemicals

Wood can be treated using chemicals in order to improve durability. The chemicals used in the treatment of timber-based products do not tend to degrade the wood fibre and a range of available chemicals are specified in AS 1604.1-2005 *Specification for Preservative Treatment—Sawn and Round Timber*.

The effect of waterborne preservatives or other wood-swelling organic liquids, typically applied to seasoned timber to assist with chemical uptake, is to lower the mechanical properties of the wood. These properties can be regained by the removal of the liquid through redrying.

Oil-borne and solvent-based preservatives tend to have a non-appreciable effect on wood properties due to their non-swelling nature on wood. An exception to this is ammonia, which has a plasticising effect on wood, and can affect both strength and stiffness. But once it has been removed, these properties are generally regained.

However, certain chemical solutions can permanently affect wood strength properties. In general, care should be taken when using chemicals that decompose wood fibre through a process of oxidation (e.g. nitric acid) or hydrolysis.

Wood has been used extensively in cooling towers and fertiliser storage facilities due to its superior resistance to mild acids and solutions of acidic salts compared with other construction materials. Alkaline environments are more hazardous to wood fibre.

FURTHER READING

Acoustic properties

Building Research Establishment, UK (1976). Sound insulation of lightweight dwellings. *BRE Digest* no. 187.
Commonwealth Experimental Building Station (1958). Noise in buildings. *Notes on the Science of Building* no. 48.
Commonwealth Experimental Building Station (1971). Noise problems in buildings. *Notes on the Science of Building* no. 116.

Electrical resistance

AS/NZS 1080.1:1997 *Timber—Methods of Test—Moisture Content.*
Forest Products Laboratory, US Dept. of Agriculture (1999). *Wood handbook. Wood as an engineering material.* General technical report FPL-GTR-113 Madison, Wisconsin: US Dept. of Agriculture.

Thermal properties

British Standard 4016. *Building Papers (Breather Type).*
Building Research Establishment, UK (1969). Standard U-values. *BRE Digest* no. 108.
Forest Products Laboratory, US Dept. of Agriculture (1999). *Wood handbook. Wood as an engineering material.* General technical report FPL-GTR-113 Madison, Wisconsin: US Dept. of Agriculture.

Chemical properties

AS 1604.1:2005 *Specification for Preservative Treatment—Sawn and Round Timber.*

Chapter 5

Corrosion aspects of wood use

Most structural materials suffer some deterioration when in contact with the more reactive chemical solutions and fumes. In general, wood is superior to the common metals in resistance to mild acidic conditions but inferior in regard to alkalis. It gives a reasonable performance under moderately acid and alkaline conditions (between, say, pH 2 and pH 10) provided the temperature is in the normal atmospheric range.

Resistance to chemical attack is greater in softwoods than in hardwoods. Softwoods usually have a lower hemicellulose and higher lignin content so are basically more able to resist attack, but ease of penetration of the wood is also of practical importance. Sapwood, because of its permeability, has lower resistance, while the heartwood of dense hardwoods can give almost equal performance to that of softwoods, at least in coping with acidic conditions. Resin has some inhibiting effect on penetration and degradation so softwoods with considerable resin content, such as Douglas fir and slash pine, usually have good resistance to chemicals if free of sapwood. Timber with knots, checks or splits should be avoided in applications requiring optimum resistance to corrosive agents.

Strongly oxidising chemicals, such as nitric acid, potassium permanganate, chromic acid and hydrogen peroxide, have a destructive effect if contact is prolonged. Hydrogen sulfide and carbon dioxide are not corrosive to wood but flue gases containing sulfur dioxide can be very corrosive. Organic acids are much less destructive than inorganic acids. Alcohols and refined petroleum oils are not destructive.

Wood is commonly used for vats and tanks for chemical storage, for mixing equipment and for the structural members of buildings where corrosive vapours are present, such as swimming pools and fertiliser storage. The use of epoxy coatings and fibreglass liners is a common way of giving extra protection.

Wood components are frequently held together by steel nails. Iron salts are often strongly acidic so when moisture is present for long periods, iron can have a hydrolysing action on the enclosing wood. In boats, for example, the wood around rusting nails is often discoloured and softened, a condition sometimes described as 'nail sickness'. Such deterioration is most noticeable in species that are strongly acidic or high in tannins, such as eucalypts, redwood and European oak.

Staining by alkalis

Species liberally endowed with polyphenolic extractives are very prone to staining by alkalis. For example, fire doors made with a fibre-cement infill and eucalypt veneer facing can suffer staining if there is enough residual dampness in the infill to cause outward migration of alkali. Alkaline adhesives, such as casein, can cause stains that are difficult to remove if the top veneer is thin.

Alkaline vapours can produce staining too. This factor can be put to use in providing a decorative brown colour to eucalypts; the wood surface is exposed to ammonia vapour in a closed container as the final step in its preparation before the application of a protective finish.

Effect of seaside atmosphere

Surface degradation of tile battens and rafters in unsarked roofs is observed occasionally in dwellings built close to the sea. A fuzz of orange-brown fibrous material is often observed on Douglas fir rafters in sea-front houses in the Sydney area. It may reach a depth of 5 mm after 16 years' exposure. It appears that the formation of salt crystals causes mechanical disruption of the wood fibres. Something similar occurs occasionally on the internal surfaces of boats when continual evaporation leads to a build-up of salt, and on cooling tower components when water with a lot of dissolved salts is involved.

Effect of solvents

Due to its complex polymeric nature the basic substance of wood is very resistant to solvents, but some of the extractives are easily dissolved. The rate of removal of extractives will depend on the particle size of the pieces of wood being extracted and the temperature of the solvent. Heating with high-temperature steam will also remove a lot of the hemicelluloses, while alcohol–water mixes at high temperatures have some solvent action on lignin.

Effect of oxidising agents

Strong oxidising agents, such as potassium permanganate, chromic acid, hydrogen peroxide and nitric acid, attack both the lignin and polysaccharides. High concentrations of oxidising agent at elevated temperatures will completely destroy wood's complex structure. Dilute solutions of oxidising agents are used for bleaching purposes (e.g. chlorine, sodium hypochlorite, hydrogen peroxide).

The use of chlorine in the circulating water in cooling towers to control the growth of algae must be carefully controlled to prevent damage to the wood and the concentration should be maintained below one part per million.

Natural acidity of wood

Wood is almost always somewhat acidic. Aqueous extracts that were obtained by shaking wood particles with water were used for the determination of acidity, which is listed in Table 5.1. Acidity and alkalinity are expressed scientifically in terms of pH value. A full explanation of the meaning of pH and its relation to the concentration of hydrogen ions is out of place here (consult a chemistry reference book) but in simple terms a pH of 0 is extremely acid, 7 is neutral and 14 is extremely alkaline. The scale of progression between these numbers is logarithmic (i.e. a change of 1 unit indicates a tenfold change). The pH figure is generally characteristic of a species, but the heartwood is generally slightly more acidic than the sapwood.

The pH figures recorded for a range of local and imported species are given in Table 5.1. The number of samples tested varied considerably betweens species so the figures quoted should be treated as a guideline only.

Corrosion of metals by wood

The pH figure gives only a general indication of a wood's relative corrosiveness; the actual effect of a particular species will depend on the types of acidic material present, moisture content and preservative treatment. Seasoned timber is seldom corrosive but the acidic constituents are likely to be more reactive when the timber becomes wet or if it is used when unseasoned, at which time it may also contain a small amount of acetic acid. When the pH is below about 4.3, steel's rate of corrosion when in contact with *damp* timber increases very considerably and the effect is often noticed on nails. Aluminium, copper, brass, bronze and galvanised steel are much more resistant than steel to wood acids, although aluminium can undergo considerable pitting when in contact with the moist wood of highly acidic species.

Sometimes logs become contaminated with salt, either through immersion in sea water or by exposure to salt spray. Salt is sometimes used overseas in the seasoning of species prone to checking because its hygroscopic nature slows down the rate of surface drying. However, it does increase the risk of subsequent corrosion. Salt is very corrosive to iron and steel when the wood becomes damp, as is likely to occur because of the attraction of moisture by salt.

Metal corrosion is a process of oxidation—moisture and oxygen have to be present on the surface of the metal before it can occur. Corrosion can be arrested if a thin film of oxide forms on the surface but if some acidic substance is present to keep a fresh metal surface exposed, it will continue unchecked.

When corrosion of iron and steel occurs, the wood in contact with the metal gradually loses much of its tensile strength, for rusting metal catalyses the oxidation of the polysaccharides of the wood.

Table 5.1 pH values for a range of local and imported woods

Species	pH	Species	pH
Alder, brown	5.0	Kapur	3.2–3.7
Ash, alpine	3.6	Karri	4.1
Ash, Crow's	5.1	Kauri	5.1
Ash, English	3.5–5.3	Kempas	3.6–4.6
Ash, mountain	4.5	Keruing	5.1
Ash, silver	5.1	Larch, European	4.0
Ash, silvertop	3.5	Mahogany, African	4.5–5.1
Balsa	5.4–7.2	Mahogany, brush	5.1
Baltic, red	4.3–4.6	Mahogany, red	2.4–3.4
Baltic, white	4.0–5.0	Mahogany, rose	4.0
Bean, black	3.8–5.2	Mahogany, white	3.9
Beech, European	4.5–6.1	Maple, rose	5.5
Beech, negrohead	4.6–5.1	Maple, sugar	5.0–5.8
Beech, silky	5.7	Meranti, red, light	4.3–6.1
Beech, white	4.6–5.0	Meranti, red, dark	3.9–5.3
Birch, white	3.9–4.9	Merbau	4.3
Blackbutt	3.4	Mersawa	4.3–4.6
Bloodwood, red	3.6	Messmate	3.2
Bollywood	3.9	Oak, European	3.3–5.2
Box, brush	3.9–4.6	Oak, Japanese	3.2–4.7
Box, grey	3.5	Oak, silky, mountain	4.1
Brownbarrel	3.3	Oak, tulip, blush	5.2
Carabeen, yellow	4.4	Pine, CCA-treated H5	5.1
Cedar, red, western	2.9–4.0	Pine, CCA-treated H3	4.8
Chestnut	3.6	Pine, hoop	5.2
Coachwood	5.0	Pine, Huon	4.5
Cypress, white	5.7	Pine, LOSP tin-treated	4.6
Elm	6.0–7.2	Pine, maritime	3.8
Fir, Douglas	3.1–4.4	Pine, Parana	5.2–8.8
Geronggang	2.6	Pine, radiata	4.0–4.8
Gum, blue, Sydney	3.6–4.2	Poplar	4.6–5.6
Gum, grey	3.8	Ramin	5.2
Gum, red, forest	3.7	Sapele	5.3–4.6
Gum, spotted	4.6–5.0	Sassafras	5.5
Hemlock, western	4.8–5.4	Seraya, white	5.0–5.5
Hickory	5.2	Spruce, Sitka	3.4–5.5
Ironbark, grey	3.7	Sycamore	4.2–6.0
Ironbark, red, narrow-leaved	3.7	Tallowwood	3.6–3.8
Iroko	5.2–7.2	Teak	4.5
Jarrah	3.0–3.7	Turpentine	3.6–3.9
Jelutong	4.6	Yellowwood	4.9–5.2

CCA = copper–chrome–arsenic. LOSP = light organic solvent-borne preservative.

Corrosion of fasteners in treated timber

Most oil-based or light organic solvent-based preservative treatments do not have any significant effect on corrosion. Some timber preservative treatments do, however, increase the rate of corrosion of metal fasteners that are in direct contact with preservative-treated timber. This increase in rate can usually be attributed to the presence of 'salts' or the dissimilar nature of the metals in the preservative, such as copper, and possible higher moisture contents present in treated timber.

Common preservative treatments, such as copper–chrome–arsenic (CCA), can increase the rate of corrosion of galvanised fasteners by up to twofold (Plate 19). Recent research indicates that some of the newer preservative treatments, such as ammoniacal copper quaternary (ACQ) and copper azole, will be more than twice as corrosive as CCA.

For galvanised steel fasteners, corrosion protection is directly proportional to the thickness or weight of the galvanised coating. For normal environments where the moisture content of the timber, including CCA-treated timber, would rarely exceed about 18 per cent, the minimum recommended weight of galvanising on 'light' metal connectors, straps and so on has typically been specified as Z275 (275 gm/m^2) and for hot-dipped galvanised bolts and heavier connectors, at about 450 gm/m^2.

For more corrosive environments or when timber treatments are more corrosive, consideration should be given to the use of stainless steel fasteners, the use of heavier galvanising, or supplementary protection of the fastener by application of epoxy paints or plastic coatings or sleeves.

Corrosion at metal fixings in boats

To avoid the risk of corrosion it is important to use the same metal, or very similar metals, throughout the vessel or to provide careful insulation of the metals from each other. The electrical system should be checked regularly to ensure that there are no leakages of current, which will promote electrochemical attack of the metals.

The strongly electrolytic salts in sea water provide ideal conditions for the corrosion of dissimilar metals in boats as they act as the poles of a galvanic cell. Acid is produced at the anode and alkali at the cathode. The more electropositive metal acts as the cathode, where the alkali formed damages the wood more quickly than the acid does at the anode. Copper fixings are commonly used in boats and because of copper's highly electropositive character, it is generally the cathode. The alkali that forms around it under active electrolysis can soften the wood and lead to a weakening of the grip of the copper fastenings.

Corrosion of metals by wood vapours

Wood is used very extensively in the manufacture of containers for the conveyance of goods; sometimes it is used in a seasoned condition, sometimes not. If valuable metallic equipment is to be stored in closed containers for a considerable period, it is important to ensure that the container is made from seasoned timber or the equipment is given special surface treatment.

Corrosion of metals is aided by a high relative humidity in the surrounding air and the rate of corrosion increases rapidly once the relative humidity exceeds 80 per cent.

The risk of corrosion will obviously depend on the conditions of exposure of the container. Storage in the hot sun, in ships' holds in tropical conditions or in defence stockpiles in jungle areas obviously presents conditions of considerable hazard.

Long storage in unfavourable conditions could cause some hydrolysis of hemicelluloses, resulting in the formation of acetic acid, which will attack metals. If susceptible equipment is to be stored for long periods, it is wise to wrap it in impermeable bags or provide protective surface coatings. With regard to this latter point, softwood of high resin content, and hence high in volatile turpentine, should be kiln-dried to drive off the turpentine, which can have some solvent action on protective coatings.

Salt water penetration of immersed logs

In parts of the world, logs are sometimes transported by towing them through harbour waters to the site of the sawmill or veneer mill and sometimes they may remain stored in such salty water for many weeks. Salt is a very strong electrolyte so its presence in quantity in the timber can affect its electrical insulation value and its ability to take radiofrequency curing of adhesives, as well as making it hygroscopic and corrosive to metal fixings.

Penetration of the heartwood is very slight but the sapwood of softwoods has been found to have increased levels of salt after 6 months storage in sea water; about half of this amount is taken up in the first few weeks. The outer 5 mm of the sapwood may have between 4 and 7 per cent of salt. Subsequent soaking of the logs in fresh water is ineffective in removing the salt. The presence of bark on the log cannot be relied on to stop the penetration, although it will have some retarding effect.

As with treated timber, moisture meter methods of determining the moisture content of timber and veneer cut from such logs may give quite unreliable results.

FURTHER READING

American Wood Preservers Institute (1971). Treated timber in corrosive environments. *Wood Preserving* 49(11): 13–17.

Baker, A. J. (1974). Degradation of wood by products of metal corrosion. USDA Forest Service research paper FPL 229.

Experimental Building Station (1977). Cathodic protection. *Notes on the Science of Building* no. 149.

Farmer, R. H. (1962). Corrosion of metals in association with wood. *Wood* 27(11): 443–6.

Pinion, L. C. (1970). The degradation of wood by metal fastenings and fittings. UK Forest Products Research Laboratory. *Timberlab Papers* no. 27.

Simpson Strong-Tie (2004). Preservative treated wood. Technical bulletin. Dublin, CA: Simpson Strong-Tie Co. Inc. <www.strongtie.com>.

Chapter 6

Timber processing and products

A multiplicity of processes is available to convert logs to useable and valuable timber and timber products. These processes can vary significantly in their form and sophistication, from basic techniques, such as debarking and docking to length, to sawing or peeling or further breakdown of the wood into strands, chips or fibres followed by reconstitution.

For most operations, processing usually starts in the forest, with the output and end products from the forest being dictated by demand, species and log quality. Once felled, trees will normally be assessed, graded and docked into logs for conversion using different processes depending upon their shape, form and quality. Logs may be earmarked as girders or poles, or for sawing or peeling, or if of low quality, to be converted to chip, strand or fibre for reconstitution into structural and panel products.

The following briefly describes the most common processes and products.

Round timber

There are many uses for timber that do not involve the longitudinal sawing of the log section. Very large quantities of timber are used each year in the form of round timber for bridge girders, poles for electricity and telephone services, building poles, retaining walls and landscaping applications. Timber piling is another common use for round timber for supporting wharves, as well as providing the foundations for buildings on land that has been filled or has poor load-bearing properties. Round fence posts, pergolas and playground equipment in preservative-treated plantation pine are also common applications across Australia.

Poles

The wood quality of poles required for power and communication purposes is dealt with in AS 2209-1994 *Timber—Poles for Overhead Lines*, which provides grading rules for three categories: poles intended for use without full-length preservative treatment; hardwood poles intended for use after full-length preservative treatment; and softwood poles intended for use after full-length preservative treatment. A list of acceptable species is given for each category.

If the narrow band of sapwood on durable poles is not preservative-treated, it will eventually decay so its width is ignored in making calculations of the mechanical strength of the pole. In order to make full use of timber resources it is now common practice to impregnate the sapwood on the naturally durable species also with preservatives so as to take advantage of the full cross-section in engineering calculations of the pole size required. Alternatively, untreated sapwood can be removed to ensure that it does not become unsightly when it decays and to provide a continuous firm footing when embedded in the ground. In removing the sapwood from the pole it is undesirable to shave off large portions of natural bumps to make the pole more symmetrical as this will weaken the pole.

When the less durable species are to be treated, all sapwood should be retained to provide as thick a shell of treatment as possible, even if this does mean that the shape is not as regular as one might wish. AS 2209-1994 specifies minimum thickness requirements for sapwood on poles intended for preservative treatment. The Standard specifies greater thickness of treatable sapwood for the less durable species and the minimum charge retentions for a range of acceptable preservative chemicals.

The Standard provides for two grades of straightness, 'select' and 'standard', which take into account sweep, crooks and kinks; interpretation is made easy by diagrams. 'Select' grade straightness should not be specified except for poles in important public areas where aesthetic considerations have to be paramount.

The amount of taper to be expected averages about 8 mm per metre of length. Young trees are usually very slender with a large height-to-diameter ratio, as also are trees from high quality forests, although some species (e.g. blackbutt) are inclined to have a considerable butt swell.

Ground-line diameter is the critical factor in pole performance. AS 1720.1-1997: *Timber Structure—Design Methods* provides typical structural design rules for poles and round timber and applies additional modifications if the poles or round timber have been trimmed or shaved or are of small diameter or from immature trees. Other Australian Standards provide specific design guidelines for special applications, such as power poles, piles and retaining walls.

All poles, even those that have been given approved preservative impregnation, may need some supplementary ground-line treatment at perhaps 4- or 5-year intervals, especially in the more tropical areas. A lot of research has been carried out on improving ground-line treatments and also in non-destructive test methods for the determination of decay or termite attack in the interior of the pole during its service to ensure that poles do not fail unexpectedly or, on the other hand, are not removed unnecessarily because of mere suspicion of internal deficiencies. The traditional method of assessment has been a visual assessment by experienced examiners or mechanical proof testing. New techniques include the use of sound waves, X-rays, pulsed electric currents and thermal imaging, which all apply a form of energy that distinguishes sound timber from decayed material and voids.

Enclosure of a pole, or post, in concrete is an undesirable practice because it encourages decay. There may be instances, as in unstable soil, where such a procedure is undertaken to provide additional mechanical support, but the presence of the concrete tends to retain moisture and makes it difficult to carry out supplementary ground-line treatment of the soil around the pole.

If such concrete encasement is unavoidable, the concrete should be a 'no fines' mix (i.e. concrete with aggregate and sand) to enable better drainage away from the pole, the drainage of the area should be good, and the runoff of water from the pole should be prevented from running down the inevitable gap between wood and concrete, which can be 'caulked' and maintained. Ensuring that the concrete collar is about 100 mm below ground level will lessen the risk of water entering that gap.

The tops of all poles, treated or not, should be fitted with a metal cap to prevent water entry into the absorbent end-grain and any shaved nodes or branch stubs should be treated with a supplementary preservative and sealed to prevent water entry into end-grain of the branch stub.

Piles

In addition to their widespread use for the support of wharves, piles are commonly used to provide the foundations of buildings erected on sites where the bearing quality of the ground is unreliable.

When embedded in ground below the water table, piles will last virtually indefinitely, even if untreated. If the tops protrude above the water table, they will be at risk of decay and termite attack, so some protective treatment is needed. Except for a few species, such as turpentine, which is used for marine piles, land and marine piles should be preservative-treated in accordance with AS 1604.1-2005 *Specification for Preservative Treatment—Sawn and Round Timber*. Timber piles are ideally suited to highly corrosive sites, such as where acid sulfate soils are encountered. For these highly acidic sites, oil-borne treatments, such as pigment-emulsified creosote (PEC), should be specified as acidic environments may affect waterborne treatments.

When driving piles, it is desirable to fit a circular ring of metal around the top to limit the extent of splitting caused by the many blows of the pile driver. When the damaged area is cut off, the freshly exposed surface should be treated with an appropriate preservative oil or a gel containing fungicide and insecticide.

AS 3818.3-2001 *Timber—Heavy Structural Products—Visually Graded—Piles*, which applies to both treated and untreated hardwood piles and treated softwood piles, provides relevant grade descriptions and specifications in addition to species information.

Detailed information on timber in marine applications can be obtained from *Marine Borers and Timber Piling Options* by L. J. Cookson (see further reading).

Hewn timber

'Hewn' means that the timber is shaped with a 'board-axe'. In years gone by, hewn timber was preferred over sawn timber for exterior purposes partly because the blow of the axe blade was claimed to compact the surface and close the pores of the wood against moisture entry (in contrast with the woolly surface imparted by a saw cut), but the main reason for a preference for hewn timber seems to be that the operator would be sure to pick straight-grained timber to make the task easier. Railway sleepers, bridge girders and other large structural members were generally hewn until the advance of mechanisation overwhelmed the craft of the 'axeman'.

Sawn timber

Many types of saws and sawing patterns are used to convert round timber into sawn square and rectangular sections. The saw types and techniques used will vary depending upon species, log size, throughput, end products and cross-sections required.

Examples of different types of saws include single and twin circular saws (for breaking down large diameter logs), band saws, twin edger saws, gang saws (multiple circular saws) and frame saws (multiple reciprocating vertical blades).

Methods of sawing

The simplest method of cutting up a log is to 'spot' (cut a small amount off) one side to provide a level base for the log and then, after turning it onto this base, to make a series of parallel cuts without any further turning of the log. This is known as 'sawing through and through'. Gang saws carry out this operation with one pass of the log through the saws. This is a common method for fast large-scale production, but it lacks flexibility and is not suited to the production of varied sizes and qualities. It is quite unsuitable for processing logs with a large central pipe, and, owing to the mixture of grain directions obtained, a large amount of seasoning faults (e.g. warp, twist, etc.) may occur. 'Through and through' sawing is often used with logs of small size and good form, producing standard lines.

Hardwoods, which vary greatly in log diameter and may have a large central pipe, require methods of 'sawing around' the major defects by altering the position of the log during sawing to permit the separation of sapwood from heartwood, clear portions from knotty portions, and sound timber from areas of decay. There are two main methods of sawing around the defect:

- back-sawing (back-cutting, tangential cutting)
- quarter-sawing (quarter cutting, radial cutting).

Back-sawing is the most common method in Australia and aims at the production of boards with faces roughly tangential to the annual growth and at right angles to the rays. In practice, timber is regarded as back-sawn if the growth rings meet the face of the board at an angle less than 45°.

Back-sawing is flexible and enables high-grade timber to be obtained from low-quality logs. It generally gives a higher recovery of timber than quarter-sawing, a greater speed of production, and is a simpler milling

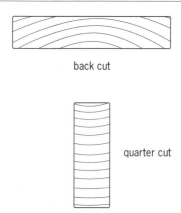

back cut

quarter cut

Fig. 6.1 Back-cut and quarter-cut timber

operation. Knots, if present, show in round form, not as a spike, and ring shakes, gum pockets and resin pockets may be cut out in one board instead of affecting a number of boards. The proportion of wide boards will also be greater than from a similar sized log when quarter-sawn.

Quarter-sawing aims at producing as many boards as possible with their faces parallel to the rays. Timber is called 'fully quarter-sawn' when the growth rings show an angle not less than 80° to the face of the board. For normal milling, an angle not less than 45° is acceptable in quarter-sawn material. Quarter-sawing has a number of advantages.

1. It may give a better appearance to a hardwood by showing prominent ray figure, or the stripe or ribbon effect of interlocking grain; however, in those species (softwood or hardwood) with pronounced growth rings the back-cut surface is usually more decorative.
2. Because quarter-sawn boards shrink less in width there will be a less noticeable movement in service, which may be of importance for such applications as ship's decking. The quarter-sawn boards of some species wear considerably better than back-sawn boards.
3. The gum veins that are commonly found in the eucalypts may show on the back-sawn boards as shallow but wide and unsightly blotches; on quarter-sawn faces the same veins may show as narrow lines, quite acceptable in appearance.
4. Quarter-sawn material is generally less prone to cupping, warping and checking.
5. Hardwoods that are prone to collapse during the seasoning process can be more successfully reconditioned if quarter-sawn, as the back-sawn material, unless carefully controlled during drying, can tend to form many surface checks.

Scantling and boards

The cross-sections produced by sawing are usually categorised as either scantling and framing or boards. These products may be further sorted, graded and processed (dried, dressed, remachined, etc.) depending upon the final product destination. Sizes produced 'green off saw' will be targeted to enable final end-product dimensions to be achieved and the initial sawn size will need to take into consideration subsequent shrinkage due to seasoning and reduction in dimensions due to dressing or planing.

The usual nominal dimensions of unseasoned sawn hardwood and softwood will have thicknesses of about 16, 25, 38, 50 and 75 mm, with widths (depths) of 38, 50, 75, 100, 125, 150 and so on to 250 mm. Typical seasoned dressed framing (softwood or hardwood) dimensions are a thickness of 35 and 45 mm and width (depth) of 70, 90, 120, 140, 170, 190 and 240 mm.

Board products are usually graded visually in accordance with relevant Australian or company standards, which take into consideration aesthetic as well as any structural requirements depending upon the product, such as flooring, lining, cladding, mouldings or furniture stock. For structural timbers, grading requirements are covered in Chapter 3.

Manufactured products

Nail-laminated and nail-plated sections

Because the maximum dimensions of seasoned structural timber are limited, larger cross-sections can be built up using nail-laminating and nail-plating technology.

Vertical nail-laminated beams can be made by nailing together thinner solid sections to achieve a section with equivalent structural properties of a full solid section of the same overall dimensions. AS 1684.2–4-1999 *Residential Timber-Framed Construction* provides guidance on nail sizes and spacing for vertically laminated beams.

Nailplate-joined timber members are produced by joining small sections of seasoned timber together using *pressed in, toothed nail-plates* that are similar in nature to truss nailplates. The final beam sections

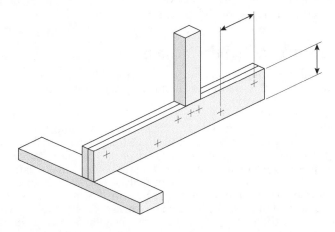

Fig. 6.2 Vertical nail lamination

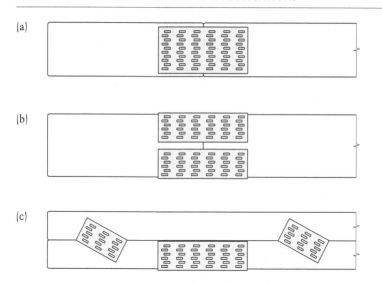

Fig. 6.3 Examples of nailplate-joined beams: (a) butt-joined single plate; (b) butt-joined double wrap around plate; (c) built-up butt-joined multiple diagonal plates

can be built up by joining pieces of timber one on top of the other and also by plating together butt joints. As nailplate joining technology is proprietary, structural capacity and allowable spans are provided by the individual manufacturers. AS 4446-1999 *Manufacture of Nailplate-Joined Timber Products* provides guidance on materials, quality, manufacture and tolerances.

Nail-plate-joined members are not suitable for use in external applications, such as deck joists and bearers, because changing moisture content in the timber may cause the nailplates to become dislodged, with a subsequent loss of structural integrity.

Glued laminated timber (glulam)

Glued laminated timber, sometimes referred to as glulam, is an engineered structural material consisting of a number of graded, seasoned and mostly finger-jointed laminations, bonded with a proven structural adhesive to form a solid member of cross-section, length and shape limited only by manufacturing, transport and handling capabilities. Lamination has the benefit of using smaller pieces of timber which, when glued together, may produce a member of higher grade than the individual pieces.

It is possible to manufacture a glued laminated timber beam with higher strength laminates in areas of high stress, such as in the top or bottom of beams, and lower strength laminates in the areas of low stress. Steel and fibre can be incorporated in areas of high tensile stress and may be positioned either parallel or perpendicular to the laminate direction.

Glued laminated timber can be custom-built to almost any size, shape and length, including curved, tapered or profiled cross-section, however, a range of standard sizes is available. The product can be used in almost any type of buildings, from simple dwellings to major public buildings and even bridges. Its strength, stability, chemical and fire resistance, and its almost limitless range of sizes and shapes, makes it one of the most versatile building products available today.

Glued laminated timber is manufactured in accordance with AS/NZS 1328.1:1998 *Glued Laminated Structural Timber—Performance Requirements and Minimum Production Requirements* and standard grades are set out in AS/NZS 1720-1997 *Timber Structures—Design Methods*. These grades have been developed with a suite of structural properties that are different from the 'F' ratings used on solid timber and the use of 'F' ratings to grade this product is therefore inappropriate. Modulus of elasticity (*MoE*) is the structural property that generally governs the design of a beam and, for this reason, the industry has adopted a descriptor based on the *E* value of the grade (i.e. GL18 means it has an *E* value of 18 500 MPa).

Laminated veneer lumber (LVL) and laminated strand lumber (LSL)

LVL and LSL are engineered structural materials that are manufactured by bonding wood veneers or strands together with a structural adhesive to form a solid member of end-sections and length limited only by manufacturing, transport and handling capabilities. The grain direction of each veneer or strand is usually oriented parallel to the length of the piece but may be cross-banded for speciality applications. Its laminated structure disperses strength-reducing characteristics more evenly, giving LVL and LSL higher bending strength and stiffness than the equivalent solid timber section of the same species. LVL and LSL are manufactured as seasoned product.

The main use of these products is in residential and industrial buildings as floor joists, lintels, purlins, roof truss components, portal frames and so on. The product can be cut to a variety of shapes and facilitates structural innovation using angular and curved forms.

LVL and LSL are produced as billets 1.2 m wide and 2.4 m wide. Structural member sizes are resawn from the billets in a range of standard widths, depending on the individual manufacturer. Other sizes are available to order. Curved shapes can be manufactured, provided the curved profile can be cut from the production 'billets'.

Commonly available stock widths and depths are as follows but advice should be sought from individual manufacturers prior to specification:

- depths: 95, 130, 150, 170, 200, 240, 241, 300, 302, 356, 360, 400, 406, 457 mm
- widths: 36, 44, 45, 63, 68, 75, 89, 90 mm (other widths can be created by laminating pieces together)
- lengths up to 12 m are available (more from some manufacturers).

Each manufacturer designs and tests products in accordance with AS/NZS 4063:1992 *Timber—Stress-Graded—In-Grade Strength and Stiffness Evaluation* to determine their design properties. This engineering data is available from the relevant manufacturer, together with span tables for common applications.

LVL and LSL are generally not considered an appearance product, as glue lines are often quite visible. However, they may be coated with an opaque finish after a light sanding if the unfinished appearance is not acceptable in visually exposed applications.

Not all LVL and LSL are the same. When a design is based on a particular size and brand of the product, substitution with another brand should not be made without engineering advice. Product-specific information, including member span tables, is available from individual manufacturers.

Parallel strand lumber (PSL)

Parallel strand lumber (PSL) is a high-strength proprietary structural composite timber product manufactured by gluing strands of wood together under pressure.

The initial steps of PSL manufacture are similar to those used in the manufacture of plywood. Logs are turned on a lathe to create veneer and the veneer sheets are dried. The veneer sheets are clipped into long narrow strands of wood up to 2.4 m in length and about 12 mm in width. Strength-reducing characteristics are evenly dispersed, giving the product higher bending strength and stiffness than the equivalent solid timber section of the same species. PSL is manufactured as a seasoned product.

The strands are coated with an exterior-type adhesive (phenol-formaldehyde), which is laid up with the strands oriented to the length of the member, and formed into a continuous billet that is fed into a belt press. Under pressure and microwave-generated heat, the glue is cured to produce a finished continuous billet about 300–500 mm in cross-section.

The billet is then cross-cut to desired lengths, rip sawn to produce stock dimensions or custom sizes, and sanded down to finish dimensions. Larger dimensions can be produced by edge gluing billets together using techniques that are common to those used for the manufacture of glued laminated timber.

As it is a glued-manufactured product, PSL can be made in long lengths but it is usually limited to 20 m by transportation constraints. Currently, PSL is imported into Australia, mainly from North America, and is a proprietary technology protected by world patents owned by the manufacture.

PSL is well suited for use as columns and beams for post and beam construction, and for beams and lintels. It is used for large members in residential construction and as intermediate and large members in commercial building construction.

PSL readily accepts preservative treatment and a very high degree of penetration and therefore protection is possible. PSL exhibits the dark glue line of glued laminated timber except that the glue lines are much more numerous. It can be machined, stained and finished using the techniques applicable to sawn lumber.

The stock sizes available for PSL are intended to be compatible with established timber framing materials and standard dimensions. PSL beams are available in thicknesses of 63, 89, 133 and 178 mm but 63 and 89 mm are most likely to be stocked in Australia. The width (depth) range of beams varies from 95 to 480 mm.

I-beams

I-beams are 'I'-shaped, engineered, wood-based structural members. They are made up of a top and bottom flange of graded solid timber, LVL or LSL with a vertical web of structural plywood, oriented strand board (OSB) or hardboard. The flanges resist bending, tension and compressive stresses and the web provides the necessary shear performance. I-beams are relatively light in weight and offer strength, versatility and economy for use in residential and light commercial applications, such as floor joists, rafters and purlins. They are ideal for long spans and are readily available. Their strength to weight ratio makes them ideal for long spans and provides economical solutions for floor and roof structures. The design of the product enables larger holes to be made in the web to accommodate building services (e.g. waste pipes) than can be made in sawn timber.

The sizes vary in both width (depth) and thickness between individual manufacturers. Stock items are straight, with no camber and are available in lengths up to 12 m but may be longer from some manufacturers.

There are no grades for the product as each manufacturer has designed and tested their range of sizes to determine their design properties. This engineering data is available from the relevant manufacturer, together with span tables for common uses.

I-beams are not what can be described as appearance products, because the glue lines are often quite visible, both in flanges and webs. However, when exposed to view they may be coated with an opaque finish if their unfinished appearance is not preferred. Advances in modern adhesive technology may, in the future, achieve 'wood tone' glue lines that will enhance appearance.

I-beams are generally not suitable for weather-exposed applications, however, short-term exposure during construction is not detrimental. Most can be made termite resistant by preservative treatment to H2 level.

I-beams have the same practical workability characteristics as solid timber, however, because of their specific characteristics and configuration, product-specific practices need to be applied. These may vary between manufacturers and therefore reference should be made to the individual manufacturers' recommended practices. When a design is based on a particular size and brand of the product, substitution with another brand should not be made without engineering advice.

Plywood and reconstituted timber products

Chapters 9 and 10 deal in detail with plywood and reconstituted timber products.

FURTHER READING

Cookson, L. J. (1986). Marine borers and timber piling options. Research review 1986. Melbourne: CSIRO Division of Chemical and Wood Technology.

Hartley, J. N. (1976). An aspect of the conversion of fast grown eucalypts. Reprint 76 WT. Sydney: Forestry Commission of NSW.

McMahon, T. A. (1975). The mechanical design of trees. *Sci Am* 233(1): 93–102.

Waugh, G. (1980). The effect of log size on the economics of sawing regrowth eucalypts. Melbourne: CSIRO Division of Building Research.

Williston, E. M. (1976). *Lumber manufacturing: the design and operation of sawmills and planer mills*. San Francisco: Miller Freeman.

Chapter 7

Drying of wood

The living tree is dependent on the presence of a large quantity of water in its tissues to enable the soil nutrients to be conveyed to the leaves for photosynthesis and for the products so formed to be delivered to the regions of cell growth. Trees may contain water in quantities from 40 per cent to even 200 per cent of the dry mass of wood substance, depending on the species. Dense hardwoods have relatively low 'green' (i.e. as in the living tree) moisture contents but young softwood sapwood (e.g. of radiata pine) may have a moisture content exceeding 200 per cent. Sapwood, as the region of active nutrient transportation, usually has considerably higher moisture content than heartwood, but because of the ease of movement of water between its constituent cells it dries out at a faster rate than heartwood.

In the tree and in the freshly felled green log the walls of the wood cells are saturated with water and the space inside the cells also contains a lot of water. When the wood starts to dry, the water within the cavity is lost first and only when most of this has dried out does the water combined in the cell wall start to evaporate. This transition stage is described as the *fibre saturation point*, while the process of drying moisture out of wood until its moisture content is in balance with the normal humidity levels of the surrounding atmosphere is often called *seasoning*.

Consequences of water loss

Drying is much more rapid from the ends than from the sides of a piece of timber. As each cell dries below the fibre saturation point the cell wall begins to lose water and start to shrink. A moisture gradient develops between the outside of the log or piece of timber and its inner layers, and the shrinkage causes internal stresses that may be strong enough to produce surface checks, end splits and even the large internal checks commonly described as 'honeycombing'. The more rapid the loss of water, the greater the risk of such degrade.

In addition to the stress created by the moisture gradient there is also the stress produced by the uneven loss of dimension by the cell. The shrinkage in the direction tangential to the growth rings is, in most species, about twice that in the radial direction or the direction of the rays, largely due to the restraining effect of the rays on movement in the direction of their length. Shrinkage in the longitudinal direction (i.e. in the length of the tree) is very much less, at least in straight-grained timber free of reaction wood. As a rough guide, the relationship of the tangential to radial to longitudinal shrinkage is about 100:50:1.

The amount of shrinkage is relatively steady, or linear, between the fibre saturation point and the *equilibrium moisture content*. The equilibrium moisture content is the moisture content that timber approaches under set conditions of humidity and temperature. If the relative humidity of the surrounding air is 60 per cent, then the moisture content of the timber will be about 11 per cent. The humidity in the surrounding air will usually be in a continual state of change but not so much that it will affect the moisture content of the wood by more than a few percentage points. Figure 7.1 gives an indication of the approximate equilibrium moisture content for various temperatures and relative humidity levels. The actual figure will vary between species. It is apparent that for the normal range of temperature and humidity, 'dry' timber will have a moisture content between about 8 per cent and 16 per cent (based on the oven-dry mass of the wood substance) depending on the local climatic conditions and seasonal variations.

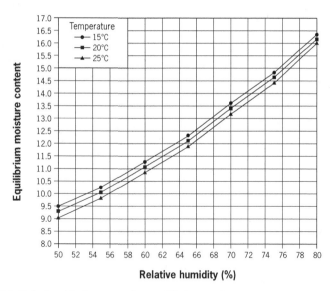

Fig. 7.1 Relationship between the equilibrium moisture content, temperature and humidity

Under set temperature and humidity conditions, wood that is losing moisture will reach a slightly higher moisture content than wood that is absorbing moisture. This is known as the *hysteresis* effect and is a characteristic of wood-based materials.

It will take considerable time for the sawn timber to reach a moisture content close to the equilibrium moisture content, depending on the species, the thickness of the piece, the initial moisture content and the conditions of exposure. The unsawn log may never become seasoned, except for the outer layers, and in fact conditions will favour its decay.

A decision as to whether a stack of timber is seasoned or not cannot be based on the time it has been stacked undergoing drying. When seasoned timber is required, the moisture content range desired should be specified and accurate test methods should be used to check its moisture content. When moisture meters are used, appropriate corrections for the species must be applied and the limitations of the meter taken into consideration. In critical applications oven-dry testing of samples in a laboratory-type environment can provide results that are more accurate.

Reasons for drying

It is important for many end uses that the moisture content of the timber should be stable and close to the equilibrium moisture content of the local atmosphere of where it is to be used. This will ensure that in-service movement is small and mainly associated with climatic variations. For other purposes it may be necessary for some initial drying. For example, timber that is to be impregnated with preservatives may need some drying before the treatment process is carried out. Unseasoned timber is appreciably heavier than seasoned material, so drying facilitates handling and reduces freight charges.

Some species stain readily in the sapwood if the outside surface is not dried quickly. Rapid drying will also check invasion of the unseasoned material by bostrychid borers. If timber remains in a damp condition for long periods, it is also in danger of decay. Timber surfaces that are to be painted must be in a dry state if paint coatings are to adhere properly and give satisfactory service.

An important consideration is that relatively defect-free timber of most species is considerably stronger in most mechanical properties when dried. Compression strength may be increased as much as 90 per cent and bending strength by 60 per cent, but the modulus of elasticity is unlikely to increase by more than 25 per cent. The increase in strength that occurs more than compensates for the inevitable loss of dimension.

Effects of the drying process

Each species has characteristic combinations of cell types and sizes, which have a direct effect on the speed with which the wood can be seasoned. Wood with large rays is difficult to dry without degrade since the ray tissue is at right angles to the vessels and fibres and shrinks at a different rate, so there is a strong tendency for radial checking to occur. Generally dense species, although relatively low in initial moisture content, are difficult to dry because of severe and uneven shrinkage stresses, so surface checking and splitting are common. Softwoods are generally of lower density and more uniform in structure than the hardwoods and have very narrow rays, so are usually easier to dry.

The water within the cell cavity ('free water') evaporates quite rapidly, but that within the cell walls ('combined water') is more difficult to remove. If all the free water throughout the piece of timber dried out first, seasoning would be a relatively easy process. Unfortunately, what happens is that the free water in the outer layers evaporates quickly, and the combined water in these layers starts to dry out long before all the free water in the inner zones has had time to come to the surface and evaporate. As a result, the outer wood shrinks while the inner layers are still fully extended, thus creating very considerable stresses in the outer layers.

Uneven drying causes most of the losses in seasoning, and it is obvious that great care is necessary in the early stages of the process. If freshly sawn timber is left exposed to the hot sun at the sawmill or on the building site, the all-too-frequent result is that the exposed surface checks severely. A *check* may be defined as a separation of fibres along the grain, producing a crack that does not extend from one surface to another. If the crack does extend from one surface to another, it is called a *split*.

Because of the generally much greater shrinkage in the tangential direction than in the radial direction, back-sawn boards will tend to cup away from the face nearest the heart of the log because the other face represents a greater amount of the higher shrinkage tangential cut. In a quarter-sawn board, which has its face parallel to the rays, the greater shrinkage will be in its thickness and it will tend to remain flat; quarter-sawn material usually shows less response to variations in humidity and so tends to give a more stable product.

Unless a square section is cut with the sides virtually parallel and perpendicular to the rays it will tend to become diamond-shaped as it dries. The relationship between tangential and radial shrinkage will also ensure that a section that is round in green timber will be slightly oval after seasoning.

Moisture moves much more quickly along the grain than across it, at a rate said to be between 10 to 25 times faster. Moisture movement in the radial direction is aided by the rays and is twice to four times faster than in the tangential direction.

For timber to be considered satisfactorily seasoned, the difference in percentage of moisture content between the outer layers of the cross-section (the *case*) and the moisture content of the central part of the cross-section (the *core*) should not be more than a few per cent. For timbers over 50 mm thick this ideal state may be very hard to achieve in practice.

To determine such moisture gradients during the seasoning process, particularly in hardwoods, test samples are cut and their moisture contents are usually determined by the oven-dry method. An indication of the moisture gradients in semiseasoned timber can be obtained with the resistance-type moisture meters by varying the depth of penetration of the electrodes.

Collapse

In some species high surface tension in the cell walls during the early stages of drying can cause these walls to buckle, or *collapse*, which is evidenced by an uneven and greater than normal shrinkage of the piece of timber whose radial surface may have an undulating or *washboarding* appearance (Plate 20). A steaming treatment (known as *reconditioning*) near the end of the drying period will usually restore the cross-section almost to the shape that it would have reached if this abnormal form of shrinkage had not occurred. However, there is the possibility that some internal checking, or *honeycombing*, may remain as evidence of the occurrence of collapse (Plate 21).

Collapse is common in cool-climate eucalypts and in the central core of regrowth eucalypts even in coastal areas; rainforest species may also be affected but usually in a relatively minor way. It will be noted that in listing the amount of shrinkage many publications give both the 'before reconditioning' and 'after reconditioning' figures, which is indicative of the amount of collapse that is likely to occur. Exposure of susceptible timber to severe conditions in the early stages of drying increases the likelihood of collapse occurring and makes remedial measures more difficult. Collapse is complete by the time the fibre saturation point has been reached.

Methods of drying

Drying methods often differ between softwoods and hardwoods and are also influenced by the end use. For structural applications drying conditions can be harsher and greater variation in the moisture distribution can be tolerated. The drying temperature for structural softwoods is often very high, whereas for structural hardwoods lower temperatures are necessary. Appearance products, such as flooring or furniture stock, require gentler drying and particularly with hardwoods, periods of air drying or time in a predrier is necessary prior to final kiln drying.

Air drying

Drying requires an efficient circulation of air throughout the stack in sufficient quantity to dry the material as fast as is consistent with an economic minimum degrade. As the temperature of air rises its power to absorb moisture increases, while the wood's power to hold onto water diminishes with its rise in temperature.

The amount of water vapour contained in air is indicated by its *absolute humidity*. The drying power of air or the amount of water it can continue to absorb until saturation is referred to as its *relative humidity* and is of more interest to the timber processor. Relative humidity is defined as the amount of moisture in air at a given temperature compared with the amount it will hold at the same temperature if fully saturated; hence it is expressed as a percentage.

Wood is a hygroscopic (i.e. water attracting) material and even when seasoned will quickly absorb or release moisture according to its environment unless restrained by materials impregnated in the wood or to some degree by surface coatings. These substances or coatings are, however, unlikely to prevent moisture changes if a differential is maintained for a considerable period. When water evaporates from the unseasoned surface, the surrounding air cools and contracts, which makes it denser and it falls to a lower level. If timber is stacked in such a manner as to enable a free circulation around each piece, a continuous movement of air will be induced and this is the basis of natural air drying, which is still the most common method.

To help this natural circulation, stacks should not be too wide (say, approximately 1 m) and foundations should be level, of durable material and high enough (at least 400 mm from the ground) to permit rapid discharge of the descending moisture-laden air. There should be a good current of air through the yard, with stacks of timber so oriented that all get their share of the prevailing breezes. A space of at least 600 mm between rows is necessary for access to locate the sample boards required to monitor the drying process. Excessive drying out of the ends of the boards should be prevented by end coating with a sealer.

To provide space for air circulation, and also to assist in keeping the timber straight and flat during drying, boards are separated by *stickers* or *stripping pieces*, which should be arranged carefully in vertical alignment in the stack. The stickers should be of seasoned wood, of uniform thickness (generally about 20 mm) and perhaps 38 mm wide. They should be relatively narrow, as wide stickers cause staining, uneven drying and result in additional stresses.

Stickers can be reused many times. Their spacing will be governed by the thickness and species of timber being dried. Those species that distort readily may need a spacing, for 25-mm thick timber, of 350–450 mm, while others will dry satisfactorily with stickers at 900-mm spacing. The stacks should have all the board ends flush, as overhanging ends will distort and be wasted. Uneven lengths can be taken up in the body of the stack.

Green timber is pliable and easily distorted by uneven loading. If it is held straight and flat by uniformly sized stickers in vertical alignment and by the weight of material above until it has dried, it will tend to maintain this good shape so long as it remains dry.

Covers or roofs on the stacks plus some restraining weights, such as blocks of concrete with pockets for forklift or gantry loading, will save the top layers from degrade and restrict moisture penetration into the stack. Roofs should project far enough to ensure that rain falls clear of the stack. The covers should be of simple and rugged construction, able to withstand frequent handling.

Air drying is a quite suitable method of drying but its rate is largely at the mercy of the weather and in some climates high-density hardwoods will not dry adequately for internal use. Material that is 25 mm thick may take 3–9 months to air dry. Air drying can only reduce the moisture content to near the prevailing equilibrium moisture content (emc) of the drying facility, which will often not meet the requirements of the end user unless the facility is located in a naturally dry locality. For this reason kiln drying may be needed to reach the required dryness.

Kiln drying

The use of kilns fitted with mechanical ventilation and heat and humidity control permits accurate control of the conditions required for drying and it is much faster and predictable, taking a matter of hours for some softwoods to approximately a week for higher density hardwoods that have initially been dried to below fibre saturation point (around 25 per cent moisture content for most species). Many softwoods can be economically kiln-dried immediately after sawing, a desirable way of avoiding bluestain damage. Kiln-drying schedules, representing the most suitable combination of temperature and relative humidity, have been determined for many species and thicknesses and are available from research organisations and other publications (e.g. *Australian Timber Seasoning Manual*).

Although there is no real difference in quality between dried and kiln-dried material, the ability to have a planned output while minimising stock levels has resulted in kilns providing the preferred drying option. Due to the increased cost and difficulty in drying material thicker than 50 mm, such material is seldom available as a seasoned product. Kilns permit greater control over heat and humidity relationships and so are very valuable in seasoning difficult species, but they do need skilled operators, even with automatic controls, to make sure that drying conditions are maintained at a consistent level throughout the kiln. Kilns are often built from sandwich-insulated panels of aluminium skins with high-temperature insulation between. However, there are also kilns being built from aerated concrete panels, and in the case of low-temperature solar kilns, various types of plastic skin are used. Steam, hot water, hot oil, gas and solar energy provide heating, and saturated steam or water sprays provide humidification.

Kilns usually have a series of fans above the stack; the air enters at one side of the stack and is forced across the width of the stack, a baffle being placed on the top of the timber to prevent short-circuiting of the air current. The direction of the air current is reversed at regular intervals, and vents are provided to enable some of the moisture-laden air to be expelled and fresh air to be admitted. Control of the drying operation is based on two thermometers, the *dry bulb thermometer*, which gives a direct measure of the heat in the kiln, and the *wet bulb thermometer*, which records the amount of cooling due to evaporation of water from the wet bulb, thus giving a measure of the humidity conditions in the kiln. When both wet and dry bulb readings are available, the relative humidity can be obtained from tables in books on kiln drying. Some lower temperature kilns use relative humidity sensors instead of wet bulb thermometers.

Measurement of the progress of drying of hardwoods is usually done by the regular weighing of *sample boards*, which are short pieces of timber representative of the condition of the stack and which have been carefully end-coated so that they will not dry faster than the rest of the load in the kiln. The results of the weighings enable the moisture content to be calculated. In order to gather these boards it is necessary to provide small inspection doors in the kiln. Alternatively, and particularly with softwoods, electrodes can be embedded in sample boards and linked to an external moisture meter or plates can be inserted into the stack to measure moisture content by a change in capacitance through the stack. Other methods, including the temperature drop across the stack (which reduces as the timber dries), have also been investigated and in some facilities a combination of approaches is used.

Drying times vary considerably. Elevated temperatures with the correct airflow reduce drying times but inevitably create considerable drying stresses, so it is a common practice at the end of kiln drying to give the stack a *high humidity treatment*, which makes the timber more pliable and relieves the stresses. Drying to a low average moisture and providing a high humidity treatment not only relieves drying stress, but provides a tighter drying distribution at the correct average moisture content.

Presteaming

Some species in appropriately fitted kilns benefit from presteaming for 2–4 hours before drying begins, particularly some of the collapse-prone ash eucalypts. Steaming can increase moisture conductivity in the tangential direction and reduce the magnitude of the moisture gradient, leading to improved recovery of collapse. It appears to loosen the bond between the border and torus of the aspirated pits of the cells, thus improving permeability. Temperatures between about 80°C and 100°C are normally used for presteaming and steam is injected into the kiln. Alternatively, for some species, kilns are heated up with their vents closed to allow the humidity to build up, and this has a similar effect to presteaming.

Predriers

An improvement on the normal air-drying procedure for hardwoods, but without the careful control of conditions that kilns can offer, is given by the predrier, which is cheaper to operate than a kiln. It usually consists of a large enclosure containing a number of parallel lines of timber stacks and is fitted with fans that blow air at a rate of 1–2 m/s. A small amount of heat is provided on a continuous basis. The predrier serves as a very useful alternative to air drying in bringing the moisture content down to the fibre saturation point, after which the stacks are transferred to the normal kiln. Green 25-mm thick hardwood generally spends 20–30 days in the predrier compared with 4–6 months in the air-drying yard. It has the merit of needing comparatively little land space, is not affected by weather conditions, and provides the flexibility often required in adequately fulfilling the demands of the market. It can be used for round as well as sawn timber.

Most of the denser hardwoods are dried by partial air drying, or drying in the predrier, down to 20–25 per cent, with the kiln being used only for the final stages, with accompanying stress relief by high humidity treatment, or reconditioning if collapse has been considerable.

Conventional and high-temperature drying

Conventional kiln drying uses temperatures below the boiling point of water. For many hardwoods and appearance softwood products, kiln temperatures up to about 70°C are commonly used. Kilns may be heated by steam, hot oil or hot water flowing through heat exchanges, with the energy being provided by wood waste firing or gas burning. Humidification is provided through boiling water baths, saturated steam injection, mist water sprays or a combination of steam and water sprays.

High-temperature drying that is common with plantation softwoods involves the use of temperatures well above boiling point. High-temperature drying is undertaken at different temperatures in different operations and depends on the species being dried and the design of the drying equipment. Temperatures of 120–140°C are common. Some slash pine is dried at temperatures up to 200°C in just a few hours. For high-temperature kilns the means of heating and humidification are the same as for conventional kilns.

The juvenile inner core of softwoods is inclined to have material with pronounced spiral grain, which can produce excessive twisting, spring and bow in the sawn timber. If the temperature of the wood is raised well above boiling point at the stage when its moisture content is high, the various wood components are softened. Lignin, the essential binding material in wood, starts to soften at about 90°C. If this softening process is carried out under considerable restraint imposed by heavy stack weighting and the timber is brought to a seasoned state under such restraint, a much more suitable product is obtained.

The use of this high-temperature drying technique has meant that plantation thinnings, formerly regarded as suitable only for reconstituted products or case manufacture, can be transformed into structural framing. Some loss of strength can result from the use of high temperatures, but it is not of significance in house framing. Drying at high temperature tends to reduce the hygroscopicity of wood and this marginally improves its dimensional stability in service. The success of the process does appear to depend on bringing the kiln charge down to a lower moisture content than would normally be sought (perhaps to 10 per cent), in order to obtain a satisfactorily narrow range of moisture contents within the kiln charge. Higher final moisture contents tend to give steep moisture content gradients.

Stack restraint is usually provided by concrete slabs that are about 200 mm thick and fitted with pockets for forklift or gantry loading, but they lose effectiveness if the timber is not sawn to an even thickness, with a tolerance of no more than ±1.5 mm, and stacked with accurately thicknessed stickers. If these precautions are not taken, the looseness of the stack will still permit a large measure of twisting to occur.

Reconditioning

The reconditioning chamber, used to recondition the stack or to apply high humidity treatments at the end of drying, is essentially a sealed box with a steam line into a water trough; the use of the kiln itself for the process is also done, however, this can be undesirable because it can cause accelerated corrosion of the fans and other equipment.

The process is used to recover collapse in some hardwoods, relieve drying stresses and balance out moisture contents. Collapse recovery necessitates temperatures above 90°C, at which the wood plasticises. Stress relief is obtained through the process of creep and moisture contents are evened out partly by the steam condensing and wetting the timber surface and partly by diffusion.

Solar drying

Even 0.01 per cent of the solar energy reaching the earth's surface would be enough to fulfil all of humanity's energy needs, so there is a great incentive to tap into more of this abundant resource. However, since it is available only when the sun is shining and is reduced considerably by cloud cover, there is the problem of providing a suitable method of storing the energy so that it can be made available whenever it is required. Solar collectors for the provision of hot water are now a common sight on Australian roofs, but even they have to be fitted with a booster permitting the use of another source of energy during cloudy or wintry weather.

The use of solar energy to provide the heat for kiln operation has seen many designs being developed from various states and many solar-powered kiln facilities are now operating. Due to dependence on the sun, it is also common for kilns to be gas assisted. Some kilns utilise double transparent skins for insulation purposes, while others have the solar collector separated from the insulated drying chamber, so that temperature loss during the night is minimised.

In many instances with these kilns the temperature rises slowly throughout the drying process. This is accompanied by a relatively rapid increase in relative humidity during the initial stages of drying followed by a gradual decrease in humidity till the end of drying. As a result of this gentle process, good quality product can be produced, although it takes significantly longer than in a conventional kiln. Preliminary air drying to the fibre saturation point is beneficial to reduce drying times.

Dehumidification drying

The heat pump principle used in air-conditioners has been applied to the drying of timber. Moisture evaporated from the timber by a flow of warm air is removed in part by condensing it on the evaporator coils of a refrigeration circuit and the condensed water is then drained away. Kilns also vent to reduce humidity. The heat obtained in condensing the moisture is transferred to the refrigerant, which is compressed and passes through hot coils, reheating the airstream. Because of the temperature limitations of the most commonly available refrigerants, the operating temperature of the kiln is usually limited to about 60°C.

These types of kilns are still operating but their popularity has reduced in recent years. Although heat pumps make efficient use of electricity and can utilise off-peak electricity, they can still be relatively expensive to run, particularly if supplementary electric heaters are used to boost temperatures. Due to the low operating temperatures, drying is relatively slow and preliminary air drying is very beneficial to reduce processing times. Over the years maintenance has proved to be high, resulting in an increased use of stainless steel in driers to overcome the corrosion problems associated with the condensed water. Drying conditions in these kilns are mild and good quality product can be produced.

Vacuum drying

In a vacuum, the boiling point of water is reduced and the use of vacuum driers therefore provides conditions of rapid drying at moderate temperatures. Some heat does need to be provided to the chamber and various methods have been employed, including hot water platens, steam and radiofrequency. This type of kiln has the potential for producing high-quality timber in both board and larger end-sections. Capital and energy costs are high and therefore the output from these kilns is destined for high-value products. This type of kiln is starting to be introduced into Australia and showing some good results.

Microwave pretreatment

In recent years there has been considerable interest and Australian research into microwave modification of wood and the beneficial effects it can have to reduce drying times. Recent research indicates that, after microwave treatment, unseasoned sawn hardwood boards may be dried in less than 10 days without the need for initial predrying in a predrier or by air drying. The process can also enhance various properties, including stability and strength. Introduction of the technology will be capital intensive but significant benefits in increased productivity, higher quality and reduced stock holdings is expected to more than offset this.

Chemical seasoning

When timber is required to be completely free of surface checks for articles of high commercial value that are able to carry the cost of the extra work involved (e.g. rifle butts, carvings, golf club heads), the soaking of the timber in a chemical that is hygroscopic (i.e. moisture attracting) will slow down the rate of water loss and thus reduce the risk of a high moisture gradient with its accompanying increase in stresses. Such a treatment must be started as soon as possible after the green timber is cut before even minute checks have started to form. In the case of large turnery articles, it may be desirable to work them roughly to shape before treatment.

Chemicals commonly used are urea, polyethylene glycol and sodium chloride (common salt). The first two also have some 'bulking' action in that they replace some of the combined water in the cell walls and prevent the wood shrinking to its normal extent. This 'anti-shrink' property is undesirable with species that are susceptible to collapse as it is likely to increase the tension stresses in such wood. Common salt is preferred in these cases but it does have the drawback of presenting a corrosion hazard to subsequent metal fixings. With all these chemicals there is the risk of temporary 'blooming' (whitening) of finishes in periods of high humidity if the layer of treated timber is not removed by the manufacturing operations. Polyethylene glycol tends to retard the drying of finishes; polyurethanes are said to be least affected.

The chemical is applied either by soaking the timber in an aqueous solution of moderate concentration for about one day per 25 mm of thickness or by a momentary dip in a saturated solution. The timber is then set aside in a drying stack well protected from weather and strong breezes until seasoned. The ultimate equilibrium moisture content reached will be slightly higher than that normally expected.

An alternative method of inhibiting checking by reducing moisture gradients is to create a surface skin that will retard the rate of drying. Sodium alginate, a derivative of seaweed, provides such a skin. The freshly cut green timber is dipped in a 2 per cent aqueous solution and then stripped out in stacks in the normal way, taking care that the alginate is not washed off by exposure to rain.

Microcrystalline wax, emulsified with water and applied by spraying, dipping or brushing, presents a further alternative.

Common forms of seasoning degrade

Bow, spring and twist have already been described on pages 32–33, however, there are a range of other characteristics that affect drying quality, some of which are outlined below. Other publications, such as AS/NZS 4787:2001 *Timber—Assessment of Drying Quality*, provide comprehensive information on aspects relating to moisture distribution, as well as on methods to assess the quality of the dried product. Other factors influencing the quality of the dried product are listed below.

Surface checking

The breaks in the surface layers, known as checks, occur in the early stages of drying and are due to the excessive moisture gradient at that time. The initial loss of moisture needs to be slow and at a steady rate, achieved by such measures as:

1. keeping the freshly sawn timber sheltered from hot sunlight
2. using stack covers to keep the rain out of the stack
3. providing removable screens to deflect strong winds or sunlight from the sides and ends of the stack in the early stages of drying
4. applying coatings of a proprietary end seal, bituminous paint, wax, grease or a quick-drying paint to the end-grain.

Checks develop along lines of weakness in the surface, such as the ends of the rays. This factor, combined with the greater intensity of tangential shrinkage, causes them to be much more common on back-sawn than on quarter-sawn surfaces.

Surface checks of considerable width in the early stages of drying will frequently close tightly when the whole cross-section of the piece has seasoned.

Internal checks

Also known as honeycombing when severe, internal checks are not visible on the surface but are exposed when the piece is cross-cut. They are quite common in species prone to collapse or high shrinkage.

Splits

These are checks that have become so extensive as to extend to the adjacent or opposite surfaces of the piece of timber.

Cupping

This is most commonly observed in wide boards and is the term applied to a curvature across the grain that causes the board to be concave on one side and convex on the other. It is generally restricted to back-sawn material, the concave side being that which is further from the heart of the tree.

Residual drying stress

During the initial stages of drying when the case is drier than the core, stresses develop initially with the case in tension and the core in compression. The case is prevented from normal shrinkage about the higher moisture content core and this results in tension stresses developing in the case. As drying continues and the core dries, its shrinkage is now restrained by the oversized outer case. At the conclusion of drying a stress reversal develops where the case is now in compression and the core is in tension. As a result of this a piece of timber can have a relatively even moisture content through the piece but can have severe residual drying stresses. Such a piece of timber, if moulded or ripped down its length, will create boards that are cupped and bowed. Care during drying and appropriate final steaming minimises these stresses. When more severe this is often referred to as 'case hardening'.

Discolouration

Discolouration relates to a change in colour that may occur during the drying process. Discolouration generally occurs from chemical reactions between chemicals in wood, including sugars, sap and extractives, and the atmosphere. It is of importance with appearance products and can result in dark or light bands where drying strips or stickers were present. This is often referred to as sticker stain.

Determination of moisture content

Timber cannot be assumed to be in a seasoned condition just because it has been in the drying stack for a long period or because it feels dry to the touch. Accurate determination will save much recrimination and disappointment.

The most accurate method is to cut a cross-section about 15 mm long at least 500 mm from the end of the piece to obtain a representative result for that piece, weigh it and heat it in an oven maintained at 103 ± 2°C until no further loss of weight occurs (usually within 24 hours but it can take longer for high-density species).

The moisture content of timber is conventionally expressed as a percentage of the oven-dry weight (i.e. actual wood substance) and is calculated thus:

$$\text{Percentage moisture content} = \frac{\text{weight of moisture}}{\text{oven-dry weight}} \times 100$$

$$= \frac{\text{original weight} - \text{oven-dry weight}}{\text{oven-dry weight}} \times 100$$

Because of the time taken to carry out the above method and the necessary destruction of some timber it is more customary to use a battery-operated *moisture meter*. One type of meter works on the basis that oven-dry wood is a good insulator but electrical resistance falls rapidly as the moisture content increases. The relationship between electrical resistance and moisture content is not identical for all species, so it is necessary to know the name of the species being tested and refer the results obtained with the meter to correction tables (see AS/NZS 1080.1:1997 *Timber—Methods of Test—Moisture Content* and Appendix 2) to adjust for the species, since most meters have been calibrated for mature Douglas fir (Oregon). The meter has a lead fitted with pins, which are driven into the surface so as to measure resistance. Timbers such as silver ash, basswood, calophyllum, white cheesewood, keruing, Philippine mahogany, meranti, ramin, taun, terminalia and yasi-yasi give such variable results that they have not been listed in Appendix 2.

It is important to bear in mind that the correction figures are only for solid timber. The adhesives and additives in reconstituted wood products mean different electrical conductivity

It is also important to remember that the correction figures represent averages and a variation of 1 or 2 per cent each way in the actual moisture content of a particular specimen is possible.

The species correction figures are to be applied after corrections have been made for other factors, such as:

1. *Temperature.* The meters are generally calibrated at a temperature of about 21°C. A correction of ±1.5 per cent should be made for every 11°C respectively above or below 21°C.
2. *Thickness.* The normal blades or needles fitted to the hammer attached to the meter are meant for testing timber of a thickness between 6 mm and 30 mm. For thicker material, ordinary steel nails can be driven into the wood to reach the centre of the cross-section; they should be spaced apart to match the distance between the electrodes, which are then placed in position on top of them in order to take a reading.
3. *Treated timbers.* Timber treated with oil-based preservatives may give readings slightly lower than the real moisture content. The water-borne preservatives generally make the wood more conductive of electric current, so readings are generally higher than the true figure, of the order of 1–4 per cent.

Special needle electrodes are used for measuring the moisture content of veneers.

Capacitance-type moisture meters measure an electrical property called the 'dielectric constant'. In so doing, an electric field produced by the meter and the presence of the timber on which the meter is positioned form a 'capacitor' type of arrangement. The electric field can penetrate deep into the timber but meter readings are biased towards moisture in the surface layers. Both the moisture content and the density of the timber affect this electrical property. The effective range of capacitance meters is from approximately 0 to 30 per cent moisture content. The more sophisticated meters can be adjusted for timbers of different densities. Less expensive meters do not have density compensation and for these meters corrections to meter readings must be applied based on the density of the species being tested. Such meters are usually preset to be more suited to softwoods and lower density hardwoods and this can cause limitations with higher density species (i.e. large correction factors are necessary).

Moisture meters provide a good guide to the moisture content in timber, however, they also need to be used with common sense and care as many factors can affect readings. In certain cases, the more accurate method involving oven drying may be desirable as a check on results obtained with the meter.

Publication of shrinkage figures

In order to compare readily the difference in shrinkage behaviour between species, figures are published for the shrinkage between the green condition and a moisture content of 12 per cent, a figure fairly representative of seasoned timber in dwellings. Considerable within-species variability in shrinkage occurs because of differing degrees of wood maturity and environmental effects, so the figures for shrinkage that are given in the species descriptions are merely a guideline figure from which considerable variations will occur in practice.

Movement of timber in service

Because of the time and cost involved in their drying, large structural sections are generally used in the unseasoned condition (unless the product is laminated), so designers and users should keep in mind the possible effects of shrinkage. Shrinkage in length is generally not significant but reduction in other dimensions may be as much as 8–10 per cent of initial green size. Positioning of fixings should take into account this movement to avoid distortion and uneven transference of loads.

Positioning of nails in green framework is of importance in reducing cracking to a minimum. For example, when nailing the studs in the corners of a room, the nails holding the studs to the plates should be very close to the corner so that shrinkage will occur towards rather than away from the joint.

The use of insufficiently seasoned timber can mar the appearance of a job, but timber that has been overdried can cause even more concern. Overdried flooring boards have been known to crack walls or lift tent-like (peak) from the flooring joists when they swell to return to equilibrium.

A thorough understanding of the wood–water relationship is essential for efficient use of wood as a structural and decorative medium. The speed of change in moisture content is greater in thinner material. With the same thickness, movement generally shows up more quickly in the species of lower density. Material of 38 mm thickness and over does not show the effect of rapid changes in humidity level. Because of the slow transfusion of moisture through the wood, the core of the timber will take a considerable time to reach equilibrium with changed atmospheric conditions and so is seldom affected by short-term weather fluctuations; the lower amount of movement of large sections is due to the restraining influence of the unaffected core.

Although low-density timbers generally have an appreciably lower movement per 1 per cent change in moisture content, this advantage over the dense timbers tends to be counterbalanced by their greater short-term susceptibility to large moisture content movements through greater sensitivity to humidity variations.

When working with internal timbers, knowledge of the movement (shrinkage or swelling) that can be expected due to small changes in moisture content can be useful. Figures for different species have been published for both the tangential and radial directions. Many timbers are predominantly back-sawn and some publications only publish the 'unit tangential movement' (UTM). This is the percentage dimensional change in a particular species for a 1 per cent change in moisture content, occurring in the moisture content range from 3 per cent to fibre saturation point. For example, brush box has a published UTM of 0.38. Therefore, a 3 per cent increase in moisture content could be expected to cause an 80 mm wide back-sawn floorboard to increase in size by 0.38 × 3 per cent × 80 /100 = 0.91 mm. Care is necessary when using these figures as they are averages from a particular study, most boards are not fully back-sawn and in timber floors other effects, including the fitting and restraint provided by adjacent boards, can lead to analysis errors. It has also been shown that the growing locality and age of the tree can significantly affect in-service movements.

Shrinkage of large structural members

In the normal framework where studs are located at 450–600 mm centres, the size of members is generally small so when green timber is used the subsequent shrinkage is relatively slight. When post and beam construction is used, involving few but large section members or where, for example, large openings have to be spanned in normal house framing, the large green cross-sectional sizes will normally result in considerable shrinkage in the initial months of service.

Seasoned timber will seldom be available in large cross-sections, except from demolition contractors, or in the form of laminated members obtained by bonding together small sections of seasoned material. If only green timber is available for the job, it is essential to limit the consequences of shrinkage by careful design.

Because of the considerable difference between radial and tangential shrinkage, it is important when using large sections as flooring supports that they be of similar cut (e.g. *all* quarter-sawn or *all* back-sawn) so that an even surface will be maintained.

Joists are usually placed directly on top of bearers; if both are of considerable depth of section, the total amount of vertical shrinkage that may occur could be quite large so it may be worthwhile to consider infilling the joists *between* the bearers and supporting their ends on a batten fixed to the lower part of the bearer. Also, if joists are of deep section, it is desirable to seat the joists on the bottom plate, rather than vice versa. In brick veneer construction, sills should have a clearance of about 20 mm from the brickwork to allow for shrinkage when unseasoned framework is used.

Unsightly gaps sometimes open up where the skirting meets the floor as a result of large shrinkage in the under-floor timbers. One way to meet the problem is to use a double skirting, the inner member being fixed to the wall and the outer one to the floor.

All end-grain should receive an adequate protective coating to restrain sudden changes in the moisture content of the timber adjacent to the ends.

Care of seasoned material on the building site

It is a costly process to season timber so it is important to protect it from the weather during the construction of the building.

Flooring that is to be clear finished should be brought to the site only when the dwelling is watertight and cement render and plaster work have dried out thoroughly.

Seasoned material should *not* be stored in a shed where humid conditions prevail (e.g. with earth floor and little ventilation). If there is a risk of rain, delivery trucks should be covered in order to prevent seasoned timber products and packaging from getting wet. It is preferable that seasoned timber is delivered just prior to it being used irrespective of whether it is used internally or externally. Houses built for sale are sometimes left closed up for months in hot summer weather with the sun streaming in the uncovered windows. Areas of considerable shrinkage will then show up in the severely exposed areas of flooring. The remedy is proper protection against such abnormal conditions.

The use of water-repellent dips for window joinery and external mouldings is a worthwhile interim protection against excessive uptake of moisture while the timber awaits the attention of the painter.

Large sizes of structural timber are usually unseasoned and thus prone to considerable surface checking if left lying on the site fully exposed to the hot sun. While this may be of little concern if they are to be covered later by wallboard and so on, those that will be on show deserve careful stacking to assist drying out and avoid distortion. Sealing of end-grain would be worthwhile.

Roof trusses should be stacked on a level area to avoid imposing on the nailplates stresses for which they were not designed. Seasoned timber is often used for their construction and it is a most unfortunate waste of resources when such material is dumped in wet grass or mud on the building site and then left without cover for weeks before installation.

What is the right moisture content to specify?

For some uses seasoned timber is not required. Hardwoods, cypress and Douglas fir are used in the unseasoned condition for building framework, mainly because scantling sizes take a considerable time to season, seasoning increases costs and the hardwoods are more difficult to nail when seasoned. Other softwood framing is sold in the seasoned state because of its ease of seasoning and the extra strength given to it by drying. For furniture, joinery and similar finished work, seasoned material is essential; the equilibrium moisture content figures for a district will indicate the moisture content to seek but in many areas the difference between summer and winter figures may be considerable; one must aim for the average figure. Air-conditioned buildings are a further complication and it is desirable to ascertain the operating temperatures and humidity to be used; from them it will be possible to calculate the moisture content range that the timber will experience. It must also be considered that domestic air-conditioning may only be used intermittently.

Australian Standards usually require dressed timbers for decorative purposes to have an average moisture content of between 9 and 14 per cent at the time of delivery. This does not mean that timber that meets the relevant Standard in this regard will necessarily have an appropriate moisture content for immediate fixing on a particular job. For example, flooring supplied at, say, 12 per cent average moisture content would be in an unsuitable condition for a best-quality appearance feature floor if immediately nailed down in a locality where the humidity levels are such that 9 per cent moisture content is the in-service average. Similarly, if flooring is supplied at an average of 11 per cent moisture content and the average in-service moisture content is 15 per cent, then due allowance is necessary to accommodate the expansion that will occur in such a climate. It may be possible to loosely stack the timber, allowing airflow through it, in the in-service environment to acclimatise it for a period of a few weeks, however, commonsense must prevail. If acclimatising is undertaken during weather conditions that are going to promote moisture loss, when it is intended that average moisture content of timber is to increase during the period, then more damage can be done than if it is not acclimatised at all. Similarly, some high-density species are very slow to respond and will absorb or lose moisture very slowly. Clearly, some judgment is necessary. Adjusting cramping pressures in floors and allowing regularly spaced small gaps at board edges across the floor can also be an effective way of accommodating future movement.

FURTHER READING

Australian/New Zealand Standard (1997). AS/NZS 1080.1:1997 *Timber— Methods of Test—Moisture Content.*

Australian/New Zealand Standard (2001). AS/NZS 4787: 2001 *Timber— Assessment of Drying Quality.*

Blakemore, Philip. (2003). The use of hand-held electrical moisture meters with commercially important Australian hardwoods. Melbourne: Forest and Wood Product Research and Development Corporation (FWPRDC), project no. PN01.1306.

Harrison, J. W., Nassif, N. M., Hartley, J. N. (1970). Methods of determining the moisture content of wood. Tech. pubn 13. Sydney: Forestry Commission of NSW.

Haslett, A. N. (1998). Drying radiata pine in New Zealand. FRI bulletin no. 206. New Zealand Forest Research Institute Ltd.

Hildebrand, R. (ed.) (1970). *Kiln drying of sawn timber.* Oberboihingen, Germany: Hildebrand.

Ministry of Forestry (1996). Producing quality kiln dried timber in New Zealand. Ministry of Forestry and New Zealand Forest Research Institute Ltd.

Nolan, G., Innes, T., Redman A., McGavin, R. (2003). Australian hardwood drying best practice manual. Melbourne: FWPRDC, project no. PN01.1307.

TRADAC (1995). *Timber seasoning*. Brisbane: Timber Research and Development Advisory Council of Queensland.

Waterson, Grahame C. (ed.) (1997). *Australian timber seasoning manual.* Launceston, Tas.: AFARDI.

Chapter 8

The joining of timber components

The choice of the most appropriate method of joining pieces of timber depends on a number of factors, including the quality of finish, loads, environmental service conditions, cost considerations and construction processes. A range of alternatives is available, including fasteners such as nails, nailplates, screws, bolts, split ring connectors, shear plate connectors and dowelled fin plate connectors, and various adhesives. In general, the simpler the joint, the better it is.

On-site connections frequently rely on mechanical fasteners for the principal load-carrying system. Adhesives are used in the industry in the manufacture of wood products. In these applications, the adhesive is applied in a factory setting.

Adhesives

Adhesives are substances that hold the surfaces of materials together by either chemical or physical forces, or both.

Adhesives are used in the production of timber panel products, such as particleboard, plywood and medium-density fibreboard (MDF). They are also used to produce structural glued laminated beams, laminated veneer lumber (LVL), box and I beams. The adhesive must be appropriately durable for the service conditions, and in structural applications perform like solid timber. The choice of adhesive for a particular application is dependent upon the performance required (structural or non-structural), cost, ease of use and durability.

Adhesives can also be used for on-site fastening, such as gluing of timber flooring to the substructure, or gluing wall panelling to frames. In these cases, an elastomeric adhesive is more desirable so that any movement in the elements can be accommodated by the glue.

Careful preparation of the wood surface is essential. It should be freshly dressed, smooth and accurately cut to provide a close-fitting junction. Some adhesives have good gap-filling properties, while others are rendered ineffective by the same gap, so this characteristic should always be kept in mind when choosing the appropriate bonding agent.

The quality of a glued connection is a function of a number of different parameters. Many of these are specified by the adhesive manufacturer, but some of them must be established by controlled experiment for different applications. The parameters include:

- *Species.* Some timber species may contain resins, waxes, oils, gums or tannins, which may make them difficult to bond with some adhesives. The density of timber also has an impact on the ease of gluing. High-density hardwoods require more accurate machining to deliver closely matched surfaces for the bond.
- *Surface quality.* A good-quality bond generally requires freshly machined surfaces that are free from tears, glazing or burning. There should be no contamination of the surfaces to be bonded by dust (including sawdust), oils or greases, including those naturally occurring on the skin.
- *Moisture content.* For most adhesives, the timber moisture content at the time of bonding is crucial. For most formaldehyde and epoxy adhesives, the moisture content must be between 6 per cent and 12 per cent. Many thermoplastic adhesives, such as polyvinyl acetate (PVA), will tolerate moisture contents up to 17 per cent. Care should be taken to have similar moisture contents in the pieces across the glued joint so that the dry-out rates are similar in both pieces.
- *Timber treatments.* Treatments, such as preservative treatments, fungicides, and fire retardants, can all affect the chemistry of the wood–adhesive interface. Advice should be sought as to whether the treatment should be carried out before or after gluing.
- *Adhesive mix.* A number of glues incorporate two or more components that must be mixed prior to application. Binders, fillers, hardeners, extenders or solvents should all be accurately measured and thoroughly combined. The viscosity of the mix is very important as it affects both the flow of adhesive into the joint, and its response to pressure. The *pot life* is the maximum duration that the glue can be mixed before it is used. It is published by the manufacturer and is different to the 'assembly times' (see below).
- *Temperature of mix.* Manufacturers specify a range of temperatures for successful gluing. Depending on the season, this may require heating or cooling of the glue during mixing.
- *Adhesive application rate.* While it is obvious that insufficient glue at the joint can lead to a weak connection, too much glue can also weaken the joint. Excessive glue can either hold the connection apart under pressure, or bleed out of the joint. Either case can cause a weak joint. The manufacturer's recommended spread rate should be used, unless experiment shows that better results can be achieved under different conditions.
- *Open assembly time.* The time between the application of the glue and the closing of the joint is the open assembly time. In that time, some glues develop a 'tackiness' that is necessary to achieve a good bond. In these cases, closing the joint too quickly can reduce the strength of the connection. If the open assembly time is too great, then most glues will start to harden and have reduced effectiveness.
- *Closed assembly time.* The time between closure of the joint and the application of pressure or curing is the closed assembly time. Again, a range of times is published for each glue.

- *Pressure.* Pressure brings the mating surfaces into close contact. Pressure across the glue line is particularly necessary when using an adhesive with poor gap-filling properties. Glue manufacturers publish a range of confining pressures and also indicate whether the pressure must be maintained during the curing period.
- *Curing.* The process of holding the glued joint together under pressure or temperature for a period while the bond is established is called curing. It may be a multistage process, with high pressure for the first period, and then no external pressure for a further time. Care should be taken not to load the joint if it needs to be moved during the curing period. Each adhesive has an optimum range of curing temperature and clamping pressure, which is stipulated by the manufacturer; a pressure of 700–1500 kPa is common.

Appropriate protective clothing should be worn by all people handling glue, or timber with wet glue. When handling adhesives containing formaldehyde or hardeners, which can be irritating to the skin, it is desirable to use a barrier cream or gloves. Inhalation of formaldehyde should be avoided. All glues may cause injury to the eyes, so protective goggles should be worn.

The efficiency of glued joints is usually assessed by examining the amount of wood failure when the joint is fractured. If the failure of the joint is in the wood, then the glue is clearly stronger than the wood and it has structural potential. However, if in nearly all cases, the failure is through the glue line, then the wood is clearly stronger than the glue, and the glue cannot be relied upon as a structural element.

Types of adhesive

Adhesives may be divided into three groups: those of *animal origin*, and those of synthetic origin, which are either *thermosetting* or *thermoplastic*. Thermosetting types are converted into an insoluble state by chemical reaction, whereas thermoplastic types undergo a physical change only, which is reversible.

Adhesives of animal origin

A generation ago the main bonding agent for internal use was animal glue, which was derived from hides and bones. It was easy to handle, although it set quickly on cooling and was only suitable for joins of small surface area; gap-filling properties were good. It has now virtually vanished from use and the only natural adhesive still in common use is *casein*.

Casein has good heat resistance, even up to 70°C, and long assembly times are possible. Its good gap-filling properties are also an advantage. Some suitable applications are for sandwich panel construction, flush doors and attachment of laminates where they are not exposed to the elements.

Casein has only fair resistance to moisture and because of its protein nature it is susceptible to fungal attack under damp conditions; because of this its use is best reserved for internal joins and away from tropical conditions.

Adhesives of synthetic origin that are thermosetting

Thermosetting adhesives are converted into an insoluble state by a chemical reaction, with or without the application of heat, and the change is irreversible. They are favoured for strong structural joins and for the bonding of wood particles to produce reconstituted wood products, such as particleboard. The main types in common use are urea formaldehyde, melamine formaldehyde, phenol formaldehyde, resorcinol formaldehyde, tannin formaldehyde, isocyanates and epoxies. Fillers and extenders are often added. Fillers improve joint-filling properties and can have some adhesive force. Extenders have no adhesive force.

Formaldehyde is a vital constituent of many thermosetting adhesives. It is available in three forms: formalin, an aqueous solution that is not easy to use in practice; paraformaldehyde, a solid form that makes for ease of preparation of the adhesive for sale but which is becoming increasingly expensive; and as urea formaldehyde syrup, in which the urea acts virtually as a carrier.

Urea formaldehyde   Urea formaldehyde is a very commonly used adhesive in the manufacture of internal particleboard, which is widely used in furniture and kitchen cupboard production, and also for plywood. It is available either as a creamy liquid or white powder, to which a hardener is added just before use. Wheat flour extender is often incorporated but the amount should be strictly controlled to avoid weakening the bond. Assembly time varies with the hardener used but is usually up to half an hour. The joint requires pressure for several days at room temperature but the time can be reduced very considerably by raising the temperature. Gap-filling properties are relatively poor.

It is not suitable for use at temperatures below about 13°C, nor is it waterproof. Prolonged exposure to elevated temperatures and high humidity weakens the glue so it is not a desirable adhesive for tropical conditions, nor is it advocated for structural joints where very long-term durability is essential to the integrity of the structure. There is some doubt as to its merit as an adhesive for timber that has been treated with preservatives.

Melamine formaldehyde   This adhesive is usually sold as a white powder and a hardener is added at the time it is mixed with water. Sometimes up to 50 per cent of urea is added to reduce the cost. Melamine formaldehyde produces a water-resistant glue line but it does not have the same waterproof nature as a phenolic-type adhesive.

Since heat in excess of 70°C is required for proper curing of the bond, melamine adhesives are essentially for factory use. They respond well to the use of radiofrequency heating and this combination is a favoured one for scarf joints and finger joints (Plate 22) where a rapid cure is desirable to overcome handling difficulties with the product.

The glue line is pale in colour in contrast with the phenolic types and provides a very strong bond, except in the case of timber previously treated with preservatives.

Phenol formaldehyde   Phenol formaldehyde adhesives usually require elevated temperatures (e.g. about 130°C) for curing so their use is confined to factory production, especially of waterproof plywood and structural particleboard, and for the bonding of metal to wood.

They are available in the form of a brown liquid or powder or thin sheets of solid material. Gap-filling properties are not very good but the glue line has excellent resistance to fungal attack and weathering.

Veneer treated with boron salts for immunisation against borers is difficult to glue with phenolics.

Resorcinol formaldehyde   Resorcinol formaldehyde adhesives provide a very efficient waterproof bond, impervious to fungal and insect attack, and with the added advantage of curing at normal warm weather temperatures.

Several variants are available commercially; one formulation is essentially resorcinol and formaldehyde, another contains a minor amount of the cheaper phenol, while in a third variant the amount of phenol is dominant. An increase in the phenol content requires an increase in the temperature required for curing.

Resorcinol adhesives are sold as a two-component system consisting of a brown liquid, the resorcinol plus some formaldehyde, and a brown-coloured powdered hardener containing additional formaldehyde and catalyst. Mixing causes a rise in temperature that is good for fast curing but shortens assembly time so it may sometimes be necessary to precool the resorcinol. In general, though, a temperature of at least 21°C is needed for effective bonding, so the factory may require supplementary heating in winter.

If it is cured at high temperatures (above 90°C), a thickener is often added to prevent excessive wood penetration arising from the reduced viscosity.

Gap-filling properties are good and it is the most outstanding adhesive for exposed conditions and for long-life structural components, such as glued laminated arches. Pressure must be maintained for several hours for the glue line to cure adequately.

Unless elevated curing temperatures are used, the bonded material should be set aside for several days before further processing.

The efficiency of phenol resorcinol adhesives in bonding timber that has been impregnated with copper-chrome-arsenic (CCA) preservatives can be improved very considerably by brushing the surface with sodium hydroxide solution.

Tannin formaldehyde   The bark of many tree species is rich in polyphenolic compounds, which are reactive with formaldehyde to form a good-quality waterproof bond. Tannin adhesives are dark in colour. Some phenolic resin may be added for improved bond quality. A filler may also be included to minimise the loss of adhesive due to penetration of the wood, and to increase gap-filling properties. The rate of reaction can be varied by adding salts of zinc, copper, chromium and aluminium.

Epoxy adhesives   Epoxies are formed by reacting epichlorhydrin with bis-phenol in the presence of sodium hydroxide, and are used as a two-pack system with a separate hardener, usually a polyamine.

The two liquids react to form a clear solid without any evolution of solvent so there is a minimum of shrinkage and excellent gap-filling behaviour. The pot life can be varied considerably by the choice of hardener.

Resistance to heat and chemicals is very good. The glue line is usually less strong than the wood so epoxies are not recommended for highly stressed joins. They are very good for bonding metals to concrete or wood.

Two-part polyurethane adhesives These adhesives consist of an isocyanate part and an alcohol-based part. They react together to produce a polyurethane resin. They have good strength but may not be very weather resistant. They have some gap-filling properties. This type of adhesive is undergoing continued development, and manufacturers should be consulted for properties, mixing and application requirements.

They have been used successfully in Europe for a number of years in metal-to-wood bonds where the service conditions are somewhat protected.

One-part polyurethane adhesives The active ingredient in this adhesive is an isocyanate, and it reacts with the moisture in the wood. These adhesives are similar in strength to the two-part polyurethanes, but do not have the same gap-filling properties. There is a considerable range in durability properties, with limited weather resistance indicated.

Emulsion polymer isocyanate adhesives This is a two-pack system, with one part, an emulsified polymer (e.g. PVA) and the second an emulsified isocyanate. Working properties are much the same as for the PVA adhesives, but when the glue line dries, the isocyanate is released and acts as a cross-linker. There are reports of high durability and strength with this type of adhesive but development of it and appropriate tests for its durability is relatively new.

Adhesives of synthetic origin that are thermoplastic

Thermoplastic adhesives are usually in the completely reacted condition when purchased and the bonding action results from physical, either through loss of solvent or solidification on cooling, not chemical, change. Physical changes involving melting or dissolving with solvent can reverse the bonding process. Most of the thermoplastic types tend to deform under stress or elevated temperature, a form of behaviour referred to as *creep*. The most common examples of thermoplastic adhesive are PVA emulsions, elastomers (a term embracing mastics and contact adhesives) and hot melts.

1. *PVA emulsions.* These thick white liquids are made by polymerising vinyl acetate alone or with other polymers, the adhesive being suspended in a protective colloid. Usually they are in a form ready for immediate use, although cross-linked types are produced in two or more component systems and can be used as hot-setting adhesives cured by dielectric heating.

Most PVAs are cured at normal room temperature and set rapidly, some of the water dissipating into the wood; well-seasoned wood is essential. Assembly time is very short (10–20 minutes) so this adhesive is not suited to bonding large areas. Temperatures below 21°C should be avoided when a strong bond is required. Although gap-filling properties are good, firm and rapidly applied pressure is important in securing a good-quality join.

Because of their ease of application and colourless glue line, PVAs are in very common use in general joinery and furniture workshops but are not favoured for highly stressed connections because of the potential to creep, which is increased if high temperatures are likely to occur for an extended period. PVA adhesives have high initial strength but resistance to moist conditions is quite poor; the cross-linked types have an improved performance.

2. *Contact adhesive.* Elastomeric adhesives contain an elastic material of natural or synthetic rubber so the glue line is relatively non-rigid; the stronger types are the contact adhesives.

Contact adhesive is spread on both surfaces and much of the solvent is allowed to evaporate before the surfaces are brought together. If the glue soaks into the wood quickly, a second coat may be needed to secure sufficient film thickness.

The solvent is usually very volatile, presenting some fire hazard and toxicity, so the work area needs to be well ventilated and free of flame sources. Products soluble in water have been developed but are slower to grip and of lesser strength. Normal warm weather temperatures of 21–32°C give the best results.

Because of the instantaneous grip of contact adhesives, the bringing of the surfaces together needs careful planning to avoid mismatching. Some brief application of pressure, even if only by block and hammer or manual roller, is needed. Gap-filling properties are good.

A common use for contact adhesives is the application of sheet laminates to counter tops.

3. *Mastics.* Elastomeric adhesives without the instantaneous grip of the contact types are commonly used, often in conjunction with nails, for fixing sheet flooring to joists and wallboards to studs. They help to stiffen a floor and reduce the likelihood of squeaking, while on walls they reduce the number of nails required and so help to reduce the risk of nail popping.

Mastics are usually applied to only one of the surfaces and evaporation of the solvents before bringing the two together is less important. The temperature of the operation is less critical and even winter conditions can be accommodated if not below freezing point.

The adhesive is usually supplied in a cartridge and is applied using a caulking gun. Its thick consistency gives it good gap-filling properties. When fixing flooring, the joists need to be seasoned and level. At least the surface should have a moisture content suitable to adhesives in general. If tongued and grooved panels are being attached to walls, a bead of the mastic should be placed in the groove.

AS 2329-1999 *Mastic Adhesives for Fixing Wallboards* describes mastic adhesives for internal attachment of hardboard, particleboard, plywood and asbestos cement panels to wood and metal framing.

4. *Hot melts.* Hot melts are formulated from vinyl polymers, rubbers and other natural or synthetic resins and sold in ribbon, sheet or pellet form. The adhesive is applied by equipment that is specially designed for melting and spreading it. While not of much current application to timber members, they are a valuable adhesive in the packaging industry; they can be used for bonding laminates, particularly edges.

Hot melts are usually applied at temperatures above 120°C to just one of the surfaces, but contact between the surfaces must occur within a few seconds because the adhesive will set very quickly on the other cooler surface. Because of this the general temperature of the workshop should be above 20°C. Hot melts have generally poor resistance to solvents or heat above 50°C.

Load capacity of structural connections

For structural connections, AS 1720.1-1997 *Timber Structures—Design Methods* classifies the most commonly used species into six joint groups for the purpose of joint design. It also provides tables of basic lateral and withdrawal loads for nails, screws and bolts for each joint group and for various sized fasteners. The requirements for detailing of joints are also given.

Joint strength is related to the density of the timber, not its grade. Each species is classified into different joint groups on the basis of its density. Seasoned timber uses the series JD1 (strongest) to JD6. Unseasoned timber uses the series J1 (strongest) to J6. Special consideration must be given to the design of connections for unseasoned timber, as splitting may occur as the timber dries in service, inducing increased stress around the connection.

Connectors transfer loads within a structure from one member to another, and can be differentiated according to the way in which the force is transferred between the members. Type 1 connections transfer force using shear in the connector or fastener. Type 2 connections transfer load by axial force in the fastener.

Type 1 connections

In type 1 connections, force is transferred by bearing between the timber and the connector, and across the shear plane between the timber members by shear in the fastener. The force is then transferred by bearing from the connector to the other member. Failure occurs when the fastener causes crushing in the wood immediately next to the shank. Eventually, the fastener will either break or cause fracture of the wood nearby, causing separation of the joint.

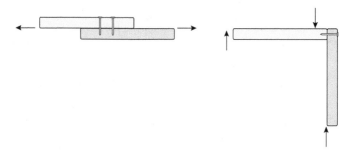

Fig. 8.1 Type 1 mechanical connections

Type 2 connections

The fasteners in type 2 connections are in tension, and failure occurs when the force holding the fastener in the members is insufficient to resist the forces acting on the connection. The fastener remains straight and simply slides past the wood as it pulls out of the timber member. The capacity of fasteners driven into end-grain is generally less than the capacity of fasteners driven into side grain.

The capacity of the joint or connection is dependent on the joint strength of the timber, the type and stiffness of the fastener, and the geometry of the connection.

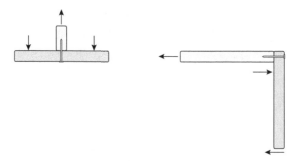

Fig. 8.2 Type 2 mechanical connections

Fasteners

Nails

The most common, easy to install and cost-effective method of joining pieces of timber together in general building construction is by the use of steel nails of various diameters or gauges, lengths, and types of point, head and shank.

Where no predrilling of timber is required, gun-driven nails can be used efficiently, and provide an effective connection between two pieces of timber. Nails are quick and easy to install, and the use of a large number of them will spread the load over a large area and bridge any weaknesses in the member and produce a resilient connection.

When nails are driven into timber, they do not cut or break the fibres; they simply push the timber fibres apart. The tensile or bending strength of the timber remains unaffected as no cross-section is removed. However, processes such as predrilling holes, which cut or remove timber fibres, reduce the strength of the timber.

Composition of nails

Most nails are made of cold-drawn, low-carbon steel, either plain or galvanised. However, nails of copper, aluminium and stainless steel are sometimes used to prevent corrosion or staining. Aluminium nails are easily bent during driving and are rather weak in shear, but because they do not stain they can be useful for fixing external cladding and joinery. In extremely corrosive conditions, such as a very salty atmosphere, monel metal (copper–nickel alloy) may be necessary.

The denser species of timber need stronger nails, either of heavier gauge or hardened. High-carbon steel nails are sometimes used for the extra hardness required to obtain easy penetration of hardwoods and even masonry but their brittle nature dictates extra care when driving them.

Type of point

Using a blunt, dump, chisel or flat-point nail can reduce the danger of splitting the timber (as when laying cypress flooring or nailing into hardwoods). This is because these nails punch through the fibres rather than forcing them apart. The damage to the wood fibres during driving may reduce withdrawal resistance.

Type of head

Selection of head type, bullet head or flat head, is a compromise between the low visual impact of the bullet-head nail (easily hidden with putty or filler), and the reduced risk of pull-through with a flat-head nail. Flat-head nails are commonly used in attaching cladding and in fixing particleboard flooring when heavy traffic and vibration may cause bullet-head nails to pull through and so lead to squeaking of the flooring.

Form of the shank

Increasing use is being made of spirally grooved, annular grooved, helically threaded and other variations from the normal straight smooth shank. The withdrawal resistance is superior under changing ambient moisture conditions. Their use goes some way to overcoming the problem of nail 'popping' in unseasoned timber. Nail popping is related to the length of the nail and the amount of shrinkage of the timber. In green timber it is advisable to use the shortest nail practicable. Ring shank nails are often used in softwood, and screw shank nails in hardwood. Screw shank nails are particularly effective against shock loads, and are widely used in applications such as flooring, panelling, gusset plates, cladding, roofing and plasterboard.

Penetration of nails

Nails should penetrate into the second member of the joint for at least half the length of the nail in dense hardwood timbers and two-thirds in softwoods.

It is advisable to avoid nailing close to edges and ends, and near knots. If the species of timber tends to split, it is important to predrill holes in the timber before nailing.

Withdrawal resistance

The amount of friction developed between the nail shank and the timber fibres determines the withdrawal strength of the nail. The withdrawal strength of a nail is governed by the factors listed below.

Surface condition A number of proprietary products using glue coatings to enhance withdrawal resistance of nails are available.

Galvanised nails are often used to avoid staining and prolong the life of the nail in corrosive environments. If evenly distributed, the zinc coating on the nail can increase withdrawal resistance but if large irregularities are present on the surface of the nails, this tends to reduce the withdrawal resistance.

Direction of driving Nails driven perpendicular to the grain of the wood may have at least twice the withdrawal resistance of nails driven parallel to the grain (i.e. into the end-grain), but the angle at which the nail is driven has less effect in high-density timbers than in low-density timbers. Skew nailing (i.e. driving at an angle) increases the withdrawal resistance slightly, but nails that will be loaded laterally should not be driven on the slant unless the direction of the load will tighten the joint.

The effect of direction of driving is modelled in AS 1720.1-1997 *Timber Structures—Design Methods* for structural nailed connections.

Length of time the nail is in the timber joint Nails driven into green timber and pulled before seasoning occurs have about the same withdrawal resistance as nails driven into seasoned timber and withdrawn soon after driving. Smooth shank nails driven into green timber that has then had time to season or into seasoned timber that has been subject to weather extremes lose a considerable part of their withdrawal resistance.

Even in seasoned timber protected from the weather there is some reduction in withdrawal resistance with the passage of time, but if the nail rusts slightly in the timber, there may be a considerable increase in withdrawal resistance.

Predrilling of nail holes Nails driven into holes that have been predrilled (to reduce the danger of splitting) to a diameter slightly smaller than that of the nail have somewhat higher withdrawal resistance that those driven without predrilling. The capacity of a nail is not affected by the predrilling of holes so long as the hole diameter is less than 80 per cent of the nail diameter.

Clinching of the nails Withdrawal resistance can be increased considerably by this practice, which involves the bending over of the protruding end of the nail, but the extent of the increase will be affected by the moisture content of the timber, the species, the size of the nail and the direction of the clinching in relation to the grain of the timber.

The use of clinched nails in green timber that is then seasoned before testing can give up to four times as much resistance as ordinary nailing. Nails clinched across the grain have about 20 per cent more resistance than along the grain.

Resistance to lateral displacement

Nails can be very effectively used in transmitting lateral loads. AS1720.1-1997 *Timber Structures—Design Methods* allows calculation of design capacity of nailed joints, and presents some geometric requirements for structural connections.

For satisfactory lateral resistance, nails should be placed as far away from the ends and edges of the piece as practical considerations permit and the placement of the nails in relation to each other is important in restraining splitting tendencies.

The resistance to lateral displacement of nails in side grain is virtually the same irrespective of whether the load is applied parallel or perpendicular to the grain or whether the nail is driven into the back-sawn or quarter-sawn surface.

When nails are driven into end-grain, their resistance to lateral displacement is about two-thirds that for nails in side grain.

Skew nailing or toenailing

When nailing building framework together it is common practice to skew nail through the end or edge of a piece to attach it to a main structural member, and this is sometimes referred to as 'toenailing'. The maximum strength of such joints may be obtained by:

- using the largest nail that will not cause splitting
- making the distance between the end of the piece and the point of the nail entry one-third the length of the nail
- driving the nail in at a slope of 30° to the piece.

Engineering requirements

AS 1720.1-1997 *Timber Structures—Design Methods* provides design data on nailed joints, giving permissible loads, nail lengths, edge and end distances, spacing between nails and withdrawal loads.

Nailing of plywood

Because of plywood's alternating bands of grain direction, it is less inclined to split than solid timber of the same species when nailed close to the edge.

The nail withdrawal resistance of plywood is somewhat less (15–30 per cent) than that of solid timber of the same species, mainly due to the presence of peeler checks.

Steel fixing plates

Slotted plates are available for use in conjunction with nails for firmly connecting butted end joins, eliminating halving and lapping.

Nailplates

Nailplates are rectangular plates of galvanised steel, with prongs stamped from the plate (toothed plate connectors), which are used to join timber of the same thickness (Plate 23).

Nailplates are available in a wide range of sizes and are most commonly used to hold roof truss components together. The large number of steel shanks in the nailplates transfer load from one timber member into the light-gauge steel plate across the discontinuity between the members and into the other piece of timber. Nailplates can effectively reduce the tendency for timber to split, as all of the nail shanks are held in position and cannot move sideways. This means that they can be installed much closer to the ends and edges of timber members than normal nails. Nailplates can also be used on the end-grain of poles and on large-sized timber members to restrict splitting.

Generally, the prongs on the plates are forced into the timber by special hydraulic presses, so are most suited to installation in a factory. Nailplates are often used in prefabricated trusses and built-up beams. Lateral strength is good but there is limited resistance to direct withdrawal. The fire resistance of joints made with nailplate connectors is much poorer than those made with ordinary nails.

Nailplates are proprietary products and so design information for them is not included in AS1720.1-1997 *Timber Structures—Design Methods*. Because the load capacity varies with the thickness of the plate, the length of the nails and the pattern of the nails, each product has its own design information.

Nailplated trusses

Nailplated trusses are prefabricated in a factory environment in which the presses and cutting of elements can be carefully controlled. Truss manufacturers generally have design programs that match the selection of nails and member sizes to the structural loads that the truss must carry.

The wood into which the plates are pressed must be free of large knots in order for the connection to have the specified capacity.

Nailplated roof trusses are designed to deflect slightly under the load of the completed roof but to bear only on the external walls; internal walls should be at least 12 mm lower. The extra height in the external walls is often provided by doubling the top plate or using a deeper section of top plate. If there is a 50-mm gap, ceiling battens can be run continuously across internal partitions. Truss spans are measured from the external edges of the top plate.

To provide some stiffening to the internal walls and the bottom chords of the trusses it is usual to fit metal brackets to connect them; the nails to the chords ride in vertical slots for freedom of movement in that direction. To accommodate this freedom of movement, cornices are fixed only to the ceiling and are free to slide down the walls.

The trusses should bear on the external wall plate directly over the studs to ensure proper transference of the roof load. The use of trusses entails greater attention to lintels, which should be seasoned and able to support the concentrated loading without significant deflection.

A strong junction between the truss and the supporting wall plate is most important, particularly in windy locations, and is usually achieved by the use of galvanised angle plates, which enable nails to be driven into the wood at right angles to the grain for maximum holding power.

Diagonal bracing of the top chords is necessary to prevent buckling and to stiffen up what is a relatively light assembly. Such bracing should run from near the apex down to the wall plate.

The nailplates enable a single thickness of wood to be chosen for the entire truss, and the truss is quite slender. It is essential that trusses are handled carefully between manufacture and final assembly as a roof. They should be stacked so as to remain flat. AS 4440-2004 *Installation of Nailplated Timber Roof Trusses* outlines the requirements for stabilisation of the trusses to prevent buckling during lifting and while temporarily supported in the structure.

Staples

Machine-driven staples of bright steel are commonly used in conjunction with mastic adhesives for fixing wallboards in position and in the production of the cheaper lines of furniture.

Nail lamination

Nails can be used instead of adhesives to join segments of timber together to form a large section beam. Pieces nailed together side by side (i.e. vertical lamination) can form beams as strong and stiff as solid beams.

When making the vertical laminates, each lamination should be full length. Nails should be not less than 2.8 mm diameter and at least 50 mm long, with the protruding ends clinched (i.e. bent back at right angles). The distance between nails should be not less than twice the thickness of the timber, with alternate nails staggered vertically and with additional nails at points of load concentration. So that each lamination can carry its share of the load, the bottom surface on bearing points must be level. Equal load sharing will also be better achieved by all timber being of the same species and of a similar cut (e.g. all radial or all tangential).

Horizontal lamination can be used for top plates to increase thickness, but in order to make a member with the same strength as the solid member with the same cross-section, a very large number of nails is required. In general, horizontal laminating is not very effective.

Other metal fasteners

Screws

Screws are suitable for either type 1 or type 2 connections. They are installed into a drilled hole with a diameter the same as the root diameter of the screw. The threads along the shank of the screw cut into the wood fibres and form a mechanical bond with the timber. Screws have considerably greater resistance to withdrawal than similar sized nails but the lateral load capacities are similar to those for an equal diameter of nail. The resistance to withdrawal is due to the interlocking of the metal thread with the timber fibres. Failure of a screwed connection occurs when either the screw fractures in tension, or it pulls out the plug of wood fibres attached to the metal thread of the screw shank.

Drilling a hole in order to install screws removes wood fibres and reduces the cross-section of the timber at that point. This slightly reduces the strength of the timber in tension.

Screws can be removed easily and reinserted without significant loss of holding power, but are seldom used for structural work. Penetration into the second component should be at least seven times the screw diameter.

Screws are available in steel, galvanised steel, brass, chromium-plated, aluminium and stainless steel and with various head shapes.

Type 17 screws are now commonly used and are self-drilling screws with a hardened drill bit as the lowest part of the shank. They have the same capacity as normal screws. They can be a cost-effective alternative to normal screws as they can be installed in a one-step operation using a powerful low-speed drill.

AS 1720.1-1997 *Timber Structures—Design Methods* provides information on permissible loads, spacing and withdrawal loads. These capacities and requirements apply equally to wood screws and type 17 screws.

Bolts

Bolts are available in a range of sizes and grades, and are specified by diameter, length and grade. The most commonly used sizes for structural timber are M10, M12, M16, M20 and M24. They are installed into predrilled holes with large washers under both the bolt head and nut to ensure that there is adequate bearing on the timber to transfer forces from the bolt to the timber members without crushing.

Bolts have larger diameter shanks and hence a higher capacity than screws and nails, so fewer bolts are required in a connection. However, the installation of bolts is more complex and labour intensive and therefore more expensive than nailed or screwed connections.

Steel bolts are used for assembly work, large trusses, bridge girders and the like where thick sections have to be held together. Such thick sections are seldom in a seasoned condition when first installed so it is an important maintenance procedure for the bolts to be tightened regularly in the first few years of service. Washers should always be installed to spread the load. Bolts, nuts and washers should be galvanised if they are likely to become wet in service. In some situations, helical washers can be used to accommodate some or all of the shrinkage of the timber member.

Capacity of bolted connections

Because bolts transfer load between pieces of timber using bearing, they have different capacities if the load is applied parallel to the grain and if the load is applied perpendicular to the grain.

AS1720.1-1997 *Timber Structures—Design Methods* provides information on the capacity of bolts both perpendicular and parallel to the grain, and the size of washer required at each end. The Standard also provides information on geometric requirements for bolted connections.

Coach screws

Coach screws have similar behaviour to bolts. Instead of screwing into a nut, a coach screw screws into timber. Its capacity in type 1 connections is very similar to the capacity of a similar sized bolt, and its capacity in a type 2 connection is modelled on screw behaviour. Their capacities are also presented in AS1720.1-1997 *Timber Structures—Design Methods*.

Steel shear plates

In order to provide an efficient transfer of load from a steel member to one of timber, shear plates can be fitted into a groove cut in the timber and the load is then transferred with the aid of a bolt, which holds the components together. These connectors can be used to transmit larger loads than bolts or nails, but care needs to be taken to prevent splitting in service.

Split ring connectors

One way of spreading the load when transferring it from one timber component to another is by means of a steel ring sprung into grooves cut in the faces of the two components, the join being held together with a bolt, but the ring carries the load. It has been claimed that one ring of 60 mm is as strong as three 19-mm bolts.

AS1720.1-1997 *Timber Structures—Design Methods* provides the essential design detail for the use of split ring connectors, shear plate connectors and toothed metal plate connectors.

FURTHER READING

Australian Standard. (1997). AS 1720.1 *Timber Structures—Design Methods*.

Adhesives

Australian Standard. (1999). AS 2329-1999 *Mastic Adhesives for Fixing Wallboards*.

Booth, C. C. (1979). A guide to building construction adhesives. *Adhesives Age* 22(2): 31–7.

Canadian Forestry Service (1972). Strength of glue lines. *Research News* 15(1).

Chugg, W. A. (1964). *Glulam: the theory and practice of the manufacture of glued laminated timber structures*. London: Benn.

CIB W80/RILEM 71-PSL. (1987). *Prediction of service life of building materials and components*. CIB publication 96.

CSIRO Division of Forest Production. (1960). Wood adhesives: a summary of their properties and uses. *Trade Circ* 49.

Fox, S. P. (1974). Residual strength of fire-damaged laminated beams. *For Prod J* 24(1): 48–50.

Gillespie, R. H., Countryman, D., Blomquist, R. F. (1978). *Adhesives in building construction.* Agriculture handbook 516. US Dept Ag. For. Service.

Hall, R. B., Leonard, J. H., Nicholls, G. A. (1960). Bonding particleboards with bark extracts. *For Prod J* 10(5): 263–72.

Houwink, R. and Salomon, G. (eds). (1965). *Adhesion and adhesives.* Vol. 1: *Adhesives.* Vol. 2: *Applications.* Netherlands: Elsevier.

Plomley, K. F. (1966). Tannin-formaldehyde adhesives for wood: wattle tannin adhesives. Tech. paper 39. Melbourne: CSIRO Division of Forest Production.

Raknes, E. (1995). Adhesives (Ch A12). In: *Timber engineering step 1.* Netherlands: Centrum Hout.

Skeist, I. (ed.) (1963). *Handbook of adhesives.* London: Reinhold.

Strickler, M. D. (1980). Finger-jointed dimension lumber. *For Prod J* 30(9): 51–6.

Vick, C. B. (1980). Structural bonding of CCA-treated wood for foundation systems. *For Prod J* 30(9): 25–32.

Watson, A. J. and Higgins, H. G. (1950). Suitability of Australian timbers for veneer. CSIRO bulletin 260.

Wood, W. G. and Mills, A. C. (1975). Penetration end joints. *For Prod J* 25(5): 51–6.

Yoshida, H. (1986). Bond durability of water-based polymer isocyanate adhesives (API resins) for wood. (Japanese with English summary.) *J Jap Wood Res Soc* 32(6): 432.

Nails and other fixings

Australian Standard. (2004). AS 4440 *Installation of Nailplated Timber Roof Trusses.*

CSIRO Division of Building Research. (1973). Keep your roof on. Seminar papers.

Hirst, K. (1972). Application of gluing pressure by nails or staples. *CSIRO Forest Production Newsletter* 388: 5–8.

Keating, W. G. (1973). Nail laminating. *CSIRO Forest Production Newsletter* 393: 3–4.

Leicester, R. H., Seath, C. A., Pham, L. (1979). The fire resistance of metal connectors. Topic 2/12. 19th Forest Production Research Conference. Melbourne: CSIRO Division of Building Research.

Longworth, J. and McMullin, A. E. (1963). Effect of moisture content on strength of bolted connections. *For Prod J* 13(3): 104–7.

Mack, J. J. (1978). The grouping of species for the design of timber joints with particular application to nailed joints. Tech. paper (2nd series) 26. Melbourne: CSIRO Division of Building Research.

Mack, J. J. (1978). The establishment of lateral working loads for nailed joints for Australian conditions. Tech. paper (2nd series) 27. Melbourne: CSIRO Division of Building Research.

Mack, J. J. (1979). The withdrawal resistance of plain steel nails and screws in Australian timbers. Tech. paper (2nd series) 30. Melbourne: CSIRO Division of Building Research.

National Association of Forest Industries (1989). Timber data file J1. Timber joints design—1. Design principles. Canberra: NAFI.

National Association of Forest Industries (1989). Timber data file J2. Timber joints design—2. Nails, staples and screws. Canberra: NAFI.

National Association of Forest Industries (1989). Timber data file J3. Timber joints design—3. Bolts, coach screws and timber connectors. Canberra: NAFI.

National Association of Forest Industries (1989). Timber data file J4. Timber joints design—4. Fabricated metal connectors. Canberra: NAFI.

Stern, E. G. (1967). Effects of bradding and clinching of points of plain shank and helically threaded nails. Virginia Polytechnic Institute.

Stern, E. G., et al. (1974). Mechanical fastening of wood. A review of the state of the art. Madison, USA: For. Prod. Res. Soc.

Chapter 9

Plywood and laminated veneer lumber

Plywood and laminated veneer lumber (LVL) are products manufactured from an assembly of veneers (thin sheets of wood of uniform thickness) bonded together to form a panel or beam. In plywood, the veneers are usually assembled with the grain direction in one veneer being at right angles to that in the adjacent veneer to form a panel, while in LVL the veneers are usually jointed and laid end to end to form a beam.

In the case of plywood, the much greater strength of timber along the grain than across the grain (25 to 40 times as much) makes it worthwhile to cut logs into veneers and then alternate the grain direction in each successive layer before bonding the veneers together. To ensure a stable balanced construction free of warping tendencies, an odd number of veneers is used (e.g. 3-ply, 5-ply, 7-ply) and the grain of the face and back veneers is parallel. The crossing of the grain at right angles tends to equalise the strength in all directions and the uniformity increases with the number of plies used.

For special purposes, such as when it is required for bent work at tight radii, plywood is sometimes laid with the grain of the individual veneers running in the same direction.

In addition to the rearrangement of strength properties that plywood permits, it also provides greater stability by utilising timber's very low longitudinal movement to restrain the normal lateral movement that occurs with changes in moisture content.

Because of the stresses that can be created thereby, it is essential that good-quality adhesives be selected and carefully applied. In general, coarse-textured species (e.g. *Shorea* sp. from South-East Asia) do not give a very strong glue line because of the possibility of tearing out of the fibres when under load. Such species are satisfactory for non-structural use, as in panelling and furniture, but for structural purposes involving considerable stress, as in plywood for boats, species with a fine-textured surface are more suitable.

In the case of LVL, the veneering process significantly improves the structural properties of LVL over the parent wood due to the randomisation of defects. Defects (such as knots), when peeled into veneer, which is then assembled into LVL, are no longer concentrated in one location. In sawn timber all of the strength-reducing effect of a defect is concentrated around the one cross-sectional area of the beam, but in LVL the effect is distributed in the beam effectively, increasing the proportion of 'good wood' at any cross-section. This process can increase strength properties by 250 per cent and stiffness by 50 per cent when compared with solid timber from the same resource. LVL is usually manufactured in a continuous process, enabling the production of beams of very long length in thickness up to 105 mm and width up to 1200 mm. The available length is only limited by transport constraints.

Manufacture of plywood

The veneer from which plywood is formed is obtained by either rotating the log against a long knife edge (rotary cut), so that the veneer comes away from the knife in a long ribbon that is later cut into suitable widths for processing, or by slicing, in which relatively narrow widths are cut from segments of log, usually in an endeavour to obtain decorative effects from particular characteristics of the wood. Before the veneer is cut the log is usually heated in hot water or steam to soften it.

Rotary cut material constitutes the majority of veneer production because of the simplicity and speed of the operation, but some species give their best appearance on the quarter-cut face (e.g. silky oak, Queensland maple, Queensland walnut) so it is then necessary to slice the veneer from log sections that have been cut to develop the best figure. The resultant sheets of veneer are kept in sequence to facilitate the subsequent matching of panels. The term 'crown cut' is often given to veneer sliced from a billet to yield a succession of veneers that are all parallel to the axis of the billet. They are kept in sequence as cutting proceeds.

Another method, known as semirotary cutting, involves the peeling of quartered log segments set up eccentrically on a rotary lathe. It is possible to obtain a fully quarter-cut figure if the log flitch is carefully positioned.

One of the main problems in producing good veneer is to minimise the breaking effect of the knife edge, which produces a 'tight' side and a 'slack' side. In the thicker veneers there is a tendency for minute fractures, known as 'peeler checks', to show up after the application of finish coatings or after a period of use.

The thickness of the veneer usually ranges from about 0.3 mm to 6 mm, the thicker material generally being used for the inner veneers, while face material, which should have a minimum of peeler checks, is usually of thin veneer, especially when expensive, very decorative veneer is involved.

Veneering makes it possible to obtain decorative effects that are not available in solid timber. The effect can be matched and repeated a number of times; irregular growths and gnarled stumps can provide beautiful figured veneer, yet the same logs would be worthless for sawing into solid timber because of the difficulty of seasoning satisfactorily such unevenly grown material. Veneering permits the use of expensive rare woods without exorbitant cost for the finished article. Wide panels can be made up free of joins or with veneers matched to provide an unbroken appearance and panels can be as long as 15 m. Veneering also permits the use of decorative species whose density or workability would rule

113

them out for use as solid panelling. As well as the use of veneers to form plywood, they are used for facing blockboard and particleboard.

Fancy veneers for special figure effects may be cut from roots or gnarled trunks, but for the normal run of production the plywood manufacturer looks for straight cylindrical logs with sound heart and as free as possible from defects.

The veneers are dried, edge-glued and taped together in sheets of the required size, coated with adhesive, assembled to provide the requisite thickness and pressed in large, heated hydraulic presses that are capable of handling a large number of plywood assemblies at the one time. The plywood sheets are trimmed to size and sanded ready for market.

Movement in plywood

The alternating change in direction of the grain of the veneers makes plywood resistant to splitting and puncturing and it is very strong in relation to its density. Fixings may be driven through plywood relatively close to its edges because of its enhanced resistance to 'pull-through'. Changes in thickness in plywood due to moisture content variation are approximately the same as for solid timber of the same species but other dimensional changes are much lower than that of the solid timber.

A comparison between the shrinkage of solid timber and plywood of the same species, expressed as a percentage variation in dimension per 1 per cent moisture content change, is shown in Table 9.1.

Table 9.1 Comparison of shrinkages

	Plywood (5 mm 3-ply)		Solid timber	
	Along the grain of face plies	Across the grain of face plies	Radial	Tangential
Hoop pine	0.010	0.014	0.17	0.22
Coachwood	0.015	0.021	0.19	0.29
Silver ash	0.014	0.023	0.20	0.27

Blockboard

Blockboard is the term applied to the composite board product that is made by applying one or more veneers to each face of a core of narrow (say about 25 mm) timber strips. The terms 'solid core' and 'core stock' are also applied to such material. One advantage of blockboard over conventional plywood (multi-ply) is that it enables more efficient dowelling when joining segments together and provides a better base for the attachment of hinges. Careful attention to the moisture content of the core material is important for satisfactory performance, as is also the alternating of the growth ring direction in adjacent pieces. Blockboard is used mainly for internal applications since its core is normally of species that are not durable under long-term exposure. Its most frequent application is for office partitions, wall panelling and doors. Care must be taken when assembling solid core doors to avoid spiral-grained material in the blockboard. If the door is subjected to a change in moisture content after it has been installed, the door is very likely to twist when the blockboard is of spiral-grained material.

Types of plywood

Plywood is only as good as the adhesive that is used in bonding the veneers together. Plywood that is used for the manufacture of furniture and for interior panelling does not normally require a highly water-resistant bond, but plywood that is to be exposed to the weather (e.g. in exterior doors and cladding) requires an adhesive that is undamaged by water and fungi and which is strong enough to resist the much severer stresses in the timber that are caused by the greater range of moisture content in exposed positions.

Plywood is made to conform to standards published by Standards Australia. The current standards are:

- AS/NZS 2269: 2004 *Plywood—Structural*
- AS/NZS 2270: 1999 *Plywood and Blockboard for Interior Use*
- AS/NZS 2271: 2004 *Plywood and Blockboard for Exterior Use*
- AS/NZS 2272: 1996 *Plywood—Marine.*

AS/NZS 2270 and 2271 do not apply to blockboard for door infill.

A most important consideration in choosing the right plywood for a particular use is the type of adhesive used to bond the veneers together. Bonds are classified into four types:

- *Type A*: A waterproof bond that is able to withstand exposure to the weather for a long period without deterioration. Phenol formaldehyde, resorcinol formaldehyde and tannin formaldehyde adhesives can provide such a bond.
- *Type B*: A waterproof bond but one that is subject to deterioration after several years' continuous exposure to the weather. This bond is suitable for use in plywood for concrete formwork and for permanent applications where only occasional exposure to wet weather is involved, such as in exterior doors. Melamine urea formaldehyde adhesives are commonly used.
- *Type C*: A bond that can withstand occasional dampness, and suitable for general internal plywood. Extended urea formaldehyde is used.
- *Type D*: A bond that is only suitable for internal conditions completely free of dampness. Highly extended urea formaldehyde is the most commonly used adhesive.

Although the use of a durable adhesive provides a bond of long-term effectiveness, it does not imply that the veneers being bonded together will have any long-term durability. For example, if plywood is to be used for a marine craft and will experience service conditions that are liable to encourage decay, then it will also be necessary to ensure that the veneers are of a durable species or that the plywood be impregnated with a non-leachable preservative. The term *waterproof plywood* is often misunderstood. It doesn't necessarily mean that the plywood is waterproof but rather that the glue is waterproof.

A brief summary of the main features of the Standards listed above is as follows:

1. AS/NZS 2269: 2004 *Plywood—Structural.* This standard applies to plywood that is made of hardwood or softwood veneers or both. The quality of the veneer is judged from the finished sheet. Five veneer qualities (A, S, B, C and D) are described: quality A is suitable for clear finishing; S is a 'special' grade suitable for clear finishing but permitting natural characteristics that are promoted as decorative features; B is suitable for painting with pigmented paint; C is suitable for presenting a solid face; and D allows open defects, such as holes, splits and joins, between individual pieces of veneer.

   Only one bond quality, type A, is allowed. A wide range of stress grades determined through in-grade testing, the use of stiffness graded veneer or machine stress grading, from F7 to F34, is possible. The most common stress grades are F8 to F22. The moisture content of the plywood is required to be within the range 10–15 per cent for sheets up to 7 mm thick, and 8–15 per cent for thicker material. Tolerances on the ordered size are provided for both sanded and unsanded sheets.

   Sapwood that is susceptible to lyctid borer attack must be immunised or excluded. Other preservative treatments against insect and fungal attack are subject to special ordering, as is fire-retardant treatment. Each sheet is required to be branded with the manufacturer's mark, the word 'structural' or product description, the grade of the outer plies (face first, back last, e.g. CC, CD or DD), the bond type of the glue line (A), an indication of the stress grade, and branding in accordance with AS/NZS 1604.3: 2004 *Specification for Preservative Treatment—Plywood* if it is preservative-treated.

2. AS/NZS 2270: 1999 *Plywood and Blockboard for Interior Use.* This Standard applies to material for non-structural uses, such as internal wall panelling, furniture and so on in locations that are protected fully from dampness.

   Three appearance grades of face veneer—S (decorative), A and B—are described as well as two grades of back veneer (C and D) so that there are six possible combinations of face and back veneer. Plywood with lower quality back veneer would be quite adequate for wall panelling, for example.

   The Standard gives allowable tolerances on dimensions, the quality of surface finish in relation to machining, and branding requirements. In regard to the latter, each sheet is required to show the manufacturer's identity, the word 'interior' or product description, the grade of the outer plies (face first, back last, so SC, SD, AC, AD, BC or BD), the bond type of the glue line (usually D but C is also provided for), and branding in accordance with AS/NZS 1604.3 if sapwood is preservative-treated against lyctid or termite attack.

   Moisture content at the time of dispatch is limited to the range 8–15 per cent.

3. AS/NZS 2271: 2004 *Plywood and Blockboard for Exterior Use.* This Standard applies to material that is used for external cladding or for internal locations that are subject to occasional dampness. Three

face veneer grades (S, A and B) and two back veneer grades (C and D) are described, giving a possible six appearance grades of exterior plywood. The Standard provides allowable tolerances on dimensions, requirements for smoothness of surface finish, and moisture content limits at the time of dispatch (8–15 per cent).

Sapwood is allowed; if it is subject to lyctid borer attack it has to be immunised but other preservative treatment is subject to special ordering. However, since all sapwood is of low durability when subject to damp conditions, further consideration of this aspect is desirable by the specifier, who would be wise to require the elimination of all sapwood or to require its treatment with non-leachable preservative if the conditions of use indicate potentially long periods of dampness.

Each sheet has to be branded with the manufacturer's identity, the word 'exterior' or product description, the grade of the outer veneers (face first, back last, i.e. SC, SD, AC, AD, BC or BD), the type of glue bond (A or B), and the branding requirements of AS/NZS 1604.3 if immunisation or preservative treatment has been carried out.

4. AS/NZS 2272: 1996 *Plywood—Marine*. This Standard provides for plywood that is suitable for use in marine craft and boatbuilding. Only one bond quality, type A, is allowed and there is only one grade. The range of allowable species is limited; permitted species must meet the following criteria:

(a)   dried density: 450–720 kg/m^3.
(b)   tangential shrinkage (green to 12 per cent moisture content): no more than 8 per cent
(c)   Izod value (seasoned): not less than 5.5 J
(d)   modulus of rupture (seasoned): not less than 76 MPa
(e)   texture of face veneers: fine to medium.

The species currently permitted are: silver ash, white birch, blackwood, canarium, pencil cedar, coachwood, Fijian kauri, makore, Queensland maple, scented maple, celery-top pine, hoop pine, klinki pine, sapele, bolly silkwood, red silkwood, silver silkwood and teak. The following species are acceptable only as core veneers: damanu, doi, slash pine, sassafras, southern sassafras and taun.

Many of these species are not durable in damp conditions, so if marine craft are to be kept on moorings it would be very desirable to have the plywood preservative-treated against decay and insect attack. Many buyers are under the impression that the description 'marine plywood' implies the possession of good resistance to decay, which is far from the truth.

The moisture content of the plywood at the time of dispatch is required to be within the 10–15 per cent range for sheets up to 7 mm thick and the 8–15 per cent range for thicker material.

Each sheet is required to display the following information: the identity of the manufacturer, the word 'marine', the glue bond (type A bond), and the branding requirements of AS 1604.1-2005 *Specification for Preservative Treatment—Sawn and Round Timber* if any preservative treatment has been carried out.

5. AS/NZS 2098: 1996 *Methods of Test for Veneer and Plywood*. This Standard gives test methods for the determination of the: moisture content of veneer and plywood; bond quality and strength of scarf joints in plywood; resistance of glue lines to attack by microorganisms; depth of peeler checks; density of veneer and plywood; water absorption and thickness swelling; and procedures for in-grade testing of structural plywood.

Laminated veneer lumber

LVL is bonded using only type A phenolic adhesive. Veneers used in the manufacture of LVL are usually 3.0 mm thick but may be as thin as 1.0 mm and as thick as 6.0 mm. There is no standard to describe a veneer grade for LVL. Veneer of any grade may be utilised provided that it is free of active insect attack and decay and is of uniform thickness within each sheet. LVL is typically used in structural applications where the high strength and stiffness, long lengths and large section sizes are advantageous.

LVL is manufactured to AS/NZS 4357: 1995 *Structural Laminated Veneer Lumber*. This standard requires LVL products to be manufactured in accordance with a strict written manufacturing specification. This specification must define the log resource from which the LVL product is manufactured, veneer quality, veneer arrangement, thickness and jointing, and bonding, and must provide details of the manufacturing process. Product is subject to in-grade testing and reliable structural properties are determined. The standard requires LVL to be supplied to the market at a moisture content of 8–15 per cent. The requirements of dimensional shape, manufacturing, branding and ongoing structural verification are also specified.

Utilisation

The sizes of plywood sheet currently available include:

- 1800 mm × 1200 mm
- 2400 mm × 1200 mm
- 2700 mm × 1200 mm

and these are available in thicknesses of 4, 5, 6, 7, 9, 12, 15, 17, 19 and 21 mm.

When ordering, it is important to specify the size, thickness, species of face veneer, quality of veneer and quality of bond, the number of plies, the use proposed and any special finishes that are required for the surface. For structural products it is important to specify the stress grade.

When plywood is used externally it is desirable to face it with a Kraft paper (see Chapter 11) that is impregnated with phenol formaldehyde resin. This prevents the fine checking that can show in weathered rotary cut plywood and it provides a uniform surface for painting without the need for any further preparation. A surface skin of aluminium or copper is often bonded to plywood that is used in the construction of caravans, railway rolling stock, and so on.

Plywood is frequently used for concrete formwork. The face veneers, preferably of a dense species for serviceability, are often given extra protection against the chemical action of the cement by a skin of phenol formaldehyde. This product gives a smooth surface to the concrete and may withstand even 100 pours if given reasonably careful handling. As an alternative to such special surfacings, oil-based release agents, or 'form oils', can be applied but should be used sparingly and in strict compliance with the handling instructions supplied by their manufacturers.

LVL is available in lengths up to 13.2 m in standard depths of 95, 130, 150, 170, 240, 300, 360, 400 and 450 mm. Standard thicknesses include 36, 45, 63, 75 and 90 mm. When ordering, it is important to specify the structural grade as a number of different structural grades are available from different suppliers.

A number of specialty LVL products are available, such as LVL with a factory-applied water repellent (for short-term use in exposed applications, such as formwork bearers) and preservative-treated LVL to enhance termite resistance.

Handling of plywood

Plywood sheets should be stacked on a solid support and not leaned on their edges at an angle against a wall. Face veneers that are exposed unevenly to light may darken and create patterns that are indicative of the degree of cover, which can show up later when the panel is clear finished. To prevent this happening the faces should always be protected from the light before installation. Protection from the uptake of moisture is essential, as with all seasoned timber products, and plywood panels should be allowed to adjust to the conditions of the building before final fixing.

Plywood is susceptible to damage at the corners and edges of the sheets and all edges and joints require support from the underlying framework unless provided with tongues and grooves. Nailing is possible near the edges and nails should be used there at close intervals, say 150–200 mm apart. When fixing wall panelling, contact adhesives are suggested for bonding the body of the sheet to the framework to minimise nails showing on the decorative face. When dense hardwood species are used for the face veneers, splintering along the saw cut is common unless the saw is kept sharp. When using a handsaw, the face side of the sheet should be uppermost, but it should be face down if a power saw is used.

LVL should be stacked flat with bearers or supports at 3-m centres. LVL has a tendency to split when nailed on the edge so care must be taken. To avoid nail pull-out for flooring fixed onto LVL, it is recommended that deformed shank nails are used.

Sealing of end-grain

Because of the rapid uptake of moisture through end-grain and the occurrence of end-grain on all edges of plywood, more than usual care in sealing the edges is required. This is especially so with concrete formwork because of the abundance of moisture present that will tend to thicken the edges of the plywood and so cause some unevenness to the concrete surface. The adhesives used to bond the veneers would be a good sealant for the end-grain.

Plywood flooring

Plywood is used as flooring, either in large structural sheets or in small pieces as a tile laid on a subfloor. Plywood used as a structural flooring element enables speedy laying of the floor, freedom from draughts, and provides a good supporting base for sheet materials and carpet. AS 1684-1999 *Residential Timber-Framed Construction* requires structural plywood flooring to have a type A bond. Joist spacings for plywood are required to comply with the figures shown in Table 9.2. The sheets are required to be installed with the face grain at right angles to the joists and must be continuous over at least two spans for the figures in the table to apply. If supported over one span, only the spacings must be reduced by 25 per cent. Table 9.2 also assumes that the outer veneers are at least as thick as the inner veneers. Unless tongues and grooves are provided, the ends have to be supported over noggins between joists. The joins should be a close fit but the plywood should not be cramped.

Table 9.2 Joist spacings for plywood in residential flooring

Thickness of plywood (mm)	Maximum joist spacing (mm)		
	F8	F11	F14
12	400	420	440
13	430	450	480
14	460	480	510
15	480	520	540
16	510	540	570
17	540	560	600
18	560	590	620
19	590	620	660
20	610	650	680
21	640	670	710
22	660	700	740

FURTHER READING

Referenced articles

Australian Standard. (2005). AS 1604.1 *Specification for Preservative Treatment—Sawn and Round Timber.*

Australian Standard. (2004). AS/NZS 1604.3 *Specification for Preservative Treatment—Plywood.*

Australian Standard. (1999). AS 1684 *Residential Timber-Framed Construction*.

Australian Standard. (1996). AS/NZS 2098 *Methods of Test for Veneer and Plywood*.

Australian Standard. (2004). AS/NZS 2269 *Plywood—Structural*.

Australian Standard. (1999). AS/NZS 2270 *Plywood and Blockboard for Interior Use*.

Australian Standard. (2004). AS/NZS 2271 *Plywood and Blockboard for Exterior Use*.

Australian Standard. (1996). AS/NZS 2272 *Plywood—Marine*.

Australian/New Zealand Standard. (1995). AS/NZS 4357 *Structural Laminated Veneer Lumber*.

Meyer, J. A. (1982). Industrial use of wood-polymer materials: state of the art. *For Prod J* 32(1): 24–9.

Plomley, K. F. (1980). Studies by CSIRO on the adhesive bonding of high density wood species. Melbourne: CSIRO Division of Building Research.

Websites

APA—The Engineered Wood Association, viewed 1 March 2005, <http://www.apawood.org>.

Plywood Association of Australasia, viewed 1 March 2005, <http://www.paa.asn.au>.

Chapter 10

Reconstituted wood products

There are obvious limitations to the size of building components that can be made by sawing logs and the process is somewhat wasteful because of the considerable loss of wood in the form of sawdust. The desire for more complete utilisation has led to the development of large-scale industries that reduce woody material to small particles and reconstruct it into large sheets of the desired thickness. These sheet materials are easy to handle and erect, enabling large areas to be covered quickly and economically. The types of product available can be classified as wet-process fibreboards (principally softboards and hardboards), dry-process fibreboards (principally medium-density fibreboard [MDF]) and particleboards.

Wet-process fibreboard, hardboard and softboard

Wet-process fibreboard, as produced in Australia, is made from eucalypt fibres, the raw material being mostly from forest thinnings or sawmill off-cuts. These are converted into chips, which are then either heated with steam and ground up, as in the Asplund defibrator, or the material, heated under pressure, is disintegrated by a sudden release of the pressure, as in the hardboard process. The fibres are suspended in water, which gives rise to the name 'wet process'. They are fed onto an endless wire-mesh belt (hence the pattern on the backs of the hardboard sheets), the water is removed by suction, and the ribbon of board is cut into the desired lengths and stacked in a multi-opening hot press to complete the bonding process.

Hardboard can be defined as a panel material made from lignocellulosic fibres felted together and consolidated under heat and pressure. The addition of adhesives is unnecessary, so eucalypt-based hardboards have obvious advantages in view of the rapid increase in the cost of bonding agents.

Softboards

Often called 'softboard' or 'insulating board', this board is made from softwood fibres felted together but not consolidated by heat and pressure.

The board is used for wall and ceiling lining to provide acoustic and thermal insulation. Other applications are in cool-room construction, as carpet underlay and as perforated acoustic tiles. AS/NZS 1859.4:2004 *Reconstituted Wood-Based Panels—Specifications—Wet-Processed Fibreboard* covers the dimensions and tolerances of softboard and such quality determinants as bending strength, internal bond and water swelling.

Hardboards

AS/NZS 1859.4 also describes three types of hardboard:

1. Type GP hardboard is for general purposes that are not subject to weathering.
2. Type MR hardboard is promoted for use in damp areas, such as bathrooms. It is heated with linseed oil in the final stages of manufacture and sold as tempered hardboard. This treatment also increases its modulus of rupture.
3. Exterior-grade hardboard is made from selected hardwoods (spotted gum and the *Angophora* species are excluded because of some technical problems in board production). The fibres are given extra steaming to remove material that could attract fungi. A small amount of wax is added to improve the board's water-repellent properties and the curing pressure is adjusted to provide a medium-density board with enhanced stability.

The medium-density, exterior grade hardboard is a good cladding material, stable, free of edge swelling and an outstanding substrate for all types of coating. It has good resistance to impact damage and denting, is non-corrosive, has good insulating properties and is easy to cut and nail. In the past it has been marketed in the form of narrow strips to simulate weatherboard and chamferboard, but its thin profile does not make it a very appropriate substitute visually; it would seem better to take advantage of its availability in large sheets and the speed of erection that this permits and attend to the aesthetic aspect by the application of vertical battens and so on, whose location could be very flexible.

The equilibrium moisture content of hardboard is much lower than that of timber, varying between a half and three-quarters of the figures obtained for the natural wood. However, it still needs conditioning to the environment in which it is to be used before being fixed in position.

AS 1859.4 provides the definitions, dimensions and tolerances for hardboard, and the requirements for properties such as bending strength and thickness swell in water. For exterior grades it also specifies internal bond and wet bending strength.

Hardboard of appropriate type is used for prefinished panelling, sheet floor underlay, cladding, door facings, perforated display boards, eaves lining, television cabinet backs, automotive components, concrete formwork and roof and wall shingles.

Dry-process fibreboard

Dry-process fibreboards are made with a fibre mat containing only about 10 per cent moisture and do not have the same environmental problems as wet-process types concerning disposal of the waste liquor. The fibres are obtained from the timber in a similar manner to those for hardboard but bonding is achieved by the addition of synthetic resin adhesives, which are cured under heat and pressure.

A number of different classes of dry-process fibreboard are available, including ultra-low-density, low-density, medium-density and high-density classes. AS/NZS 1859.2:2004 *Reconstituted Wood-Based Panels—Specifications—Dry-Processed Fibreboard* provides all the relevant properties and specifications for the various classes. The most commonly produced and used class is MDF.

Both standard (dry use) and moisture-resistant internal grades are produced, depending on the adhesive used. Fibreboards that are based on radiata pine have a very smooth surface and are easy to work and the edges can be smoothly contoured. The material is a good substrate for high-gloss coatings and decorative overlays, and is also very attractive in its raw form with a clear finish. It has advantages over particleboard in its screw-holding ability, internal bond strength and modulus of rupture.

The properties that are required of the raw material for fibreboard are more critical than for particleboard; for example, in order to maintain appearance and machining characteristics, less bark and silica can be tolerated for fibreboard.

Fibreboard containers

An unfortunate confusion arises from the common application of the word 'fibreboard' to the cardboard-like material that constitutes the common container used especially for the conveyance of fruit and vegetables to market and for the bulk packaging of most grocery merchandise. It is often referred to as paper board.

Such material, more akin to a thick paper, is of course a very different product from the fibreboards discussed above. It is mentioned on page 387.

Particleboard

Particleboard is a panel product that is made from relatively large particles instead of fibres and is dependent for its strength and durability on the type and quantity of adhesive that is used to bond the ingredients. Other terms, such as 'chipboard', 'waferboard' and 'flakeboard', are used to describe panel products of a similar type but differing in particle size.

AS/NZS 1859.1 2004 *Reconstituted Wood-Based Panels—Specifications—Particleboard* describes three types of particleboard:

1. Standard-grade particleboard is for internal use, as in the construction of furniture (often with a veneer overlay), cupboards and shelving. Urea-formaldehyde resin is the usual binder. It is sometimes used as

a decorative wall facing but it is important that each room be faced with material from the same manufacturer, and preferably the same batch, to ensure uniformity of appearance.
2. Moisture-resistant grade particleboard is for internal use in areas of high humidity or occasional wetting, such as bathrooms and kitchens. A large proportion of particleboard is sold as low-pressure melamine-coated board, often in the form of 'whiteboard', where a white overlay colour is used.
3. High-performance grade particleboard is used in certain structural applications.

In addition, AS/NZS 1860.1: 2002 *Particleboard Flooring—Specifications* defines grades of particleboard flooring:

1. *Flooring grade class 1* is for internal flooring, and is manufactured with an adhesive that does not deteriorate in the presence of moisture or dampness. This grade is suitable for limited exposure during construction. Phenol formaldehyde and tannin formaldehyde waterproof adhesives are most commonly used. Most flooring grade particleboard production is of class 1, which is destined for use in Australian conditions.
2. *Flooring grade class 2* is for internal flooring, but only in locations where there is no risk of dampness. Urea formaldehyde is the most commonly used adhesive in its manufacture. The class 2 board is appropriate for upper-storey floors or for ground floors where permanently dry under-floor conditions are assured. It is unsuited for tropical areas of high natural humidity.

AS 1860-1998 *Installation of Particleboard Flooring* lays down the conditions for using each class of flooring, as well as providing information on the appropriate precautions to take when laying both platform and fitted flooring of particleboard. Platform flooring may be defined as flooring material that is laid into a permanently fixed position over the whole floor area as soon as the bearers and joists are in position, so as to provide a safe working platform for the various tradespeople, and to speed up the erection of the building; it necessarily involves the exposure of the flooring membrane to the risk of considerable moisture uptake from dew and rain before the building provides full protection. The use of class 1 flooring grade is essential under such conditions, but in any case no particleboard floor should be exposed to the weather for more than 2 or 3 months. Edge swelling is a characteristic of particleboard when it is exposed to moisture; the effect is limited virtually to the area within 50 mm of the edge but much of the swelling is not recoverable on drying so an appreciable amount of material may have to be sanded off at the edges to obtain a level floor if there has been a lot of exposure to the weather. This sanding is likely to expose particles of a different size to the main body of the sheet and to have some effect on appearance. If the floor is to be covered, this is not important.

Exposure of the particleboard to the weather for more than 2 or 3 months is likely to have an effect on its internal bonding strength and stiffness.

Acceptance of particleboard for flooring and exposed uses, such as cladding, will be much advanced if some inexpensive treatment can be developed to inhibit edge swelling in damp conditions.

Manufacture

Radiata pine plantation sawmill waste, such as chipped flitches, sawdust, shavings and dockings, provide most of the material used in Australia and New Zealand for particleboard production because of the ready availability and the desirably light weight of the product. However, hardwoods can be used, and in Tasmania, for example, some quantities of hardwoods are used in conjunction with radiata pine.

Chips and dockings are flaked with spinning knives into particles of two sizes for the common three-layer board: a coarse flake for the core and a finer one for the surface layers. The flakes are dried until they contain about 5 per cent moisture. Sawdust and shavings are milled and screened to produce material of uniform size and then blended with the dried flake. The combined material stream is weighed and an accurately determined quantity of adhesive is sprayed on them. It is essential that all particles be coated in order to produce a single solid mass, which will be firm under stress. The layers of sprayed particles are spread on an endless belt; the material is then cut into lengths, which are pressed between heated platens. After pressing, the board is allowed to cure for a few days and is then sanded and trimmed to size. There is a global trend towards the production of particleboard in continuous roller presses but none of this type of press is producing particleboard in Australia, although there are a number producing MDF.

The moisture content of the flakes is important to the quality of the board produced and must not exceed 10 per cent, since excessive moisture affects the hardening of the binder. The adhesive in particleboard accounts for as much as 12 per cent by weight of the finished board.

Platen-pressed boards have almost equal properties along and across the board but moisture content changes have a more marked effect on the thickness of this type of board than on an extruded board. Strength in bending and tension in the plane of the board is quite high.

Particleboard may be produced as a single-layer product, a three-layer product and a graded-density product. The *single-layer* product is a general purpose board suitable for core stock and general construction. It is usual to cross-band it first if it is to be used for carrying thin decorative veneers. The *three-layer* product has a core of rather coarse flakes and outer layers of thinner flakes bonded with a higher loading of adhesive resin, which produces hard smooth faces that are capable of taking thin decorative veneers without the need for cross-banding. This is the common type of particleboard in current production in Australia. The *graded-density* product has a gradual increase in flake size from centre to face. It, too, produces a fine uniform surface to which the thin decorative veneer can be fixed without cross-banding.

The denser faces of the three-layer and graded-density boards result in a stronger board than a uniform density board of equal thickness and mass.

The water resistance of particleboard can be improved by the addition of a limited amount of paraffin wax, which is suspended in the adhesive resin that is sprayed on the flakes.

Some of the thickness swelling of particleboard is reversible on drying but some is not; the latter is called *springback* and it is of major importance in the potential deterioration of particleboard that is exposed to water or high humidity. The amount of resin binder present is an important factor in thickness swelling.

The bending strength of pressed particleboard is much lower than that of clear timber of the same species, and its modulus of rupture is generally about 18–24 MPa. Its stiffness, as expressed by its modulus of elasticity, may be only about 2–4 GPa. Both properties are considerably improved by facing the particleboard with veneers. Both moduli are severely reduced with a rise in moisture content above normal conditions. Deflection under sustained load, or *creep* as it is called technically, is also very likely to increase to an unacceptable amount if high humidity conditions persist. Increased compaction pressure has a generally favourable effect on mechanical properties. The screw-holding ability on the edges is not very good but many kinds of hinge of attractive design are now marketed to enable screwing to be effected through the face of the board.

The considerable quantity of resin present in particleboard tends to dull cutting equipment, so workshops handling a lot of particleboard install tungsten carbide-tipped tools. Sawing and sanding do not cause many problems but it is difficult to get a smooth surface when planing because individual flakes tend to pull out.

When face veneering particleboard, it is important that the moisture content of the panel be below 7 per cent; if this rule is followed and the gluing operation is carried out with care, it may not be necessary to veneer the other side for balanced construction if the product is to be used in a mild climate. In fact, impermeable materials, for example, the melamine laminates, are commonly applied to the top surface alone without causing trouble.

Particleboard machines quite well. The edge does tend to be rough and a lot of filling is needed if a painted edge is to show, so it is common practice to cover the edge with a moulding or plastic sheeting. When used for shelving that is to carry any considerable weight, frequent supports are necessary because of the tendency for a considerable degree of creep to occur under load.

Irritant fumes from particleboard

When urea formaldehyde adhesive is used for bonding the constituents of particleboard together, small quantities of excess formaldehyde may be given off to the air. Formaldehyde emissions from particleboard are now greatly reduced by advances in adhesive technology and are one-tenth of what they were 10–15 years ago. Nevertheless, the concentration may build up inside cupboards and unventilated rooms soon after construction. Some people are sensitive to concentrations as low as 5 parts per million and their eyes and nose may experience some irritation. High temperatures, high humidity and a room or cupboard that has been kept closed for long periods immediately after installation of the particleboard may cause this trouble.

If the particleboard is sealed with paint or clear finish, the build-up of unpleasant concentrations is usually averted.

When particleboard is made with phenol formaldehyde and tannin formaldehyde binders, the quantity of formaldehyde released is much lower and the dangers of an unpleasant reaction are much less likely to occur.

Thin particleboard (3–6 mm thick) is now commonly used for internal wall panelling, drawer bottoms, and so on, in competition with hardboard and MDF.

FURTHER READING

Australian/New Zealand Standard. (2004). AS/NZS 1859.1 *Reconstituted Wood-Based Panels—Specifications—Particleboard*.

Australian/New Zealand Standard. (2004). AS/NZS 1859.2 *Reconstituted Wood-Based Panels—Specifications—Dry-Processed Fibreboard*.

Australian/New Zealand Standard. (2004). AS/NZS 1859.4 *Reconstituted Wood-Based Panels—Specifications—Wet-Processed Fibreboard*.

Australian Standard. (1998). AS 1860 *Installation of Particleboard Flooring*.

Australian/New Zealand Standard. (2002). AS/NZS 1860.1 *Particleboard Flooring—Specifications*.

Bennett, G. A. (1973). Fibre building board as a structural material. *BRE Information* IS 7/73.

Bootle, K. R. and Chapman, P. (1977). The behaviour of flooring grade particleboard of Australian origin when exposed to the weather in platform construction. Internal report. Sydney: Forestry Commission of NSW.

Borchgrevink, K. G. and Bassett, K. H. (1968). Medium density hardboard: a leading contender for the siding market. *For Prod J* 18(10): 13–17.

Deppe, H. J. and Schmidt, K. (1978). Effect of particle treatment on the surface quality of wood particleboards. *Holz als Roh-und Werkstoff* 36(8): 305–13.

Greve, D. M. (1978). Platform floor construction. Tech. note 1. Brisbane: Qld Department of Forestry.

Jenuleson, W. H. (1973). Flat sheet hardboard finishing. *For Prod J* 23(4): 26–9.

McNatt, J. D. (1980). Hardboard-webbed beams: research and application. *For Prod J* 30(10): 57–64.

Chapter 11

Pulp and paper

Products derived from wood pulp play a most important role in daily living, providing the packaging for many industrial and household purchases as well as being the basis of newspapers, magazines, books and sanitary requirements.

Historically, paper-making from wood was based essentially on the use of softwoods because their fibres are longer than those of hardwoods and easier to felt together to produce a strong sheet of paper. Australian research workers then developed satisfactory methods for converting the short fibre, lower density eucalypts into pulp and such species have provided a significant source of wood pulp for the paper industry.

Interest in the utilisation of short-fibre hardwood pulp has been worldwide and Japanese paper manufacturers have been large-scale importers of Australian eucalypts in chip form for the production of high-quality writing papers.

For economic production, pulp mills require a large quantity of relatively uniform raw material so extensive areas of forest of ready accessibility have to be on hand before the capital outlay that is involved in pulp manufacture is justified.

The early thinnings of pine plantation forests are a source of suitable softwood fibre, while wood from native forests, such as residual pulpwood and young plantation timber, provides a source of hardwood fibre.

There are a number of ways of producing pulp, which are summarised briefly in this chapter.

Mechanical pulp

Mechanical separation of the fibres is the least expensive process because nearly all of the wood is converted into pulp, with yields as high as 97 per cent. Thermomechanical methods are now the most common, involving the steaming of wood chips under pressure, which makes it possible to separate the fibres in refiners. The thermomechanical method requires only 2 or so cubic metres of pulpwood to make a tonne of newspaper, whereas chemical separation requires at least twice as much. Bleaching can be used to assist in whitening the fibres but mechanical pulping causes less effluent disposal problems than does chemical pulping.

Mechanical pulps are most suitable for newsprint and types of non-absorbent tissue that do not have to be very white or strong. Improved refining methods are extending the use of such pulps to be used for lower quality magazine papers.

Chemical and semichemical pulp

Chemical pulp

Chemical pulping methods dissolve the lignin, which binds the fibres in wood together. The chips are treated with chemicals under conditions of high temperature and pressure and give yields of 45–60 per cent of pulp. The chemical changes that occur are very complex.

One of the oldest chemical methods is the sulfite process, which uses an aqueous solution of calcium bisulfite as the pulping agent. It is used for producing high-quality bleached paper but is more limited as to suitable species than is the sulfate process (see below), which can cope with resinous species.

The chips are cooked under pressure in an acidic solution containing calcium bisulfite and free sulfur dioxide, the pH of the solution being between 1.5 and 2.3. The lignin is sulfonated and the compounds formed dissolve in the acidic solution.

Modified sulfite processes use sodium, magnesium and ammonium sulfites and bisulfites instead of the calcium bisulfite. They involve less strongly acid conditions, leading to easier recovery of chemicals and a more acceptable effluent is produced. These processes can cope with a wider range of species and generally give a greater yield of pulp but are more expensive to install and operate.

The sulfate process produces the major portion of the world's chemical pulp. The name is misleading because sulfates play no active part in the pulping reaction. Sodium sulfate is burnt with the 'spent liquor' from the process and is reduced by the carbon present, being converted into sodium sulfide. Sodium sulfide and sodium hydroxide are the active ingredients that attack the lignin.

The sulfate process differs from the sulfite process in that the solution is alkaline, not acidic, and it penetrates the wood more rapidly. It is applicable to all species—softwood and hardwood—and so has a wide industrial appeal, but it causes potential effluent disposal problems, particularly when bleached, and can release an unpleasant odour into the surrounding district unless controlled.

The pulp obtained by the sulfate process is of high strength. Such pulp is often called 'Kraft' pulp (named after the inventor). Unbleached softwood Kraft pulp is favoured for the production of wrapping papers, while bleached hardwood Kraft pulp is used for printing and writing papers.

Semichemical pulp

The use of milder conditions results in the retention of the hemicelluloses, which can be beneficial in paper-making, and enables the yield of pulp to be increased. Such processes are referred to as 'semichemical pulping';

the chemicals merely soften the wood and enable mechanical methods to convert it into fibres without much damage to them.

Any of the chemical processes can be used in such a modified way. One that is widely used is the neutral sulfite semichemical process, which is particularly suitable for pulping hardwoods. The main chemical used is sodium sulfite but sodium carbonate is added to prevent the pH of the solution dropping below the neutral point during the breakdown of the wood.

The cold soda process is another semichemical method that is frequently used on hardwoods. The chips are softened with a cold solution of between 2 and 6 per cent sodium hydroxide and then converted to fibres in a disc mill.

Bleaching

For many uses it is necessary to bleach the pulp, for which purpose chlorine, chlorine dioxide, ozone, sodium hypochlorite and hydrogen peroxide are commonly chosen.

Paper-making

The raw pulp that is obtained by the methods outlined above is subjected to mechanical beating, which increases the surface area of the fibres, increases their water-holding power and makes them more flexible. Their ability to bond together is increased, leading to a stronger paper.

In the conversion of pulp into paper, the pulp fibres in a very dilute suspension (2 per cent) in water flow onto a moving wire gauze. The water is then sucked away, sizing and filling substances are added, and the felted web is dried between heated rollers. A smooth finish is imparted with the aid of highly polished rollers called 'calenders'. The machinery is highly complex and expensive and the operation is a continuous process.

A term commonly met in references to the pulp and paper industry is the *kappa number*. The number is in the range of 10–70 for most types of wood and is established by measuring the amount of a standard potassium permanganate solution that is absorbed by the pulp being considered. Any lignin present reacts rapidly with acidified potassium permanganate, so this is an empirical test method for examining the purity of the pulp; it is also useful for indicating the amount of chlorine or chlorine compounds that are required in bleaching operations.

Tall oil

This term is commonly referred to in the paper manufacturing industry. 'Tall oil' is a by-product of the Kraft method of pulping and results from the saponification of wood extractives by the alkaline pulping liquor. The sodium salts of fatty and resin acids are deposited when the liquor is concentrated, are removed, and then treated with acid to yield a mixture of fatty and resin acids, which is crude tall oil.

Its fatty acids are used in the manufacture of alkyd resins, soaps, detergents and oil flotation agents, while the resin acids are used for making synthetic resins and paper size.

Long fibre versus short fibre pulp

Softwoods (radiata pine) have longer fibres than hardwoods (eucalypts) and the respective pulps have different properties. The advantages possessed by softwood over hardwood pulps include the following:

1. The longer fibres distribute high stress concentrations more effectively and paper produced from them has higher tearing strength. Softwood pulp may have a tear factor about 2.5 times that of hardwood pulp.
2. Paper made from softwood pulp has very much more resistance to repeated folding, but prolonged beating of the hardwood pulp will increase its interfibre bonding and lead to considerable improvement in folding endurance.
3. The speed at which the paper-making machine is run depends, to a considerable extent, on the wet web tensile strength of the pulp. The lower wet web strength of hardwoods means that there are more breaks at the wet end of the paper-making process.

On the other hand, eucalypt pulp has some advantages over softwood pulp. These include the following:

1. The shorter fibres permit a more even spread of material during production. Long fibres tend to become entangled more readily, giving a greater degree of flocculation.
2. The eucalypt fibres have a diameter of 0.015–0.025 mm, whereas in softwoods the diameter range is 0.035–0.045 mm. As the eucalypt fibres are considerably finer they can produce a paper with a smoother surface.
3. For a given tensile strength, paper made from hardwood fibres has a greater opacity than that from long-fibred softwoods.
4. The eucalypts are higher in density than softwoods and produce a more bulky sheet of paper, so a sheet of paper meeting a certain requirement as to thickness can be made from a smaller amount of fibrous material. The higher bulk is associated with higher opacity and with compressibility characteristics that make it very acceptable for printing purposes.
5. Kraft pulps from lower density eucalypts, such as alpine ash, develop better bursting strength (i.e. resistance to stretching of the paper sheet) than pine Kraft pulps. The higher density eucalypts do not have such good bursting strength because the thicker-walled fibres do not collapse as readily during pressing and drying.
6. The short-fibred pulp flows better than long-fibred pulp at the same concentration.
7. The use of species of higher density than that of softwoods provides more pulp for a given volume of logs, resulting in a saving in freight during cartage to the pulp mill. There is also the advantage that a greater mass of wood can be treated in the pressure vessels that are used for digestion.
8. Hardwoods contain less lignin than softwoods (comparative figures are about 22 per cent and 29 per cent) and this means a lower requirement of chemicals during pulping and a reduction in the time required to convert the wood into pulp.

9. Hardwoods have a higher hemicellulose content than softwoods (approximately 35 per cent as compared with 28 per cent). The hemicelluloses are valuable constituents of pulp, helping to increase yield as well as improving fibre bonding and pulp strength. The neutral sulfite semichemical process for pulp production is particularly effective with hardwoods as it favours the retention of the hemicelluloses.
10. Hardwoods are particularly sensitive to swelling agents, such as caustic soda solution, which reduces the tensile strength of the wood to a much lower figure than for softwoods. This reduction in strength permits a speedy breakdown of chips to wood fibres and is the basis of the cold soda process.

There are a few problems in the use of hardwood that should be mentioned. Hardwood pulp has a higher content of fine particles due to the greater proportion of ray and parenchyma cells and these tend to slow down the drainage of water from the pulp. This is not a very important drawback and can be improved considerably by the use of additives that prevent the aggregation of the fine material. Also, fragments of hardwood vessels may lift out of the paper during printing and so affect its appearance.

The heartwood of old hardwood trees may have extractives such as ellagic acid and gallic acid, which increase the consumption of chemicals during pulping and bleaching. Reaction between ellagic acid and the metals of the processing equipment may cause the formation of hard-to-dissolve deposits as well as discolouring the pulp. The presence of the ellagic acid also leads to high viscosity in the waste liquids, which adds to the problem of their disposal.

Eucalypts for pulp production

Desirable features include a relatively long fibre length, thinnish cell walls, low basic density, high cellulose content and low extractives content. The lower density species give better fibre-bonding properties than those of higher density.

Basic density, reflecting the thickness of the fibre wall and the number of fibres per unit mass, has an important influence on the structural and mechanical properties of the paper that is produced from eucalypt pulp.

When breaking and bursting factors are plotted graphically against basic density, they show a much greater rate of decline in strength at basic densities below about 700 kg/m^3. However, pulps made from the higher density species must be beaten to a much greater extent and consume more chemicals, so the economics of pulping them may be unfavourable unless the cost of the wood is low.

At the intermediate basic density range of about 650–700 kg/m^3 a direct economic advantage may accrue to species of higher basic density because, as mentioned previously, they occupy less space per unit of paper-making material during transportation and more material can be treated per digester charge, but in general the lower the basic density, the greater has been the acceptability of the species.

Recycling of paper products

Since paper products constitute about half the bulk of urban refuse, a vast amount of potentially reusable fibre is available for recycling. In Australia, about 60 per cent of such paper is utilised for the domestic production of paper products. For packaging and industrial papers nearly 100 per cent of the recovered paper is used, for newsprint the figure is 24.2 per cent, for printing and writing (from Kraft pulps) 6 per cent and for tissues 12.4 per cent.

Each time the fibre is repulped it suffers some mechanical damage and its strength, shrinkage characteristics and opacity change so it is usually necessary to add a considerable amount of pulp from new fibres to ensure the production of a satisfactory quality of paper.

FURTHER READING

Australian Plantation Producers and Paper Industry Council (A3P). Recovered paper usage statistics 2000–2001, viewed 25 April 2005, <http://www.apic.asn.au>.

Britt, K. W. (1964). *Handbook of pulp and paper technology*. New York: Reinhold.

Einspahr, D. W. (1976). The influence of short rotation forestry on pulp and paper quality. *Tappi* 59(10): 53–6.

Hagemeyer, R. W. (1976). Future world demand for paper and paperboard and the geography of the technical needs. *Tappi* 59(4): 46–9.

Higgins, H. G. (1970). Technical assessment of eucalypt pulps in the papermaking economy. *Appita* 23(6): 417–26.

Higham, R. R. A. (1970). *A handbook of paperboard and board*. London: Business Books.

Hillis, W. E. (1972). Properties of eucalypt woods of importance to the pulp and paper industry. *Appita* 26(2): 113–22.

Koning, J. W., Jr and Godshall, W. D. (1975). Repeated recycling of corrugated containers and its effect on strength properties. *Tappi* 58(9): 146–50.

Maddern, R. W. (1975). National recycling of waste paper in Australia. *Appita* 29(3): 196–200.

Mamers, H. (1978). The Siropulper—a new concept in wastepaper recovery. *Appita* 32(2): 124–8.

Nelson, R. B. and Aldrich, L. C. (1979). The cleaning and bleaching of pulp produced from household wastes. *Tappi* 62(9): 55–8.

Norman, N. E. (1975). Re-use of water in the pulp and paper industry. *Appita* 29(1): 36–40.

Phillips, F. H. and Garland, S. B. (1981). Paper in south-east Asia. *Appita* 34(5): 348–57.

Saul, C. M. (1979). Chemical pulp: its status and future. *Appita* 32(5): 345–50.

Stradal, M. and Roberge, N. (1979). Dry sorting: a new concept for upgrading mixed newspaper. *Tappi* 62(9): 43–6.

Smook, G. A (1992). *Handbook for pulp and paper technologists*. 3rd edn. Bellingham, WA, USA: Angus Wilde Publications.

Thoma, P. J. and Strange, J. G. (1973). Future technical needs and trends of the paper industry. *Tappi* 56(6): 48–52.

Chapter 12

Bending of wood

When a curved member is needed in the manufacture of furniture, industrial equipment or handles, a stronger component will be produced if the curve can be obtained by bending rather than sawing the required shape out of a large piece of timber. The sawing process can involve considerable waste and the shapes created will have a lot of weakening cross-grain. Alternatively, the desired curve can be formed by gluing together a number of thin sections (i.e. the process of lamination). This is a useful alternative if the timber is difficult to bend or the section size in the single piece of timber would present seasoning problems, but the visual appearance presented by the laminations can be a deterrent.

The plasticity of wood increases with rising temperature, and steam is the most practical way of achieving this for the production of bent work. Wood has elastic properties within a limited range of stress. Within this range, the removal of the stress means that the piece of timber will return to its original shape. If the piece is deformed beyond the limiting stress it will remain bent but one must be careful not to carry this deformation too far, otherwise the piece will fracture.

Heating the wood by moist steam increases its compressibility very considerably, up to 40 per cent in some cases, but its ability to stretch under tension is changed very little. Because of this it is possible to bend the heated wood to relatively sharp curves if the outer, or convex, side of the piece is held virtually constant in length by a metal strap and the deformation is limited to a shortening, under compression, on the inner, or concave, side of the bend.

Saturated exhaust steam with little, if any, extra pressure is the most effective source of heat. Dry steam may cause checking of the timber surface. Hot water will use up more energy, may cause staining, and will wet the timber too much, although it may be useful when just a small segment of a piece is to be bent.

Selection and preparation of timber for bending

Not all species of timber are suitable for bent work. In many of the species descriptions elsewhere in this book comment is made on suitability for steam bending. Even when a species is classified as suitable for bent work it is essential, if uneconomic wastage is to be avoided, to select the stock very carefully to ensure that only straight-grained material that is virtually free of all defects is used. Even small pin knots can promote buckling of the compression part of the bend. If the bend is of a comparatively shallow nature, then it is possible to relax these stringencies to some extent. Back-cut material is favoured since the rays can promote crumpling when prominent on the compression face.

The timber's moisture content may need to be higher than normal for some bends but a level in the vicinity of 20 per cent is commonly used. If the moisture content is too high, hydrostatic pressure will build up during bending and cause wrinkles to form on the concave face. If it is too low, the timber will be hard to bend and need an excessive time in the steaming cylinder.

Since saw marks may cause local concentrations of stress it is advisable to use dressed material but allow some size fullness to provide for the subsequent shrinkage and clean-up of the surface after the bending process has been accomplished.

Accurate squaring of the ends is essential to avoid failures on the tension side, which may result if the timber is not held firmly by the end stops to which the restraining strap is fitted.

To avoid the formation of end splits it is important to prevent the rapid uptake of moisture through the end-grain during the steaming operation. The usual end sealers, such as bitumen and wax, are unsuitable because of the elevated temperature but an alkyd-type varnish should be satisfactory.

The bending process

If the curve required is only a shallow one, it may be possible to achieve this without a restraining strap, but since there is a tendency for the stock to straighten out after mild bending some over-bending will probably be needed.

For the more severe bends the application of end pressure by a metal strap is required in order to avoid tension failure. The metal strap is attached

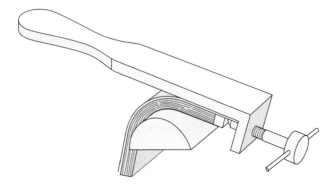

Fig. 12.1 Bending with the aid of a metal strap

to blocks that fit over the ends of the piece of timber and which have end-bearing plates, which are used not only to tighten the strap but also to release some end pressure if a buckle starts to form in the still unbent sector of the piece. A lever is attached to one end of the strap to aid in the bending of the piece around a shaped form. On the production line the bending strap is usually left on, while the ends are clamped together, enabling the stock to be removed immediately to a conditioning room, where the timber cools and sets in the new position. The conditioning period depends on the size of the timber cross-section and the amount of plasticity developed by the steaming but generally the bend has set by the time the timber's temperature falls to normal level.

The steaming chamber may be made of concrete, brick or sheet copper, with provision being made for the drainage of condensed moisture. For complicated bends, such as chair backs, hot plates with shaped platens are needed.

Treatment after bending

After the bend has set the timber usually will have to be seasoned to the equilibrium moisture content level. The drying of the bent pieces is much more difficult than for straight material, not only because of the irregular shape but because of the extra stresses developed by the bending process, so there is a high risk of surface checking. No heat treatment for stress removal can be carried out as this would affect the bend.

Behaviour in service

Bent timber will show a tendency for the curve to change with humidity conditions. High levels of humidity tend to straighten the bend, while low levels increase the tightness of the curve, so bent members need to be attached to a rigid member.

Bending of plywood

Provided the glue line is sufficiently waterproof to withstand the dampening involved, it is possible to bend relatively thin plywood successfully using somewhat similar procedures. In thicker plywood the bending can be helped by cutting narrow grooves on the concave surface perpendicular to the direction of the bend.

Use of ammonia as a plasticiser

Gaseous anhydrous ammonia has been found to be very effective at room temperature as an alternative to steam bending. Bends formed with the aid of ammonia seem to remain more stable in service. Species that are difficult to bend with the aid of steam may give a better response with ammonia, while the use of ammonia should require less force to achieve the desired bend. The unpleasant nature of the ammonia fumes would seem to be a major drawback.

Bending through lamination

Difficult bends are often more economically achieved by gluing together a number of thin sections of timber, which can be easily bent prior to gluing into the desired curve without having to resort to heat and moisture. If the laminations are thick and some prebending is required before they are glued together, it is important to dry them to equilibrium moisture content before assembly in order to secure a strong bond.

FURTHER READING

Davidson, R. W. and Baumgardt, W. G. (1970). Plasticising wood with ammonia. *For Prod J* 20(3): 19–24.

Hirst, K. (1962). Plywood bending. *Aust Timb J* 28(5): 79–85.

Chapter 13

Bleaching and stain removal

Bleaching refers to the removal of colouring materials from the surface layers of wood. It is sometimes carried out to achieve a special aesthetic effect, to match other timbers, or to remove discolourations, but it is not easy to achieve satisfactory results, particularly if large areas are involved, and should be avoided whenever possible.

The variability of the effectiveness of the chemicals used, the high labour content, the uncertain nature of the results and the fact that only a thin skin of bleached wood is produced, all point to the need to consider the value of the effort before deciding on a bleaching treatment.

Because bleaching is necessarily a surface treatment, the article has to be fully completed, or at least its components have to be ready for final assembly, before it is carried out. The surface has to be freshly prepared, free of all oil, grease, old finish or stain, which could interfere with the even penetration of the bleaching chemicals. If the timber has a natural oiliness, it would be advisable to give it a thorough rub down with methylated spirits and/or white spirit. Bleaching agents cannot be expected to make wood white but they are often able to reduce the intensity of colour very considerably.

The bleaching agents commonly used are ammonia and hydrogen peroxide, oxalic acid and sodium hypochlorite. Their effectiveness varies greatly with the species; some are virtually impossible to bleach. Unless a species' bleaching characteristics are known it is essential to try the bleach on a small specimen before proceeding any further. These chemicals have a harmful effect on exposed tissue so the eyes should be protected with goggles and the hands with thick rubber gloves. The fumes from hydrogen peroxide, ammonia and sodium hypochlorite are irritating to mucous membranes and so abundant ventilation is essential.

Methods of application

When the area to be bleached is relatively small, the bleaching solutions are usually applied with either a cotton swab, sponge or brush, taking care to use a separate applicator for each chemical solution. If it is desired to bleach large panels in a production-line setting, it is necessary to use a spray gun with stainless steel fittings that will resist the corrosive effect of the chemicals. All equipment should be washed thoroughly at the end of each period of use. Bleaching solutions should be stored in glass containers very carefully to avoid contamination. If the solutions become contaminated with metals, they may stain rather than bleach the wood.

Main bleaches used

Hydrogen peroxide, in conjunction with ammonia

Bleaches based on hydrogen peroxide have the advantage that there is no residue left in the wood to affect subsequent finishes. Concentrated ammonia solution is applied to the surface to be bleached; after it has soaked in for up to an hour, 30 per cent hydrogen peroxide (called '100 volume' peroxide commercially) is applied liberally. When the surface has dried, it is examined for the amount of bleaching. The two-stage process may need to be repeated several times.

The two solutions must never be mixed together. If bubbles appear on the timber surface when the second solution is being applied, it is an indication that the first solution has not yet dried out sufficiently.

The application of an alkaline solution preparatory to the use of the hydrogen peroxide helps to make the peroxide unstable and secures the liberation of a large amount of oxygen at a location in intimate contact with the wood cells, thus achieving a bleaching effect. Hydrogen peroxide decomposes rapidly when in contact with organic matter, metals and alkalis so careful storage, avoiding all contamination, is essential. It should also be stored in the dark since sunlight speeds its decomposition.

A 40 per cent aqueous solution of sodium hydroxide can be substituted for the ammonia solution to achieve a more powerful bleaching action but careful neutralisation of the alkali by washing down with 10 per cent oxalic acid or acetic acid, followed by water, at the end of bleaching will be needed because of the potential effect of the alkali on subsequent coating systems.

Sodium silicate and calcium hydroxide may also be used in association with hydrogen peroxide. Hydrogen peroxide bleaching is effective over a wider range of species than are oxalic acid and sodium hypochlorite.

Oxalic acid

Oxalic acid is a mild bleaching agent, which is useful for treating easily bleached species. It is easy to use, usually in the form of a 10 per cent solution in hot distilled water or methylated spirits, and should be stored in a glass or earthenware container. It tends to give timbers a pinkish tinge. Because of its very poisonous nature rubber gloves are essential when using it and a mask should be worn when carrying out subsequent sanding of the surface to avoid inhalation of the dust.

The solution is applied liberally to the freshly prepared surface, the excess is wiped off after about 15 minutes and the article allowed to dry overnight. The process may need to be repeated several times. Some authors recommend the neutralisation of the acid and/or copious washing of the surface but a more permanent bleaching effect may be secured by allowing excess acid to remain; this does mean that special care should be taken not to inhale the sanding dust. If oxalic acid has been used to remove iron stains, it seems particularly important to retain the excess acid to inhibit the return of the blue-black iron tannate colour.

Sodium hypochlorite

Sodium hypochlorite is very commonly used as a household bleach and would be the most readily procurable of the bleaching agents. It is usually sold as a 5 per cent solution, which may be diluted as much as 1:15 with distilled water, but stronger solutions will probably be required for effective action. Sodium hypochlorite tends to give a greyer result than the two bleaching agents mentioned above. Several applications may be needed, with a final washing with warm water. It should be stored in a cool dark cupboard to inhibit the release of its effective constituent, chlorine.

Sanding of bleached articles

As the bleached effect is confined to the surface layers of wood it is important that the article is allowed to dry back to equilibrium moisture content before it is very carefully sanded to remove raised grain, using the finest practicable paper. The fuzziness that sanding gives to some softwoods may sometimes be overcome by damping the surface with a small amount of methylated spirits and setting this alight. Obviously, such a step should be taken with the utmost care.

Removal of stains

Iron stains

Many species, especially hardwoods, contain a considerable amount of extractives, especially tannins, which react with iron to form blue-black iron tannate. Some softwoods, especially western red cedar and redwood, have troublesome extractives that react with iron to form dark brown stains.

Even the rapid passage of the steel saw through the log, or the veneer knife on the peeler log, will produce a blue-black colour on green eucalypt hardwoods. The presence of free moisture is necessary for such staining: there is no staining problem when processing seasoned timber. The tendency to stain when in contact with iron is not related to the acidity of the wood. Dressing of the seasoned wood will remove the stain caused by the processing of the green log but stains caused by repeated exposure of damp wood to iron, as from contact with nails or from a leaking iron roof, may penetrate very deeply and be impossible to remove.

One of the most common occurrences of iron tannate staining is on new hardwood decking. The staining is usually around the nail heads or as spotting over the surface of the deck. Such spotting usually results from the use of an angle grinder, which leaves tiny iron filings over the deck surface. As soon as the deck surface becomes sufficiently wet, iron tannates are formed. The formation of iron tannates on the deck surface can occur after the deck has been coated with a finish and the moisture in the wood migrates to the surface. It should be noted that the iron filings come from the grinding disc and not necessarily from what is being ground or cut.

It may be necessary to remove superficial staining without having to plane or sand the wood surface. Dilute acids will convert the iron tannate into a soluble form that can be washed away. Oxalic acid is often used for this purpose but it is desirable to leave the excess acid solution on the surface rather than neutralise or wash it off, otherwise it is likely that the stain may return. Because of the poisonous nature of oxalic acid it is important to exercise appropriate care in the subsequent handling of the surface.

Polyphenolic extractives from unseasoned timber often cause rapid staining of the hands but the rubbing of a cut lemon (with its citric acid content) on the affected area quickly removes the stain. The same treatment could be applied to clothes affected by superficial staining.

Alkaline surfaces stained by wood extractives

The leaching of wood extractives onto concrete, asbestos cement, brickwork and sandstone is of common occurrence during building construction. Provided the leaching is not of long continued duration, such stains will usually be bleached away by sun and rain eventually but they can be a major source of annoyance.

Eucalypt hardwoods are capable of staining wet alkaline surfaces even after many years of exposure to the weather so proper consideration should be given when designing structures to ensure that the run-off of rain from unpainted wood of species high in staining extractives does not impinge on alkaline surfaces.

If the stain is of recent origin, it can usually be removed with dilute hydrochloric or other mild acids; the excess acid should be washed off. When this operation is carried out on sandstone it may bleach some of the natural iron-derived colour of the stone but this golden tone can often be restored by judicious dabbing of the bleached area with ferric chloride solution.

Alkaline stains on wood

The alkaline nature of mortar, cement and chemicals such as ammonia can cause a brown stain to form on the wood of species rich in tannins.

This stain is not as prominent as that formed when iron is involved and is usually amenable to treatment with a dilute solution of an acid such as hydrochloric acid. The surface is first washed with water, then with the acid and finally with water to remove the acid, drying the surface each time with an absorbent cloth so that the timber will not take up a lot of moisture.

Adhesives with a strongly alkaline nature are a common source of staining (e.g. casein). A 10 per cent solution of oxalic acid in hot water is commonly used to remove such stains.

Painted surfaces stained by extractives

Storm rains can penetrate to the unpainted backs of cladding and leach extractives onto the visible painted surface. Natural finish 'stains' can also experience an extractives staining problem since the stain finish is not waterproof and the timber substrate can undergo some leaching. Timber that is to be given such stain finishes should be used in such a way that the run-off of rain does not impinge onto painted surfaces of pale colour.

Bluestain

Bluestain, which is a sap stain caused by fungal organisms that are active in unseasoned wood, is of common occurrence in many species during the warmer months. Once it is well established in the wood cells it is virtually impossible to remove by bleaching agents.

FURTHER READING

Feist, W. C. (1977). Wood surface treatments to prevent extractive staining of paints. *For Prod J* 27(5): 50–4.

Forest Products Laboratory, US Dept of Agriculture. (1967). Bleaching wood. Research note FPL 0165.

Pinion, L. C. (1973). Chemical staining in wood. *BRE information* IS 2/73.

Chapter 14

Coatings

Wood is a very durable material and certain species, under favourable conditions, can last many hundreds of years. When exposed to the weather the change in appearance of the timber surface is caused by exposure to ultraviolet (UV) light and a combination of chemical and mechanical processes occurring. This process is called weathering. Weathering is not decay and the two should not be confused. Decay results in the rapid degradation of the timber, whereas the timber beneath the weathered surface remains sound and if the weathered surface is removed the original timber colour and properties will again be open to view. Weathering results in a gradual change in the colour and texture of the timber. Initially, darker coloured timbers will often lighten and lighter coloured timbers will darken and as time progresses both will turn a silver-grey colour, but this may take up to 2 years. With weathering some erosion of the timber surfaces will also occur, more so in the softer earlywood than the latewood, and the surface will roughen.

If wood is exposed to the weather without any protective coating to inhibit water penetration, the natural colouring matter will be leached gradually from its surface cells and a greyish appearance will develop. The alternate wetting and drying of the surface will cause checking, the grain will become raised, and the surface, even if initially smooth, will become roughened.

On the other hand, wood surfaces that are protected from the weather will largely maintain their natural colour, although the effect of even diffused daylight will tend to darken light colours and bleach dark colours. Thus, the use of some form of clear finish is desirable to protect the wood surface from soiling by hands, cleaning equipment or spilt liquids. The presence of the coating also helps to stabilise the material against the dimensional changes that are produced by fluctuating atmospheric humidity levels. Coatings are not impermeable to the passage of water vapour and cannot give protection against long-term continued changes in humidity levels, but they are a valuable modifier of the normal fluctuations.

Unfortunately, no finish will keep the appearance of the wood identical to that of its freshly dressed surface because the air in the surface cells is replaced by material with a different refraction of light; the deeper the coating penetrates the wood, the greater the apparent change in colour. A rough approximation of the colour that the wood surface will acquire after a clear finish is applied is obtained by dampening a small portion with water.

Even though coatings can give a considerable amount of protection against the weathering of wood and do modify moisture content changes, they do not necessarily improve its durability against decay. Indeed, by restricting the drying out of moisture that may have entered the wood from unprotected surfaces they can sometimes increase decay hazard. Recent research has indicated that poor finishing practices can increase decay by 100 per cent. However, coatings may be considered preservatives to the extent that they prevent weathering of the surface and the development of fungal organisms, which gradually erode the surface of unprotected wood under damp conditions.

Many board walks and other similar external structures are constructed of durable hardwoods, with the sapwood preservative-treated, and these are allowed to weather naturally. Generally, the decking boards and substructures are of heavier section sizes than those used in domestic applications and, in relation to the end-section size, the effects of weathering are minimal and a long service life is achievable. In drier climates and warmer coastal areas mould growth is not generally a problem. Where end-section sizes are smaller, such as with domestic decking, and the excellent service potential is to be realised, the product should be protected from the weather by means of an appropriate coating system.

Effect of wood properties and characteristics on finishes

Wood is a very complex substance with potentially wide variations in absorption, not only between species but also within an individual piece of timber. The manufacturing process and the resulting surface to be finished also influence finishing properties. Differences that occur include grain characteristics (prominence of earlywood and latewood), wide differences in density and differences in seasonal movement, ratio of heartwood to sapwood, differences between hardwoods and softwoods, and other natural characteristics, such as extractives, gum and resin.

Moisture content

Wood needs to be relatively dry for successful painting and should not be painted if the moisture content is above 20 per cent as this can result in peeling or delamination of the finish. To enhance the service life of paint, wood is best painted when its moisture content is near that which it will average in service.

Movement characteristics (shrinkage and swelling)

Dimensional change as a result of seasonal movement from moisture uptake and loss will continually place film-forming finishes under stress. Consequently, this can contribute to the earlier failure of paint (Plates 24–27) and solid stain finishes. Penetrating stains are, however, not affected by seasonal dimensional changes. Higher density timbers are generally slower to take up or lose moisture than are less dense species and they are often subject to greater seasonal movement. They may be supplied as unseasoned product (e.g. weatherboards), in which dimensional changes are initially very high. In such applications colour-matched undercoats can mask any movement effects.

Earlywood and latewood

The presence of earlywood and latewood is often visible as distinct bands within the timber and is usually referred to as the annual growth rings. The latewood that is formed during the time of the year of slower growth is generally darker in colour, denser, smoother and harder. This is because the cells have thicker walls and the cell cavities are smaller. On painting, both paints and solid colour stains adhere well to both earlywood and latewood, however, alkyd paint systems and solid stains tend to become brittle with age, which can result in peeling initiating from the harder, smooth latewood.

Heartwood and extractives

In many species, both hardwoods and softwoods, there is a clear colour distinction between the lighter coloured sapwood beneath the bark and the darker coloured central heartwood. Heartwood is formed when extractives and other materials are deposited in the cells. Some extractives cause a natural increase in the resistance to decay and insect attack but can also cause discolouration and finishing defects in the painted surface, either at the time of painting or later on. Extractives are water-soluble and can therefore be carried to the surface when dissolved in free water. The extractives remain at the painted surface when the water evaporates, leaving a stain.

Resin

Resin is present in most *Pinus* species (softwoods) and can exude from heartwood and sapwood. It consists of a mix of turpentine and rosin, and when the turpentine evaporates the rosin solidifies. As a result, 'resin bleed' may occur through the painted surface as the resin exudes through the coating and then solidifies. In some instances, the resin bleed does not appear to damage the coating. In other instances, the resin bleed causes the coating to blister and discolour. Knots often have higher concentrations of resin and this can result in discolouration of the painted surface at the knot, which is known as knot bleed.

Special primer paints have been formulated to lessen or prevent knot show-through in the top coat of paint.

Timber characteristics

Many timber characteristics, such as knots, wavy grain and gum veins, present surface irregularities. Knots, in effect, expose end-grain in the surface of a board and end-grain is more absorbent to the coating than either back-sawn or quarter-sawn material. The presence of such characteristics, therefore, affects the paintability of the timber.

Surface roughness

The surface has a distinct effect on the durability of the coating. Coatings will tend to last longer on smooth quarter-sawn material than on smooth back-sawn material. Also, irrespective of whether the surface is quarter-sawn or back-sawn, coatings last longer on rough-sawn surfaces than on smooth surfaces.

Timber and timber product effects on finishes

The timber substrate or product that is to be finished, particularly in an exterior situation, can affect both the application and performance of the finish. Similarly, the surface texture will also have an influence. Common products with different characteristics include rough-sawn and dressed timber, plywood, finger-jointed timber, preservative-treated timber (water-borne and solvent-borne) and preprimed material.

Rough-sawn and dressed timber

The surface texture of timber affects the correct selection and application of the finish. Generally, in external situations, a rough texture enables the finish to adhere better to the surface and to form a thicker film. Consequently, the service life is longer than for dressed surfaces under the same conditions. Rough surfaces also appear to have the ability to diffuse sunlight and this may be a contributing factor in the better performance of coatings on rough surfaces.

Plywood

The surface texture, grain orientation and species all affect the finishing properties of plywood in a similar way to those of timber. However, the manufacturing process, with the veneers being peeled from the log, results in fine surface checks. These checks, particularly with the shrinking and swelling associated with weather exposure, result in early paint failure if alkyd or oil-based paints are used. Consequently, the acrylic or latex paint systems, with their greater flexibility, provide a much improved surface life. Paint quality is particularly important. For exterior cladding, plywood is generally provided with a rough-sawn surface, which also allows for better paint-holding. In exterior applications the edges of plywood sheets should be treated with a water-repellent preservative. As with solid timber, penetrating stains also perform better on a rough-sawn plywood surface than on a smooth surface.

Finger-jointed timber

Finger-jointing is the process of joining shorter lengths of timber to make longer lengths that are free of knots and other unwanted characteristics.

It involves cutting fingers in the ends of the boards and gluing the sections together. Finger-jointed timber is used in a wide variety of products for both internal and external applications. A particular board may, therefore, contain sections of timber from different trees and of different grain orientation. Due to the differential movement that is likely to occur in service, particular care is required when finishing these products. Movement, particularly with dark-coloured cladding, has resulted in paint failure at the joints. The gloss level of the coating may also differ at the joints.

Preservative-treated timber

Timber that is used in external applications often needs to be preservative-treated to prevent decay, borer and termite attack. Durable hardwoods (e.g. ironbark) that are free of sapwood do not require treatment. Water-borne treatments include ammoniacal copper quaternary (ACQ), copper azole and copper–chrome–arsenic (CCA), whereas light organic solvent-borne preservative (LOSP) treatments often contain tin and synthetic pyrethroid-based products to provide the protection. For external applications, particularly with softwoods, a water repellent may also be added to the treatment. Wood that is preservative-treated can be painted or stained, although when water repellents are used, it may be necessary to use an oil-based primer/undercoat, over which acrylic or latex finishes can be applied.

Preprimed timber

Some timber and particularly cladding, fascia and similar products may be supplied preprimed. In the past, some primers have been of low quality with poor adhesion to the timber surface, which has necessitated sanding off the primer and repriming. However, many products are now available that are preprimed with quality primers and require minimal preparation prior to the application of finishing coats. The finishing should be undertaken shortly after the installation of the preprimed timber. Recommendations are available from the Australian Paint Manufacturers' Federation.

Paints

Paint constituents

Paint usually consists of:

- pigments and extenders
- a vehicle, which conveys the other constituents to the wood surface, and which consists of the film former or binder, and the solvent or carrier
- additives—materials that are present in small quantities for the purpose of improving stability and flow, deterring fungal attack and so on.

Pigments and extenders

Pigments normally consist of very fine solids that are insoluble in the vehicle and must not settle as sediment. They provide the colour of the paint film and affect the gloss, durability, flow and various other properties, such as corrosion resistance. Increasing the percentage of pigments in paint tends to decrease gloss, flexibility and resistance to mechanical damage but provides moisture permeability and blister resistance.

Titanium dioxide is the most commonly used white pigment, having outstanding coverage and hiding power. Other pigments used include zinc oxide, antimony oxide and lithopone, which is a mix of barium sulfate and zinc sulfide. Common coloured pigments include inorganic forms of iron oxide, Prussian blue and chromium oxide.

Extenders are mixed with pigments. They are similar in nature but do not provide colour or opacity. Their purpose is to improve the strength of the film and adhesion to the surface being painted, to provide ease of sanding and to increase resistance to the destructive effects of sunlight, heat and solvents. They also improve brushing and levelling characteristics, increase wear resistance, control the degree of gloss or provide texture (as in flat finishes).

Common extenders include calcium carbonate, barium sulfate and silica compounds, such as talc, and china clay.

Vehicle

The vehicle, or liquid, portion of the paint is the carrier for the pigment. It contains a binder that is either dissolved in a solvent or dispersed in diluents and not dissolved. The binder can be thought of as the 'glue', which not only binds the pigment particles together but also to the timber surface. In addition to providing adhesion, binders are also important in terms of the toughness, hardness, flexibility, durability, gloss level and speed of drying.

Binders (resins)

There are two groups of binders—those associated with oil-based paints and those with water-based paints. Alkyd resins, which are produced from modified vegetable oils, are the major group of binders with oil-based paints. The vegetable oils may be classified as drying oils, such as tung-oil and linseed oil, semidrying oils, including sunflower, soya and safflower oils, or the non-drying castor oil.

Double bonds contained within the oils react with oxygen in the air, causing resin molecules to bridge, which results in the curing or drying of the resin. When the double bonds are more active, drying will be faster. Resins that dry more rapidly at the surface are prone to develop wrinkles in the finish and others yellow with time. Soya oil avoids these issues and is therefore predominantly used in alkyd manufacture.

Water-based resins are dispersions or emulsions in water and not solutions, unlike oil-based resins. The resins are synthetic, being either polyvinyl acetate (PVA) or acrylic. These resins exist as polymers and dry by coalescence, in which the evaporation of the water forces the polymer particles to fuse into a film, as opposed to the oxidation process that occurs with alkyds.

Solvent and carrier

The solvent is the liquid in which the pigment and binder are mixed to ensure the correct consistency for application of the paint by brush, roller, spray or dipping applications. It does not form part of the applied film as it evaporates in the drying process. In oil-based paints, turpentine-like solvents are present, and these have different drying rates, which can therefore affect application properties. In water-based paints, water is the carrier and, once evaporated, the coating provides a water-resistant film. However, moist conditions from rain or condensation that occur shortly after application will affect them.

Additives

Additives usually constitute a very small portion of the paint but are important in determining the final performance and characteristics of it. Examples of additives include silicone, which makes the paint film more resistant to marking and scratching, and zinc oxide, which makes the paint more resistant to mildew and provides UV light protection. Additives are also incorporated into water-based paints to promote a uniform film, to disperse the powders and resins and to prevent the paint from drying too quickly. In oil-based paints, additives are used to assist with the oxidation of the paint or to prevent bacterial attack.

Paint types

Acrylic paints

Acrylic or latex paints are water thinned and clean up is achieved with soap and water. They are designed for maximum resistance to weathering while not being overly rigid and will outlast alkyds in external applications. These paints are easily applied by brush or roller, painting equipment is easy to clean, and they are quick drying, usually being able to be recoated after 2 hours. They are also flexible, allowing them to stretch and contract without cracking under the seasonal movement of timber. Acrylic paints are permeable to moisture vapour, which prevents blistering, but still prevent liquid water penetration. They are available for internal and external use as primers, undercoats and finishing coats and come in a wide range of colours with sheen from flat to high gloss. In addition, they have low odour on application, are colour fast and neither 'yellow' nor chalk with time. When applying acrylics, some attention needs to be paid to their quick-drying nature. They should be applied when temperatures are above 10°C. During hot weather it is beneficial to paint the shaded areas and alternate two brushes, one of which is soaking in water.

Alkyd paints

Alkyd or oil-based paints are solvent thinned and clean up requires turpentine or mineral spirits. These paints form a tough, durable film coat and a higher gloss level can be achieved. They are resistant to oil, grease and moisture, which makes them particularly suited to trim applications and doors. However, the dry film becomes less flexible with age, which can lead to cracking and peeling. They are subject to chalking when exposed to UV light. Odour is much stronger on application and, owing to the use of solvents, they are less environmentally friendly.

Paint systems

Many pigmented paint systems for wood protection involve the application of the coating system in a three-stage process: a priming coat, an undercoat and one or two finishing coats.

Priming

New timber surfaces or those on which the paint has deteriorated require the application of a primer coat. The main function of the priming coat is to provide a strong bond between the wood substrate and the succeeding coats. It has to be water repellent and act as a sealer, and is formulated with a dull finish for the better adhesion of the succeeding coat.

Before objections were raised against the use of lead pigments on the basis of undue hazard to health, most primers where of white or red lead in raw linseed oil but now other oils, oleo-resins or even some alkyd resins are used in association with pigments other than lead. In tropical areas where fungal invasion of paints is a common problem, zinc oxide is a valuable pigment because of its fungicidal characteristics.

Because of the tendency of very absorbent species of timber to 'suck' the binder from the surface, some additional oil may be desirable in a primer for such timber, but too much of it could reduce the bonding of the primer to the surface.

Timber surfaces in an internal situation that will never be exposed to damp conditions are often undercoated without an application of primer.

Oil-borne primers are often used under water-borne top coats due to their penetration into the timber; however, fully water-borne systems are also used.

Undercoat

Undercoat is designed to have a higher degree of hiding power than the primer and the extra pigmentation helps to provide a smooth base for the finishing coat. It should also be of a colour that blends well with the finishing coat (particularly when the timber product is likely to shrink in service), have good filling and bridging properties, be easy to sand without clogging the sandpaper, and have relatively low gloss.

Finishing coats

Finishing coats are either solvent-borne enamels or water-borne emulsions, which are referred to as acrylic or latex paints.

Enamels

Full gloss enamels   These enamels are favoured when a tough, durable, washable and stain-resistant coating is required. They are designed to give freedom from brush marks. In order to achieve a high gloss, the percentage of pigment is usually lower than that in other types of paint. Other factors assisting in the provision of a high gloss are extra fineness of the pigment, the skill of the painter and the weather conditions at the time of application. Titanium dioxide is the favoured pigment for white and pastel colours because of its excellent hiding power and resistance to chalking.

The formulations for internal and external enamels differ somewhat. The range of colours is more limited for exterior use because of problems with colour fastness. The solvents that are used for the exterior paint usually have a higher boiling point for easier brushability. The internal enamels require solvents of reasonably pleasant odour and faster drying, as well as a minimal tendency to yellow with age. Red, orange and yellow colours will not perform as well as others in exposed areas because of the tendency of the pigments to fade. The problem can be mitigated to some extent by applying an additional finish coat.

Semi-gloss or satin enamels   These are usually designed for interior use on furniture and surfaces on which a high gloss is not aesthetically desirable but toughness, wear resistance and washability are required. They can be used externally but do not have the same weather resistance as the full gloss enamels.

Flat enamels   These are usually based on medium oil alkyds, dry quickly but are easy to apply, are durable and washable and have reasonably good resistance to surface mould growth. They are in direct competition with the flat latex-type finishes, which have tended to replace them.

Water-borne emulsions

The term 'emulsion' is commonly used to describe the dispersion of one liquid in another but in the paint industry it is used to describe formulations in which solid particles of polymerised organic binders are dispersed in water as fine globules. The term 'latex' is also used to describe this stable dispersion of insoluble resin particles in water. The latex usually consists of styrene-butadiene, PVA or acrylic polymers.

If a considerable degree of gloss is required, it is necessary to have a low pigment volume and the resin particles must be soft enough to flow together and envelop the particles of pigment completely. However, if they are to be used externally, they must possess a reasonable amount of hardness because otherwise dust will soon become embedded in the surface. The degree of gloss obtainable is less than that available from alkyd enamels and their poorer levelling characteristics are more likely to reveal brush marks. However, their durability is usually good, with low chalking and good colour retention.

Semi-gloss latex paints are popular for internal use because they are easier to handle than semi-gloss alkyd enamels, with fewer odours during application and less likelihood of yellowing with age. They are more serviceable than the flat latex paints as they are washable and more resistant to abrasion, but they are not as serviceable as semi-gloss enamels.

Either oil-based or acrylic primers are used under the latex paints. It may be difficult to get the water-borne finish to cover the oil-based primer evenly because of its hydrophobic nature, and when a lot of readily leached extractives are present, as is the case with eucalypt hardwoods, acrylic primers may not be fully efficient in preventing some initial brown discolouration. However, finish coats of acrylic-type formulations have now been developed to overcome some of the problems of extractive staining. With water-borne paints it may also be difficult to get an even coating on timber that has been treated with solvent-borne preservatives.

Exterior clear finishes and stains

In addition to paints, a range of exterior finishes is available, some of which allow the grain of the timber to be seen to varying degrees and others which obscure the grain in the same way that paints do. These generally come under the categories of clear finishes and stains.

Exterior clear finishes

No clear finishes that are currently available give long-term performance (greater than 18–24 months) when fully exposed to the weather; timber users eagerly await the time when a transparent finish will be available which permits a full appreciation of the beauty of wood's colour and figuring while still providing long-term protection against weathering. However, in saying this, advances have been made in recent years and a number of clear finishes that are on the market provide a reasonable service life but require more frequent maintenance than other coating systems that are available.

Many kinds of clear finishes (i.e. alkyds, phenolics, polyurethanes, acrylics) have been tried externally but none have given a satisfactory long-term service life in Australian conditions because of the severe oxidative effect of the sun's rays, which not only accelerates brittleness of the coating but also has a destructive effect on the ability of the wood surface to maintain a strong bond with the coating. This problem does not occur to anything like the same extent with pigmented paint because the pigments block the harmful rays and so protect the binder.

If clear finishes are used externally, very careful preparation of the substrate is essential. All sharp edges should be removed to ensure an even thickness of coating. The presence of holes, knots and resinous wood should be avoided. Many coats should be applied to provide good protection against the entry of moisture into the wood.

The incorporation of organic UV light absorbers, or small quantities of inorganic solids whose light refraction is such that their presence is not very noticeable, has been tried but the amount of improvement to serviceability has not been sufficient to overcome the problem.

Exterior stains

As an alternative, stain-type finishes have become increasingly popular. Even though they provide a degree of protection, they do not prevent some moisture entry to the timber surfaces to which they are applied, which are likely to develop surface checks; because of this, stain finishes are more suitable for sawn than dressed surfaces, the rough texture helping to mask the presence of the checks. Although initially they have quite good water repellency (and may have wax as an ingredient), this repellency reduces with time so that stain finishes are not a really suitable coating when dimensional stability is essential (e.g. windows), unless regularly maintained.

Because of the thinness of the finish obtained with the one or two coats that are normally applied there is little or no risk of it crazing and peeling, such as can happen with the thicker coatings that are formed by paints and varnishes. Maintenance of the surface is thus much simplified, involving merely a wash down of the old coating to remove dust, loose pigment and fungal mould, and the application of the new coat.

Stain finishes provide a relatively woody appearance if colours similar to those of the natural timber are selected and applied to a sawn timber surface. They can be used quite successfully on species (such as many of the eucalypt hardwoods) that are poor substrates for the normal painting systems because of their susceptibility to surface checking. Stain finishes do not stop all leaching of extractives and the surfaces to which they are applied should be detailed so that rain run-off does not contact pale-coloured paint, brick surfaces or concrete.

Stain finishes can be divided into three main types: semi-transparent penetrating oil stains, semi-transparent water-borne stains and solid colour or opaque oil stains.

Semi-transparent penetrating oil stains

The main constituents of semi-transparent penetrating oil stains are a drying oil (usually linseed), a fungicide to retard invasion by black surface moulds, a water repellent such as paraffin wax, and pigments, the amount of which varies considerably between products. Keeping the pigment at a low level does show the wood character to good effect but it usually reduces the durability of the finish to a level that is considerably less than that obtained with obscuring levels of pigmentation. The lightly pigmented finishes should only be selected if regular maintenance every 3 or so years is an acceptable proposition.

Linseed oil on its own is not satisfactory in providing long-term durability. Unless it is carefully applied, the oil, especially if of the 'raw' variety, tends to form sticky patches, which attract dust and are susceptible to invasion by dark-coloured surface moulds if the immediate environment is damp.

Semi-transparent water-borne stains

Semi-transparent water-borne stains are usually based on acrylic latex resins and are applied directly to the timber substrate, which usually requires minimal preparation. Although hiding the grain, they will allow the texture to be seen and provide decorative colour. Fence stains are often in this category. As a result of their low solids content, they provide limited protection.

Solid colour or opaque oil stains

The constituents of solid colour or opaque oil stains are essentially similar to those in the lightly pigmented type but instead heavily pigmented to obscure the timber's natural colouring and grain but not the texture. The increased pigment gives an improved service life and, under reasonable conditions of exposure, it may take up to 5 years before the surface develops a hungry appearance that is indicative of the need for a wash down and recoat.

Finishing exterior timber

In most instances, it is necessary to provide a proper coating system in order to achieve the expected performance from timber products used externally. Water-repellent preservatives, stains and paints all play a useful role in providing the appearance and performance that is required for external applications. Table 14.1 provides an overview of most of these coatings and some brief notes on their application.

Water repellents

A water repellent is the generic name given to a range of products that is used as a sealer beneath other coating systems. The purpose of water repellents is to change the surface nature of the timber in a way that it causes water to bead and be shed from the surface rather than be absorbed by it. Water vapour from humidity in the air will, however, pass through the water repellent and it has negligible effect on seasonal moisture content changes in timber. Water repellents substantially reduce water absorption into timber surfaces, particularly the end-grain. It is usual for water repellents to be combined with other products, such as preservatives and those that reduce mould growth. As such they are usually marketed as water-repellent preservatives.

Many applications will benefit from the application of water-repellent preservatives, particularly the more absorbent softwoods. Coating can significantly reduce surface checking, warping and possible staining from the timber. A water repellent is, however, not a long-lasting coating and therefore it generally requires other finishes to be applied over it. The reduction in shrinkage and swelling afforded by the water repellent results in less stress on paint films, which thereby enhances service life. If used as a finish (life expectancy of 1–2 years), some lightly pigmented products are available which reduce the effect of UV light, but this is still not sufficient to prevent greying. Reapplication only requires the surface to be clean and dry and is, therefore, relatively simple. Due to their water-repellent nature, water-borne finish coatings can experience adhesion problems if applied over timber that has been freshly coated with water repellents.

Table 14.1 Finish type and application

Finish type	Application
Water-repellent preservatives	Preferred as a pretreatment and effectively reduce moisture uptake and loss. Also contain preservatives that can improve durability.
Oils	Both texture and grain visible. Darken with age and require frequent maintenance.
Clear finishes	Grain highly visible. UV light inhibitors have improved durability but regular maintenance still required.
Semi-transparent stains	Solvent-borne or water-borne. Texture enhanced and grain obscured to a lesser degree than opaque stains.
Opaque stains	Generally solvent-borne. Texture remains enhanced. More durable than semi-transparent stains.
Paint primers	Applied to bare timber. Solvent-borne primers provide better penetration and water-borne primers provide better long-term flexibility. Application by brush is recommended.
Paint undercoats	Provide good opacity, high-build coating and are able to bridge checks. Water-borne undercoats have better colour matching to top coats. Solvent-borne undercoats are preferred for chalky surfaces.
Paint finishing coats	Available in various gloss levels. Solvent-borne types provide highest initial gloss levels and water-borne types provide greater long-term durability.

Water repellents may be applied by brush, but dipping is also very effective. Joints, end-grain and any areas prone to moisture uptake particularly benefit from liberal application of the water repellent. Dressed timber will only benefit from a single application and greater penetration generally occurs on rough-sawn surfaces. The more absorbent the timber, the more effective the application.

Oils

Many oil-based wood finishes are available and these, by their nature, penetrate the surface of the timber. These finishes are commonly based on oils such as linseed and tung-oil, however, they also contain other substances to prevent mildew and UV light inhibitors. Consequently, these oils should not be used in their raw state.

Application of an oil is simple and it may be applied to a clean, dry surface by brush or roller, with two to three coats initially being applied. Oil-based coatings are often chosen when it is desirable to see the grain, although they will darken the timber. Their service life is, however, relatively short and reapplication may initially be required within a year in highly exposed areas. As with other penetrating finishes, reapplication is easy, only requiring a clean dry surface.

Clear finishes

Clear finishes are often chosen because the grain and colour of the timber can be clearly seen after application. When using these finishes, careful preparation is important as sharp edges and other irregularities can cause early breakdown of the finish. Similarly, sealing of the end-grain of timber members is important to prevent moisture ingress to the timber, which can lead to breakdown of the finish. These products often dry fairly rapidly and care is also necessary to avoid lap marks that result in bands of more intense colour. A commitment to maintaining and recoating is necessary to keep the appearance good.

Semi-transparent oil-based penetrating stains

These stains are similar in some respects to water-repellent preservatives but in addition to added pigments they also contain more resin and binder. Many also contain UV light stabilisers or absorbers and fungicides. When applied to the timber, the alkyd or oil-based stains penetrate the timber to some degree and do not form a film, as with painted systems. Thus, the grain, although concealed, is also partly visible. These stains are resistant to peeling or blistering and will not trap moisture.

Service life may be as low as 2 years on dressed timber and up to 10 years on rough-sawn timber. Timber species and the initial application also influence service life. The stains are generally thin and may be applied by brush, spray or roller. When applied by brush, back brushing is necessary to prevent lap marks, and application in the shade will prevent rapid drying. For the initial two coats, the second coat should be applied while the first is still wet. About 20 minutes between applications is necessary to allow the first coat to penetrate the timber. Longer periods will be required for denser species.

Semi-transparent water-borne stains

Unlike the solvent-borne transparent stains described above, the water-borne stains do not penetrate the timber surface to the same degree. These stains form a thin film and a second coat, applied after the first has dried, is necessary to improve durability. These stains are easier to apply and less likely to form lap marks.

Solid colour or opaque oil stains

Solid colour or opaque stains are film-forming finishes that come in a wide range of colours, in oil-based or latex formulations. They are more akin to thin paints, having higher concentrations of pigment than the semi-transparent stains. As a result, they obscure the grain to provide solid colour and normally a flat finish. Being similar in nature to paints they can also be applied over previously painted surfaces without altering the texture. They provide good protection against UV light degradation and have a service life similar to that of the semi-transparent penetrating stains. Service life is also improved when applied over quality primers (latex or oil-based). Owing to the film formation they can peel from the substrate and are more affective when two to three coats are applied. They work well on rough-sawn surfaces and may also be used on smooth wood surfaces, including plywood. Unlike paint but similar to the semi-transparent stains they are subject to lap marks. This has been more of an issue with the faster drying latex formulations than the oil-based products. Application and method to prevent lap marks is the same as for semi-transparent stains.

Exterior paints

Paints are film-forming finishes that provide the most protection to timber surfaces from weather exposure. Paints contain high quantities of pigments that completely obscure the grain and are available in a wide range of colours. A service life of 10 years is not uncommon for paint systems where good-quality products have been used and the necessary preparation has been undertaken. For durability, acrylic and latex paints are preferred as they remain flexible with age, unlike oil-based paints, which tend to become brittle with time. The acrylic or latex paints are, however, more permeable to moisture than oil-based products but will still perform better over time. Paints are also available in different gloss levels. Generally, the higher gloss paints will perform better than low gloss paints, which tend to pick up dirt, more readily absorb moisture and are more prone to mould growth. Being a film-forming finish the film can blister or peel if the timber substrate is wet or becomes wet.

Wood should be protected on site from the weather prior to installation and be painted as soon as possible after installation. Any dirt and other substances must be cleaned off prior to painting and, to achieve a good service life, the following steps should be taken.

- Apply a water-repellent preservative to timber surfaces and particularly to joints and laps that are prone to holding moisture. Painting should follow once the water-repellent preservative has adequately dried, which may take from 3 days to a week of favourable weather depending on the amount applied.
- Bare timber should be primed with a quality primer, paying particular attention to joints and laps. The primer should be allowed to fully dry before applying top coats. The time will depend on the paint type and, if top coats are applied prematurely, it can add to possible issues with tannin and resin bleed (see section on discolouration later). If tannin or resin bleed are of particular concern, primers that provide improved blocking capability are available. Primers should be applied evenly and be sufficient to obscure the wood grain.
- Apply two top coats to the timber, with particular attention paid to areas of greater sun and rain exposure. Two coats over a good primer should have a service life of 10 years, whereas with a single coat the service life may be halved. Water-borne paints require temperatures to remain above 10°C for 24 hours to cure and oil-based paints should be applied when temperatures are above 4°C. Application by brush is considered to provide better long-term performance than spray or roller application. It is recommended that the first top coat be applied within 2 weeks of the primer and the second top coat within 2 weeks

of the first. Peeling between coats can occur if time frames are greater or if the surface is not adequately cleaned. Enamel paints should not be applied to cool surfaces that are likely to heat up within a few hours because blistering may occur. Dark paint colours are also more prone to blister. Paints should not be applied in the evenings if dew is likely to form.

Colour of paints and stains

Research has clearly demonstrated that lightly coloured paint and stain finishes will provide maximum long-term performance to timber that is used externally. Dark-coloured surfaces heat up significantly more than light colours and this, in turn, will cause timber to dry out more, with subsequent greater shrinkage and movement that can lead to checking and splitting. Higher temperatures also promote resin bleed in those species that are prone to it. Also, where moisture penetrates the timber, higher temperatures are more conducive to the onset and progress of decay.

Interior timber finishes

Interior timber finishes are generally more exacting with regard to appearance but are not required to withstand weather extremes. This allows a wider range of finishes that are generally very long lasting. Even so, some finishes, such as those used on timber floors, need to have good properties of wear resistance. The following sections cover transparent finishes (as may be applied to furniture), timber floor finishes and painted finishes. The range of factory applied finishes are not covered. Before looking at these areas it is important to consider the natural colour change that occurs with timber. Timber that has been recently milled will undergo a distinct colour change, which is mainly due to visible light causing the intensity to increase over the first few months. For this reason it may be prudent not to hang wall-hangings on panelling or to lay rugs on timber floors until this process has occurred.

Transparent finishes

Preparation generally consists of some or all of sanding, staining, filling and sealing, prior to final finishing.

Staining

Although many timbers are not stained, stains may be used to change the colour of the timber. This process often accentuates differences in the colour of the wood grain owing to differences in absorption of the stain. Stains are usually dyes that have been dissolved in water or solvent. Water-based stains may cause some raising of the grain in the timber, which necessitates additional sanding when the stain dries. Solvent-borne stains do not cause raising of the grain and are generally quick drying. When applied to softwoods, more stain is absorbed into the lighter coloured earlywood, which will tend to reduce the contrast in colour. In some instances bacterial infection can cause uneven uptake of the stain.

Filling and sealing

Large pores may be present in timber, particularly in hardwoods, making filling necessary prior to the application of a sealer and finishing coats. Fillers may be either transparent or coloured to accentuate the wood character and come in the form of a liquid or paste. Fillers may be applied by brush, firstly across the grain and then along the grain. After some drying has taken place the excess is wiped off across the grain, which assists in filling the pores, and then lightly wiped with the grain. The filler should then be allowed to dry thoroughly before light sanding. A sealer is then applied, which may be quicker drying shellac or lacquer, or a varnish. The sealer prevents the finish from interacting with the stain or filler beneath.

Finishing

Transparent finishes may be oils, waxes, varnishes, polyurethanes, nitrocellulose lacquers or shellacs. Oils often referred to as Danish oil may be used. These products penetrate the timber and do not create a noticeable film. They are more easily applied and the surface may be waxed. They are, however, not as resilient to soiling as the film-forming finishes. Shellac, which is applied by 'French polishing', is time consuming and although an attractive deep lustre is obtained the surface is easily affected by water. Lacquers, on the other hand, provide a hard surface but require more applications than varnishes to provide a suitable coating depth. Lacquers and varnishes that provide satin to gloss finishes are available.

Timber floor finishes

Polished timber floors have remained popular in Australia for many years and demand remains high. Although some of the more traditional floor finishes are still used, there has been substantial development in the products available, particularly with relation to water-borne products. Timber floor finishes can be categorised as oil-based finishes, composite finishes (mixes of oil-based and solvent-borne polyurethane finishes), solvent-borne polyurethane finishes and water-borne finishes. Care is required when choosing a floor finish as the appearance, wear resistance and ability to allow for the natural movement of timber differ both within and between product types. If significant movement (shrinkage and swelling) is expected after a floor is laid, owing to, for example, high seasonal moisture content changes or use of wider cover width floorboards, then a finish that can accommodate this movement should be used. Edge bonding, where the finish acts as an adhesive in board joints, can occur with some finishes and this, combined with shrinkage in the floor, can result in irregularly spaced wide gaps at board edges or splits in some boards. Oil-based, composite and water-based finishes that are applied over their specific sealers have demonstrated a better ability to accommodate individual board movement.

Research has shown that although spills may be easily mopped up off a floor, finish systems, irrespective of their type, will not significantly inhibit moisture from the air (humidity) penetrating the finish under conditions of high humidity, thereby raising the moisture content of flooring. Similarly, under conditions of low humidity, moisture is released though the coating system to the air. While the finishes do not prevent the passage of moisture from the air, they do influence the rate of that passage.

Oil-based finishes

These more traditional types of finish (alkyd/oleo-resins) are manufactured by reacting a natural oil (e.g. linseed oil and tung oil) with another chemical. Varnishes and the traditional tung oils fall within this category and are associated with the polished and waxed timber floors of the past. These types of finishes are still available but require greater regular maintenance than the other finishes. However, with the use of acrylic floor polishes, they have become easier to maintain.

Composite oil-based/solvent-borne finishes

Finishes that contain oil-based alkyds with the addition of urethanes provide reasonably good abrasion resistance. Their appearance is subdued, ranging from satin to semi-gloss. They darken with time and require more frequent maintenance, particularly in high traffic areas, than polyurethanes. Acrylic floor polishes may also be used to protect the finish.

Solvent-borne polyurethane finishes

Solvent-borne polyurethanes (one pack and two pack) were developed during the 1950s and 1960s. They provided a harder finish, generally with limited flexibility but much greater abrasion resistance. Consequently, this greatly reduces the level of routine maintenance. They currently provide some of the hardest finishes available today, with gloss levels from matt through to a very high gloss. These finishes, as with the oil-based finishes, will generally darken with time and, although hard, may scratch if care is not taken. Repairing such damage is often not as easy as with other finishes. The odour on application is also very strong with these products.

Water-borne finishes

Water-borne polyurethane/acrylic mixes and straight water-borne polyurethanes are gaining popularity in Australia. They are generally applied over a sealer (either solvent-based or water-based) that enhances the colour of the timber. Matt through to gloss finishes are available and many of these finishes do not darken significantly with time. There is little odour on application associated with water-borne finishes. A curing additive (catalyst) may or may not be used. More recently, two-pack water-borne finishes have become available.

Painting interior timber

The procedures for painting interior timber are similar to those outlined for exterior applications. However, internal paintwork on timber often requires a smooth, hard-wearing surface that can be easily cleaned and for this reason enamel paints are generally used. Timber should be sanded, primed and undercoated prior to the application of top coats. The undercoat should completely cover the timber and then be sanded prior to the application of the top coats.

Finishing timber in specific applications

For some timber applications the finishing requires special attention to ensure durability. For example, with timber decking the exposure is not only severe but the finish may also need to withstand heavy foot traffic. Similarly, in the case of traditional unseasoned hardwood weatherboards considerable shrinkage after installation can be expected. Aspects that need to be taken into consideration for these and other applications requiring specific attention are provided below.

Decking

The service environment associated with exposed timber decks is very severe. Rain wetting, with water held for periods on the flat horizontal surfaces, induces swelling and this is often followed by the severe drying effect of the sun. The finish system must be able to accommodate the movement associated with moisture uptake and loss as well as the wear associated with daily foot traffic. Surface checks and joints at board ends accumulate dirt and with the moisture held, conditions are created that facilitate the development of both mould and decay.

Many decking products also have a reeded surface on one side, which may be laid either facing up or facing down depending on the desired appearance of the deck. If laid with the reeded surface up, then film thicknesses are invariably low on the raised wearing surface. The troughs also hold moisture for longer periods and accumulate dirt.

Because of the severe conditions expected for decking, penetrating stains and oils are often used on timber decks and these provide a good solution even though regular maintenance is necessary. Decking paints and other film-forming finishes for decks are formulated to accommodate movement and to resist abrasion. Water-repellent preservatives play an important role in minimising moisture-related movement and also to provide added protection at the joints between board ends. Similarly, it is also important to reduce the decay risk between boards and joists by at least coating the joists with an oil-based primer. It is also recommended that boards be provided with one coat of the chosen finish all round prior to installation to assist in minimising moisture gradients within boards.

Cladding

Timber cladding products may be unseasoned, as in the case of weatherboards, or seasoned, as with chamferboards or shiplap. Products are available in both softwoods and hardwoods, with some softwood products being finger-jointed to provide long length, clear material. Other products may, however, contain knots.

With softwood and cypress cladding, or if a clear finish is chosen for any species of timber, boards should be sealed all round with a water-repellent preservative before installation. Some preservative-treated softwood products have water repellents included in the treatment and do not require this sealing step. Following this, one coat of the stain or clear finish should be applied all round as applicable and, for painted boards one coat all round of primer/undercoat, colour-matched to the final coat.

Some timber and particularly cladding, fascia and similar products may be supplied preprimed. In the past some primers have been of low quality with poor adhesion to the timber surface, which necessitated sanding off the primer and repriming. However, many products are now pre-primed with quality primers and require minimal preparation prior to the application of finishing coats. The finishing should be undertaken shortly after the installation of the preprimed timber.

During installation particular attention should be paid to cut ends, all of which should have a coat of water-repellent preservative, stain or colour-matched primer/undercoat applied depending on the coating system chosen. If knot bleed is of concern, then knots may be sealed with two-pack solvent-borne polyurethane or a proprietary knot sealer. Similarly, the possibility of resin bleed should be assessed in the cladding species chosen.

After installation, one or two coats of the chosen finish should be applied according to the manufacturer's recommendations. Clear finishes can benefit from a further application of water-repellent preservative prior to the application of the clear finish.

In finger-jointed product severe sun exposure can cause differential movement between the adjacent sections of board that were joined. This and a possible difference in gloss level at the finger joints may, in some instances, be noticeable after final finishing. Movement effects are much less severe when light-coloured paints and stains are chosen.

Unseasoned weatherboards will shrink after installation and their method of fixing is designed to allow this. Shrinkage in standard 180-mm wide weatherboards can be in the order of 10 mm in some boards and, as a result, some remedial touch-up work is often necessary. The amount of touch-up work can be greatly reduced if colour-matched undercoats are used. In situations where it is difficult to accommodate touch-up work at some future date, a different product may need to be considered. In some instances seasoned rebated weatherboards have been used.

Marine applications

Timber in a marine environment generally experiences harsher conditions than on land and below water it may also be attacked by marine organisms. For this reason, antifouling paints are used.

For best protection timbers should be clean and dry and, after application of a water-repellent preservative, painted with a primer and at least two coats of quality exterior marine products.

Varnishes are also often used on boat trim and again marine products that have been formulated for the harsh environment should be used. Multiple coats and frequent maintenance are necessary to achieve a lasting high-quality appearance.

Finishes for items used with food

Wooden items are often used to hold or serve food products. A finish will not only enhance the often attractive figure and grain of the wood but it also plays an important role in keeping the wood dry and in preventing checks from developing. Penetrating finishes are often preferred as they will not crack or peel, as can occur with film-forming finishes.

Penetrating finishes may include products similar to thinned varnishes, modified oils and unmodified oils of linseed or walnut. Non-drying vegetable oils have also been used but are prone to mildew and can harbour bacteria. Alternatively, paraffin wax, which is solid at room temperature, has been found to provide a simple and effective finish. Whatever finish is used, it needs to be recommended for use with foods to ensure it is not toxic.

Finish failure

Painting of exterior timber is the most common form of protection and provided the preparation and coating system has been done appropriately, then the coating should last approximately 10 years. The acrylic polymers commonly used are extremely resistant to UV light degradation and erode very slowly but noticeably faster on the sides of the building with greater exposure. Moisture and poor bonding between the coating and substrate, which can occur from relatively short periods of weather exposure, contribute to accelerated paint failure. Similarly, primer coats should not be left for long periods without the subsequent coats being applied.

In situations where repainting is necessary, intercoat peeling can occur. Intercoat peeling is the separation between two coats and is indicative of a weak bond between them. This can be caused by poor cleaning of weathered paint surfaces or to time delays as short as 2 weeks between primer and top coats.

Chalking may also occur. It is the result of the paint surface weathering and releasing particles of pigment and resin. Although all paints chalk to some extent, latex paints and those based on acrylic polymers chalk very slowly. Chalking can cause discolouration of other surfaces with rain washing. Prior to repainting, proper preparation of the surface is necessary to prevent peeling.

Interior floor finishes also experience a number of issues that become of concern to owners. Most timber floors are not finished in a factory environment and, to some degree, finish imperfections occur in all floors. Down lights and light falling at oblique angles to the floor will highlight imperfections. Some imperfections, depending on their severity, require remedial work and can be associated with rejection of the coating, delamination or variation in gloss level.

Rejection of the finish occurs if contaminants leach out of the floor and for this reason anti-rejection additives are manufactured. Delamination is usually associated with movement at board edges or ends and the coating begins to peel from the board surface.

Discolouration and moulds

Discolouration

Discolouration of timber for reasons other than those outlined below are not common but do occur. They may be associated with iron, grease or the interaction of latex 'fumes' on enamel paints. Additionally, whether it can be regarded as discolouration or not, solvent-borne internal finishes will usually darken with age. Causes of discolouration in external painted timber are generally associated with the tannins and resins occurring in some species.

Tannin discolouration

In many Australian and imported hardwoods, the heartwood contains water-soluble extractives. These are also present in significant quantities in some softwoods, such as western red cedar, and to a lesser degree in other softwoods, including Douglas fir and slash pine. Extractives provide colour and decay resistance to many timbers.

The yellowish brown discolouration that occurs from extractives through painted surfaces is generally related to moisture washing the extractives to the paint surface, where the water then evaporates and leaves a reddish brown discolouration. Water often enters the timber through surface checks, penetrating paint films or joints between members.

As the discolouration is water-soluble, it can also cause unsightly discolouration on nearby lightly coloured painted surfaces, light coloured brickwork or concrete if water carrying the discolouration falls or runs on to them.

Consequently, the more porous latex and alkyd paints should not generally be applied directly to timbers that are high in extractives. However, some tannin-blocking primers are now available, which result in the primer changing colour but prevent transfer through the top coats. A system starting with a water-repellent preservative to bare timber followed by a stain-resistant solvent-borne primer and acrylic top coats will also significantly reduce discolouration. Leaving time between coats is beneficial, whereas the application of two coats within quick succession will tend to promote tannin bleed from susceptible timber.

Resin bleed

Resin naturally occurs in some softwood species, such as radiata pine, and under certain conditions the resin can bleed through the painted surface. In timber that is treated with an LOSP or in cladding that is subject to heat build-up (dark colours and northerly facing), resin bleed is more common. External products are usually preprimed and there are often no signs of resin until after installation. Resin that does bleed through top coats may be scraped off or washed with mineral turpentine.

A hot airgun applied to areas that exhibit bleed may also be used to bring resin to the surface. Resin bleed can recur the following summer. Application of a second oil-based primer to rebind preprimed material has been shown to improve resistance to resin bleed.

In some instances the resin bleed does not appear to damage the coating. In other instances the resin bleed causes the coating to blister and discolour.

Knot bleed

Similar to resin bleed, some discolouration and resin may show through paint work at knots. Prior to painting, knots can be sealed with two-pack solvent-borne polyurethane, which is usually sufficient to prevent bleed or discolouration through the paint system.

Mould

Locations that are usually moist, such as mountainous and tropical regions, are also those areas that are more susceptible to mould and fungal growth. Mould will grow on any surface that is moist and where nutrients are available. Dust provides a source of nutrients and, for this reason, gloss surfaces that are more easily cleaned are less susceptible to mould growth. Internally, extraction fans, which remove moisture and therefore prevent condensation, can provide an effective means of control. When repainting a mould-affected surface it is necessary to clean the surface and then neutralise the mould. This involves initially washing surfaces with detergent to remove dust and grease and then sponge wiping with household bleach mixed in warm water, allowing the bleach to remain moist until the discolouration is removed. The surfaces are then washed thoroughly with clean water and dried prior to repainting. When problems with mould are greater, a fungicidal solution may be applied to the cleaned and bleached surfaces and allowed to dry before painting or mould inhibitors can be added to paints.

Lead-based paints

Timber properties

Lead, which was used extensively in paints as a pigment, presents a health hazard, particularly from inhalation of dust if sanded, and ingestion, to a lesser extent. Up until the 1950s, as much as 50 per cent lead was used in paints but by 1970 restrictions had limited it to 1 per cent. In 1992 it was further reduced to 0.25 per cent and then throughout much of Australia to a maximum of 0.1 per cent in 1997. During the early to mid 1900s white lead (lead carbonate) was the main white pigment used in both interior and exterior paints. It was used in top coats for structural timbers, door and window joinery and weatherboards. Similarly, 'pink primer' with red and white lead pigments was also used in timber priming applications, such as with weatherboards. Red lead primer was also used on timber up to the 1970s.

Lead in paint can be detected with a test kit and analytical laboratories proficient in the testing of lead are able to provide more accurate testing. If lead is present, it may be dealt with in various ways depending on the age of the house, condition of the paint and occupants in the dwelling. These may include painting over it if it is in good condition and out of reach of children, replacing some items, such as skirtings, or removing the paint. If surfaces are being disturbed during any removal or preparation work, then the work needs to be appropriately planned and safety precautions taken. Safety precautions need to include consideration of the person undertaking the work as well as the occupants, neighbours and pets.

Disposal of leftover coatings

With any coating job there is likely to be a portion of the coating purchased that is unused or leftover.

Prior to considering the disposal of leftover coatings, the options of applying a second coat over high-wear areas or storing the leftover coating for future touch-up work should be considered. Coatings are generally stable products that may be stored in their original containers in a safe place for future use. Although skins may form on the surface, which need to be removed, the coating should maintain its properties. If touch-up work is being undertaken, an area of the surface should be checked to ensure that the surface to be touched up has not had a significant colour change due to age.

FURTHER READING

Referenced

Australian/New Zealand Standard. (2000). AS/NZS 2311 *Guide to the Painting of Buildings*.

Department of Environment & Heritage—Environment Australia. (1999). *The six step guide to painting your home*. Canberra: Commonwealth of Australia.

Feist, William C. (1999). Exterior wood finishes. *Wood Design & Building* 7, 8, 9.

Forest Products Laboratory, US Department of Agriculture. (1999). *Wood handbook. Wood as an engineering material*. Chapter 15. Washington, DC: Govt Printer.

National Association of Forest Industries. (1989). Exterior finishes for timber. Timber datafile FM1. Canberra: NAFI.

Websites

Australian Paint Manufacturers' Federation, viewed 16 March 2005, <http://www.apmf.asn.au>.

Chapter 15

Destroyers of timber

If protected from weathering and mechanical damage, initially sound heartwood can last virtually indefinitely, as evidenced by the articles, thousands of years old, that have been removed from the pyramids in Egypt, or by the bloodwood log removed in 1940 from the mud 14 m below the waterline in Sydney Harbour in an 'as new' state after an estimated 20 000 years of burial.

Apart from the usual wear and tear, the factors that are likely to limit the life of wood are weathering, decay, insect attack and fire.

Weathering

Because of wood's affinity for water the surface layers readily absorb rain and dew and expand; hot sun and a lowered humidity then force this moisture out so the surface of unprotected wood is in a continual state of stress. This results, especially for those species of high shrinkage, in the development of checks and cracks. These openings gradually increase in depth and assist in the erosion of the surface.

In addition, slow erosion of the surface is also promoted by oxidative degradation caused by the ultraviolet radiation in sunlight, which attacks the wood cell's cementing material, the lignin and also, to some extent, the cellulose. The result is that the cells at the wood's surface gradually break down and soften. At this point they may also be invaded by 'soft rot' fungi, which cause even further softening. Often the softened surface layers of wood cells may slough away, exposing more cells to this slow surface breakdown; good-quality coatings will reduce the process and, if maintained, will stop it completely.

Weathering is usually a very slow process of about 0.1 mm per year but the figure varies with species, timber orientation and degree of exposure (Plate 28). The less dense wood will weather more than the denser timber and it is not uncommon, for example, to see the loss of thin-walled earlywood cells on the surface of softwoods compared with the denser latewood cells.

All wood exposed to the weather will change in colour. Generally, dark-coloured timber will lighten while light-coloured timber, such as radiata pine, will darken.

Apart from its effect on appearance weathering is seldom of major importance, but in timber that is treated with a shallow application of preservative it may eventually permit the entry of destructive agencies to the untreated timber lying beneath the skin of impregnated wood.

Decay

Decay, or rot, is caused by fungi—organisms that live on other organic matter, such as wood (Plate 29). The very fine spores of these fungi are abundant in the air and under favourable conditions of temperature and dampness and in the presence of oxygen they will attack wood, especially if it contains easily digested sugars and starches, which are commonly present in sapwood. Heartwood is less readily attacked because it contains very few readily digestible nutrients for fungi and also because of the nature of the extractives that it may contain, the amount and toxicity of which varies greatly between species.

Wood that is at a moisture content below about 20 per cent, or that is saturated with water to the point where oxygen is in restricted supply to the fungi, is not subject to fungal attack. There are exceptions, of course, and the group of fungi called 'soft rot' and some bacteria can thrive in the low oxygen conditions in saturated timber and attack the wood cells.

Soft rot and bacterial attack can develop at an accelerated rate in cooling towers and also near the ground line of poles, especially in fertilised fields in hot climates (the extra supplement of nitrogen seems to encourage attack).

Moulds and stains

Moulds are fungi of a type whose activity is confined mainly to the wood surface, although their hyphae can penetrate to some depth. They live on moist surface deposits, including wood cell sugars, that may have been produced on the surface of timber as it was milled and during drying. The fungi are termed 'lower fungi' and they are generally prolific spore producers. In addition, a mass of hyphae is sometimes seen on timber stacked for seasoning in humid climates and it can slow down the rate of drying. It is usually removed completely when the timber is dressed but the dust containing the dry spores can be very unpleasant so good ventilation in the workplace is essential. It is better to restrain the incidence of mould growth by providing stack covers to assist in the early provision of a relatively dry surface on the timber. Mould that is growing on timber surfaces is disfiguring rather than destructive to the wood.

Other so-called lower fungi cause *bluestain* or *sap stain*, which can spread rapidly through the sapwood in warm humid weather; the stain can continue to grow in cold conditions if timber is block-stacked. The stained colour is the result of pigmented fungal hyphae growing through the wood cells in search of nutrients such as simple sugars, which are contained in most sapwood parenchyma cells, notably the rays—and hence the alternative term sap stain. A blue discolouration is the most common stain but brown, yellow, orange and red stains may also appear. Unless it is very severe, bluestain has little effect on the strength of timber but it can cause an excessive uptake of solution if the timber is preservative-treated later. It is certainly undesirable aesthetically and from the marketing point of view, so most producers endeavour to minimise its occurrence. Rapid removal of the logs from the forest, followed by immediate sawing and kiln drying, usually prevent its development, since bluestain or sap stain fungi grow best at high moisture contents. If kiln drying of the green material is neither practicable nor desirable, susceptible wood can be protected by spraying or dipping in a fungicidal solution immediately after sawing. A range of modern organic fungicides are available for spray and dip application to freshly felled logs and newly milled timber. These fungicides will be rapidly washed away by rain so stack covers are essential. The same treatment will also control surface mould.

Bluestain cannot be satisfactorily removed by bleaching agents, so its control is essential for all dressed timber. If susceptible logs cannot be processed immediately after felling, it may be advantageous to store them under water sprays to keep them in a fully saturated condition, which will help to minimise attack.

Pencil streak

Dark lines and flecks are often found in association with ambrosia (pin-hole) borer damage in the following eucalypts: *Eucalyptus baxteri, camaldulensis, cameronii, campanulata, delegatensis, eugenioides, fastigata, guilfoylii, laevopinea, marginata, microcorys, muellerana, obliqua, pilularis, piperita, radiata, sieberi* and *viminalis*.

The dark deposits are present mainly in the ray parenchyma cells and may extend from the pith to the outer heartwood. Sapwood seems to be virtually free of them. The discolouration is often assumed to indicate the presence of decay but this is not so. It is caused by pioneer organisms that enter through wounds and may prepare the way for decay but it does not in itself indicate the presence of decay fungi or weaker wood.

The process of decay

Unless subject to injury, the sapwood of the living tree is not attacked by decay, but over-mature heartwood of otherwise very durable species can be subject to destruction, as can be observed in the hollow pipes of many of the eucalypts. Decay only begins in the sapwood when the moisture content in the felled tree falls to the level that is favourable to the fungi.

Decay fungi cause a significant loss in strength even in the early stages of attack when their presence is not obvious to the unaided eye; this is referred to as *incipient decay*. At a later stage the aggregations of fine strands (hyphae) may be seen to permeate the wood, which eventually becomes whitish if the fungi favour the consumption of lignin, or brown, if cellulose is favoured. White or brown surface moulds may be present, as well as fungal fruiting bodies in the form of toadstools and brackets. A simple test for the possible presence of decay is to prise out a splinter of the wood with a penknife and see if the resulting fracture is of a brittle nature. At a later stage of decay its presence will be indicated by a much easier penetration of the wood when it is jabbed, say with a screwdriver.

Dry rot and wet rot

These terms are often loosely used in reference to wood decay but they are better avoided as they tend to give an erroneous impression of the process involved. As mentioned earlier, timber must have a moisture content of above 20 per cent before there is a serious risk of decay, but this could scarcely be described as 'dry' under Australian conditions. The only true 'dry rot' is that caused by *Serpula lacrymans* (also called *Merulius lacrymans*), which is most common in Europe but sometimes found in Victoria, and which has the ability of conveying the necessary life-supporting moisture from adjacent areas onto dry timber and infecting it. Its presence is indicated by a dust of red spores. Fortunately, it has made relatively little headway in Australia.

Prevention of decay

Since the air is full of fungal spores there is no way of isolating wood from the seeds of decay so one must control the factors that enable it to become established; that is, by using wood, whenever possible, in a way that ensures that it remains in a dry condition during its service life. Proper regard for this consideration in the design of structures, in careful building and in the execution of a reasonable measure of maintenance is essential. There are some uses (timber embedded in the ground or exposed to the weather) where this requirement is obviously impossible to achieve; in such cases one must either choose a species that has high natural durability or enhance its durability by impregnating it with preservatives.

Condensation problems in buildings

The use of bathrooms, kitchens and laundries produces a lot of moisture-laden air, perhaps to the extent of at least the equivalent of 15 litres of water per day, in the atmosphere within the average house. The build-up of humidity is being increased by current attempts to make houses more energy-efficient by sealing gaps and openings in the building's skin. For example, it is now common to omit the vents that used to be a feature of the upper portions of each external wall of a room, windows are fitting more tightly and external doors are equipped with weather strips.

This means, at least in cold climates, that there is some possibility of moisture condensing inside the external wall cavities and the roof space, which might lead to such an increase in moisture content of the timber present there as to favour fungal attack, especially in non-durable species.

Water vapour travels from areas of high atmospheric humidity, as in the warm room of a house, through the wall or ceiling lining, into the much colder cavities beyond, where it may condense on the surface. If this happens on a large scale, there is some risk of distortion of the timber members due to swelling and of decay if the conditions are prolonged. If the wall or ceiling is lined with absorbent insulating material, the water vapour may condense within it and affect its efficiency.

The transmission of water vapour in this way can be prevented by the fitting of a vapour barrier, such as polyethylene sheeting or aluminium foil, on the warm side of the cavity immediately underneath the plasterboard or other wall cover. It is essential that this vapour barrier be fitted without any gaps or tears since the water vapour will find its way through such breaks.

This problem has not been of great consequence in the past except in such special circumstances as cool rooms for food storage and in dwellings in alpine climates but it is important to be aware of the potential difficulty associated with it. A number of precautions can be taken to mitigate the risk.

1. Do not vent the bathroom, kitchen or laundry into the roof space unless that area has an abundance of natural ventilation. This is seldom the case today when most roofs are sarked or fitted with aluminium foil.
2. Water vapour is rising continually from the ground under the building, even when the soil appears dry to the touch. Avoid the possibility of this vapour penetrating into the rooms either by providing abundant ventilation to the underfloor space or by laying a vapour barrier, such as polyethylene sheeting, over the soil under the building. If such sheeting is provided, the amount of ventilation needed to keep the air in the underfloor area from becoming very humid will be greatly reduced.
3. During the warmest part of the day open some of the windows to permit the dispersal of the highly humid air from within the building.

Insect attack

Even though there are many insects that use the foliage of trees as a source of food, there are only two, termites and borers, that are of importance as destroyers of the wood. In the marine environment a different range of boring organisms from those that are found on land attack wood and can be very destructive.

Termites

Termites are of common occurrence as scavengers of wood in all parts of Australia, although there are fewer species in the colder south-eastern areas (Tasmania and eastern Victoria). They are useful in the forest for speeding up the return of dead trees and fallen branches to the soil but their habit of invading buildings and surreptitiously attacking wood components makes the checking and eradication of their activity a major aspect of the pest control industry.

The term *white ant* has often been applied to termites but they are not ants and their behaviour pattern is quite different from that of ants, so that term should be avoided.

There are many different types of termite. The majority of Australian termites are grass eaters or forest floor scavengers. However, about 20 species of termites that occur in Australia are of economic importance because they feed on living and/or dead wood. Some attack only the living tree (at the inner core of over-mature heartwood), others exist in buildings without having to be in contact with the ground and live entirely within the wood (the dry-wood termites), but the most important group in regard to their potential for causing damage to buildings are the subterranean termites, which usually require ground contact to provide the necessary moisture, and travel from the nest to the source of woody food through earth-like galleries. The galleries are constructed either within the infested timber or as hollow tubes over supporting structures. The damage that is caused by all types is basically similar—a series of excavated galleries with connecting wood tissue to maintain the general shape of the wood member and with few external entry points (Plate 30). Because of the shell of untouched wood, detection is often not made until they are well established and have caused considerable damage.

Much has been said about the amount of damage that termites cause to housing in Australia. It is hard to ascertain the real picture as many competitive industries make unsubstantiated claims to promote their products or services. However, a survey conducted by the Timber Development Association of New South Wales showed that less than 0.5 per cent of householders reporting structural damage in their homes attributed it to termites. On the other hand, in Queensland, damage from termites is among the top ten reported building defects in the state. In spite of differing views from various sectors, termites are seen as a significant threat to a house structure.

The termite life cycle

Termites are social insects and each nest contains a queen and a king plus many thousands of workers and a smaller number of soldiers. The queen and king establish the nest after flying from an existing colony as reproductive alates (winged forms).

The queen often has a greatly distended abdomen due to her egg-laying activity; like the queen bee she is continuously tended by workers in her cell. Her eggs are tended by the workers and the young termites that hatch from these develop into various castes—workers, soldiers and reproductives. The workers, constituting by far the majority of the colony, are small, wingless, sightless and soft bodied but have strong jaws for attacking wood. The workers construct the nest, gather the food and feed the other members of the colony.

The soldiers, a small percentage of the colony, are sightless also but are adapted to defend the nest against invaders, such as ants. Some species of termites have soldiers with greatly enlarged jaws for attacking invaders, while others are capable of spraying invaders with a sticky material that serves to immobilise them.

The reproductive forms are tended by the workers while their wings are undeveloped; when mature the winged males and females leave the nest in a swarm, usually on humid summer evenings. When they land they shed their wings and pair together. The pair then builds a small cell in a suitable location and mate. Initially, both male and female tend the eggs and the young but the workers that are produced eventually take over this task and the queen devotes all her time to egg laying.

Dry-wood termites

Dry-wood termites are able to thrive without contact with the ground or other abundant source of moisture, which is essential for subterranean termites. They are found mostly in damp tropical climates (in Australia, on the Queensland coast) where the high equilibrium moisture content of the timber itself provides a satisfactory level of moisture.

Because of the absence of the shelter galleries of earthy material that are indicative of the presence of subterranean termites, the detection of dry-wood termites is often very difficult. As they work entirely within the wood they may be present for many years before discovery. The flight holes are small, only about 1 mm in diameter. Sometimes small pellets of frass (excreta), similar to grains of sand, fall from the holes and give a clue to their presence. Examination of the surrounding area should be made, sounding the timber with a hammer for indications of hollowness and jabbing suspected areas with a chisel in a search for hidden cavities.

There are four indigenous species in northern and eastern Australia and another four that have been introduced. The indigenous species are *Cryptotermes primus*, which is common in coastal Queensland, *C. queenslandis*, *C. gearyi* and *C. secundus*. They are found in standing trees, both living and dead, but are not a hazard to buildings. Occasional infestation of electricity transmission poles by *C. queenslandis* has occurred as far south as Sydney.

The exotic species are *C. brevis* (commonly called the West Indian dry-wood termite), *C. cynocephalus*, of minor importance in north Queensland, *C. domesticus*, widely distributed in the tropical areas of the Pacific region, and *C. dudleyi*, found on Thursday Island.

Cryptotermes brevis is the only one that is very destructive. It is likely to attack most species of seasoned wood with a density below 700 kg/m³ unless they have a relatively high durability rating. Fortunately, this termite does not fly far so its spread is usually slow, brought about mainly by the transfer of infested furniture or building material. It has caused significant damage to buildings on the coastline between Brisbane and Bundaberg, and in Brisbane in 1979 a large-scale fumigation was carried out with methyl bromide to eradicate an outbreak stemming from attack in some old public buildings.

Attack is confined mostly to the sapwood of hardwoods and softwoods and this may be prevented in building timbers by preservative treatment conforming to AS/NZS 1604 *Specification for Preservative Treatment* series.

Glyptotermes

Another group of termites with some resemblance in habits to the dry-wood types is the genus *Glyptotermes*. These termites live in small colonies in relatively moist wood without any need for ground contact. The rate of spread of attack is relatively low.

The likelihood of attack is mainly associated with mature stems of slow-growing species of eucalypt and is usually confined to the heartwood. Because of this, their presence in a stem that has been converted into a natural round pole may not be easy to detect but is more likely to be obvious if the pole is desapped.

If attack was confined to the upper reaches of the tree, the drying out of the pole is likely to reduce the moisture content of the wood to a level that would inhibit further activity, but if they are present near the butt of the pole, a sufficiently high moisture content for survival may be maintained in service. Under these conditions the pole may need to be fumigated or a suitable remedial preservative applied.

Subterranean termites

These termites seek dark humid positions for a nest, such as in an old stump or the damp, poorly ventilated foundations of a building. An earth-enclosed gallery is constructed between the nest and the timber being attacked (Plate 31), and it usually provides a readily observable indicator of their presence if access permits inspection of areas of potential hazard.

Access galleries may be built across resistant materials, including preservative-treated timber, and they can be constructed to bypass termite shields, so if regular inspections of underfloor areas are not possible, eradication by application of a remedial treatment such as Boracol or by baiting techniques may be necessary. Such treatments should be delivered only by approved pest control operators.

In recognised termite-hazard areas, the soil beneath a dwelling will require the application of an approved chemical/physical barrier during construction or before the slab or subfloor is laid. Alternatively, the building must be constructed of termite-resistant materials, such as preservative-treated timber or natural termite-resistant timbers (e.g. cypress). The Building Code of Australia (BCA) calls upon AS 3660.1-2000 *Termite Management: New Building Work* to define and detail appropriate systems of termite control, including barriers, and termite-resistant material. This includes protective measures to prevent termite ingress to the building through fine cracks, expansion joints and around plumbing fixtures. Detection of attack in buildings that are built on slab foundations without appropriate barriers may be difficult. Cavity brick (double-skin) construction provides a space where galleries can be created unobserved, so the BCA requirements must be adhered to.

When suspended timber floors are used, a dry, well-ventilated underfloor space will help to deter initial invasion but regular inspection with a light or torch at, say, half-yearly intervals is a desirable maintenance procedure. The underfloor area should be raked free of off-cuts at the conclusion of the building's construction. The underfloor area should not be used for the indiscriminate storage of junk, which is likely to encourage termite establishment and to interfere with subfloor ventilation.

Mastotermes

The most destructive termite in Australia is *Mastotermes darwiniensis*. Its occurrence is confined to north of the Tropic of Capricorn, where it is very destructive of all kinds of organic matter. In areas such as Darwin and the Pilbara region of Western Australia it is essential to thwart this rapid destroyer of wood and, again, the BCA requirements must be faithfully followed during home construction.

Termite-control measures

In all states and territories of Australia the building legislation calls up the BCA. This Code requires some form of protection *if there is a threat of termite attack*; where no threat exists, no protection is needed. Under the BCA all structural elements of a new building—the primary building elements—must be protected either by providing barriers to keep the termites out (or to force them into the open where they will be seen and remediated), or by using termite-resistant building materials, such as steel, plastic, naturally durable timber or preservative-treated timber.

The BCA calls up AS 3660.1-2000 *Termite Management: New Building Work* to define and detail appropriate systems of termite control, including barriers, and termite-resistant material. The full Standard series sets out the design and termite-management system performance requirements, guidelines for detecting and managing termite activity, and criteria for assessing the effectiveness of termite-management systems.

Barriers to prevent termite entry are of three types:

1. physical, including: stainless steel mesh or granite (or basalt) particles (graded to an appropriate size) either of which is applied beneath the concrete slab and/or around the perimeter of a dwelling and around service penetrations and termite shields on piers and in walls; and the exposed edge of the slab
2. chemical, including chlorpyrifos and bifenthrin, applied as a soil spray or reticulation system beneath the concrete foundation and/or as a perimeter barrier beneath a concrete strip
3. chemical contained within a physical matrix, including the flexible moisture barrier sheeting containing deltamethrin that may be used to cover the soil beneath the concrete foundation.

The barriers are applied as preconstruction measures. The method of installation of any barrier system is closely controlled and set down in AS 3660.1-2000 *Termite Management: New Building Work*. Protecting potential termite entry points around service penetrations, such as plumbing pipes, requires special shields that are manufactured from, for example, stainless and galvanised steel, copper, zinc and aluminium alloys.

An important physical barrier that is accepted in AS 3660.1-2000 *Termite Management: New Building Work* is the concrete slab under a dwelling. It must be designed and constructed in accordance with either the concrete structures Standard AS 3600-2001 *Concrete Structures* or the residential slabs and footings Standard AS 2870-1996 *Residential Slabs and Footings—Construction*.

A number of chemical treatments are approved for use against termites and these may be applied to timber components, as chemical barriers, termite dusts, in special baits, or in combinations of these.

Termite dusts are applied through monitoring or bait stations, or applied directly to the termites by introduction into termite foraging galleries using special puffers that are loaded with the finely divided termiticidal dust. With baiting, foraging termites are attracted to the bait station and then the aggregated termites are removed, dusted with the toxicant and then placed back in the station. The termites' own behaviour of grooming allows the toxic chemicals to be passed throughout the colony, which is ultimately eradicated.

Registered wood preservatives and remedial treatment chemicals are used for the protection of timber components of dwellings. These include copper–chrome–arsenic (CCA), ammoniacal copper quaternary (ACQ), copper azoles, creosote, and light organic solvent-borne preservative (LOSP) formulations, such as copper and zinc naphthenates, synthetic pyrethroids and tributyl tin naphthenate plus permethrin. Boron-based compounds, which are used mainly for remedial treatments, include disodium octaborate, sodium borate and/or boric acid with or without benzalkonium chloride, and sodium borate plus sodium fluoride.

Although termites may often be an unseen threat to a building's structural integrity, taking care to build in accordance with the BCA and ensuring that regular inspections and maintenance are carried out will ensure that their destructive activities are eliminated.

Borers

The presence of borer holes does not necessarily mean that active destruction is occurring or that the timber should be rejected. The first essential is to identify which borer has been responsible for the holes. Many types of beetle are likely to lay their eggs in the bark or wood. There are four stages of their life cycle—egg, larva or grub, pupa and adult beetle. It is the larval stage that does most of the boring and eating of the wood but the exit holes are usually made by the escaping adult beetle.

The main types of borer may be considered in terms of the moisture content of the timber at the time of infestation. The pin-hole or ambrosia borer attacks the tree while it is still alive but perhaps in an unhealthy state. Pin-hole borers do not attack seasoned timber. The holes usually have a dark-coloured lining, frass (larval excrement) is absent, and the holes proceed in relatively straight lines.

The jewel beetle (*Diadoxus erethurus*) will attack unhealthy or fire-damaged cypress trees. The larvae feed on the outer sapwood but may tunnel into the heartwood to pupate. Sawn timber is not reinfested but some borer holes may be present.

The bark beetle (*Ernobius mollis*), of European origin, occasionally emerges in warm weather from radiata pine building framework, core stock and furniture timber that has retained a small amount of bark, for example, around a knot, even after processing. The larvae of this beetle feed in the bark and the outer edge of sapwood of conifers. Reinfestation of the bark-covered areas can occur.

The main concern is that the newly hatched beetle may bore an escape hole through the facing material of veneer, plasterboard or carpet. Because of this it is important that the amount of bark present on wood from conifers should be kept to a minimum.

The frass-filled holes of the *Cerambycid*, or longicorn, borer are often seen in the inner bark and sapwood of trees, especially hardwoods, that have died in the forest or on logs that have been in store on the log dump for a considerable period. The holes sometimes extend into the heartwood, which is often favoured by the larva for the pupation period. Emergence is usual in the first year after attack but can occur for several years.

The longicorn beetle is large and readily distinguishable by its long antennae. The flight holes are usually oval and 7–10 mm across (Plate 32). The frass is coarse and stringy. Long periods of dry weather seem to promote attack by the beetle. Once the timber has dried no further infestation occurs.

Auger beetles (bostrychids) are another invader of recently felled logs but are of more concern than the longicorns because they often cause a significant amount of damage to the sapwood of debarked poles and piles that are undergoing a period of air drying prior to preservative treatment. They are seldom a serious problem in sawn timber unless logs have been stored in the mill yard for a considerable period. Overseas species of bostrychid (mainly *Dinoderus*) often emerge from imported bamboo furniture. The most common local bostrychids are *Mesoxylion cylindricus*, *M. collaris* and *Bostrychopsis jesuita*. Bostrychid beetles vary in length from about 6 to 20 mm and bore a hole up to 6 mm in diameter. Usually only the sapwood of hardwoods is susceptible but that of softwoods is not immune from attack. Initial attack is concentrated on the undersurface of the stacked logs or timber.

Except in tropical areas of high humidity, bostrychids do not attack seasoned timber but their larvae can continue to tunnel through it and the adult beetle may take a year or two to emerge and so may make escape holes through plasterboard walls or other cover on the structural framework.

Attack can be forestalled to a large extent if logs are debarked as soon as possible and a shell of dry wood, unattractive to them, is created on the outside. A deterrent spray or dip can be used on the fresh timber, and a boron compound would be effective. Large populations of bostrychids often result from poor yard hygiene, which is another reason for frequent disposal of all off-cuts, rejected logs and so on from the mill yard.

The main borers attacking seasoned wood are the lyctine beetles, more commonly referred to as lyctid borers (mainly *Lyctus brunneus*), which attack only starch-bearing sapwood of some hardwoods; and the *Anobium* borer, which attacks mainly softwood species, although some hardwoods are quite susceptible, and it is most commonly a problem in old furniture. Closely related to the *Anobium* is the *Calymmaderus* borer, which may attack hoop pine in semitropical climates.

The European house borer, *Hylotrupes bajulus*, a major destroyer of softwoods overseas, has not become established in Australia, although there were some instances of infestation in prefabricated housing brought to Australia in the 1950s; fortunately, whole-house fumigation with methyl bromide eradicated these outbreaks. Some instances of its importation in pine furniture from Spain have been reported but there is as yet no evidence of a second generation occurring under Australian conditions.

A fuller discussion of the most common types found in sawn timber follows.

The pin-hole borer

These borers are so described because a pin can usually be inserted (full length) into their holes. The holes are generally relatively straight and usually at right angles to the direction of the grain (Plate 33). The beetle is a forest insect that attacks the living tree. When the mature beetle bores its tunnel, it introduces a particular kind of fungal spore, which germinates and grows on the tunnel walls and provides food to sustain the hatched larva, and hence the alternative name 'ambrosia borer'. This fungal lining of the walls results in a blackish discolouration in many instances, which is a positive indicator that the damage has been done by the pin-hole borer. The larvae do not eat the wood and there is a virtual absence of frass in the tunnels.

The beetles can attack all types of tree but are more likely to select those that are unhealthy (and thus unable to put up a strong resistance to the intrusion) or the freshly felled log, which is a common occurrence in tropical areas. The ambrosial fungi require a high moisture presence for survival so attack ceases as soon as the wood begins to dry; most damage occurs in the summer months in temperate climates. The best control measure is to remove the felled log from the forest as soon as possible.

Unless attack is severe (Plate 34), as sometimes happens to eucalypts in the cooler districts of south-eastern Australia, there is usually little effect on strength but merely an aesthetic problem affecting the marketability of dressed products.

The lyctid borer

The term 'powder post borer' is sometimes applied to this borer but since it is also used in relation to the bostrychid beetles there is likely to be some confusion, so that term is best discarded.

The most common lyctid in Australia is *Lyctus brunneus* but since there are other lyctids which are not of the *Lyctus* genus the use of the word 'lyctid' is preferred to '*Lyctus*' in general descriptions. These borers are also referred to as 'lyctine beetles' in Australian Standards.

The female beetle lays her eggs in the pores of the exposed end-grain of susceptible timber when its moisture content is within the range of approximately 8–25 per cent (Plate 35). To be susceptible, timber must have pores (i.e. it must be botanically a hardwood). There must be a relatively large amount of starch present in order to sustain the growth of the larva, and only sapwood meets this requirement. In addition, the pores must be of sufficient diameter (>90 μm) for the beetle to be able to insert her egg-laying apparatus (ovipositor); many hardwoods are therefore not attacked even when their sapwood is high in starch content. In the individual species descriptions, susceptibility to lyctid attack is given where accurate information is available.

If the sapwood is high in starch, it is likely to be completely devoured, with the production of a finely powdered, cream-coloured frass. Practically all the damage is caused by the larva but the adult beetle, brown and about 3 or 4 mm long, bores the exit hole. Most activity is in the warmer months and the life cycle may be as short as 4 months but there is usually only one emergence each year. The beetles are abundant in most tropical and warm temperate climates so if susceptible sapwood is present and accessible, attack occurs within the first couple of years of service.

In Queensland and New South Wales, it was found necessary to introduce legislation (the *Timber Marketing Act 1977* in New South Wales, and the *Timber Utilization and Marketing Act 1987* in Queensland) to control the sale and use in those states of wood products containing sapwood that is susceptible to lyctid borers. Among other things, these Acts require that timber from which a long life might reasonably be expected by the purchaser (e.g. manufactured articles such as joinery, flooring, mouldings, cladding, panelling, plywood, laminated wood) shall not contain sapwood that is susceptible to attack by lyctid borers unless it has been impregnated by a preservative that is approved by the relevant forestry authority, which also lays down the required concentration of approved preservative and registers the treatment plant. In those two states importations of susceptible timber from elsewhere in Australia and from overseas also come within the ambit of the Acts.

The NSW Act is more lenient in that it does permit framing timber, which is out of sight in the finished building, to have up to 25 per cent of its perimeter in susceptible sapwood at any cross-section provided that it does not exceed 50 per cent of any face or edge at that cross-section. In part, this avoids costly wastage of those pieces of scantling with corners of sapwood but it does mean that an occasional flight hole may appear in the plasterboard lining of a room. However, the holes are easily filled and the damage is almost certain to manifest itself in the first year or two after erection.

The *Anobium* borer

Instances of *Anobium* attack are most commonly seen in Australia in old furniture and in old softwood flooring. The beetle, brown and about 4 mm long, lays her eggs in cracks and crevices and often favours the sapwood of softwoods but heartwood too can be attacked. Australian hardwoods are seldom affected but furniture-quality hardwoods of overseas origin are often susceptible. Because of this borer's association with the destruction of furniture it is often described as the 'furniture beetle'.

In New South Wales attack is seldom found west of the Great Dividing Range, and then only in the cooler uplands in fittings introduced from the coast. Attack appears unlikely in districts where the equilibrium moisture content of the wood is below 8 per cent or the relative humidity is commonly below 45 per cent. The larva dies at temperatures in excess of 29°C.

Anobium beetles have a long life cycle of between 2 and 6 years, are of sluggish habits and seldom fly far, so new infestations are usually slow to spread. Most instances of attack in dwellings can be attributed to the introduction of old furniture, pine stepladders, old packing cases and so on that are already infested (Plate 36). If such articles had been fumigated before transfer, all would have been well. It is important to remember that fumigation only kills insects that are already present and does not have any preservative effect against future invasion. Badly infested timber has a honeycombed appearance and the frass is fine but gritty. The damage is caused by the larvae but the newly developed adult beetle bores the final escape hole.

The number of reported cases of attack in Australia has been small. On the other hand, softwood flooring in houses erected in the 1920s commonly shows extensive attack.

Regular observation, particularly of radiata pine flooring (the most likely source of initial attack because of the milder temperature and higher humidity of its location), is desirable and common prudence suggests the careful inspection of old furniture at the time of introduction to the dwelling, but it would appear on present evidence that the risk of infestation is slight provided that good building procedures in regard to adequate underfloor ventilation are observed and articles infested with this borer are kept away. In the case of concrete slab construction, careful exclusion of moisture from the slab would be important to avoid dampness in the lower parts of the frame. Preservative treatment of wood against attack can be achieved by using similar methods and chemicals to those applicable to lyctid borers.

The method of treatment of infected timber will depend on the severity of the attack. If the structural member is very severely affected, it should be replaced and the infected timber burnt to destroy the active larvae. In cases of less serious attack, surface treatment with insecticides can be tried but may not be completely successful, at least from the initial effort, if the infestation extends deeply into the timber. Boron-based or permethrin-based remedial chemicals may be successfully used for this purpose and they may also be injected into the beetle's flight holes in the case of finished furniture. The flight holes should then be filled with filler or wax. Open joints and cracks should also be flooded with the boron-based or permethrin-based compound and all such locations, which are ideal places for the beetle to deposit her eggs, should be filled, in addition to the injected flight holes.

There are several beetles of occasional occurrence in houses whose presence can alarm the occupier because of their superficial resemblance to the *Anobium* beetle. One of these is the 'tobacco beetle' (*Lasioderma serricorne*), which usually infects tobacco but also attacks grain products, pepper, ginger and dried fruits; its larva is hairy. The other is the 'drug store beetle' (*Sitodrepa panicea*); this beetle has a close resemblance to the adult *Anobium* but the hood on the head is less pronounced and the larva is less hairy than that of the tobacco beetle larva. It feeds on the same kinds of household goods as the tobacco beetle. Neither of these beetles causes damage to timber.

Calymmaderus borer

Another beetle of the Anobiid family that can cause significant damage is *Calymmaderus incisus*, which confines its attack to *Araucaria* and *Agathis* species under the warm humid conditions of coastal Queensland and the far north coast of New South Wales. It is not of consequence elsewhere in Australia.

Its habits are similar to those of *Anobium* except that in addition to attacking flooring it is also found in cladding. Australian Standards require that exposed timber of the susceptible species, when used in the zone bounded by the Great Dividing Range in the west, Bundaberg in the north, Murwillumbah in the south and the Pacific Ocean, should be protected by sealing the surface with paint or varnish or by preservative treatment.

Marine borers

Marine organisms are particularly destructive of wood. While some of them use wood as a food, others bore holes in it mainly for shelter and as the wood they destroy does not pass through their digestive system the latter type are difficult to deter even by impregnating the wood with considerable quantities of chemicals.

The severity of attack varies with the temperature of the water, its salinity and the type and concentration of particular organisms found in the locality. Before using timber in sea water and river estuaries it is important to check with local marine authorities on the nature of the hazard in that area.

The marine borers can be subdivided into two groups: crustacean borers, which are many-legged, crab-like animals (e.g. *Sphaeroma* and *Limnoria*); and molluscan borers, which, like mussels and oysters, possess bivalve shells (e.g. *Teredo* and *Martesia*).

Sphaeroma have a resemblance to the common garden slater and are often called 'pill bugs' because they roll into a ball when disturbed. Their attack is confined mainly to the tidal zone on marine piling, resulting in the development of the characteristic 'hourglass' appearance of severely attacked piles. Some *Sphaeroma* do not digest the wood but merely make holes in it for shelter; they can tolerate quite a high concentration of wood preservative so the use of treated timber may be less effective than metallic sheathing or very dense wood in deterring attack. They burrow a tunnel at right angles to the wood surface and favour the more tropical waters. They can withstand considerable variation in water salinity.

Limnoria, also known as 'gribble', make long tunnels in the wood just below its surface and digest most of the wood removed. They are deterred by low temperature and reduced salinity but have a high tolerance towards creosote. The natural resistance of timber to *Limnoria* is low except for a few species of high density and with considerable extractives and silica content.

The *Teredo* borers are also called 'shipworm' or 'cobra' (Plate 37). They invade wood only during their larval stage, when they are free to swim. The larvae make a small entry hole into the timber by using their shells as a rasp. The adults remain in the tunnels they create and grow to a considerable length, even in excess of 1.5 m. Wood is a major component of the diet so chemical preservatives can have a considerable deterrent effect.

Martesia are like mussels in appearance. They feed on plankton and use the timber only as shelter, forming an egg-shaped cavity in the wood. Since wood is not their food, preservatives have little deterrent effect.

It will be apparent that because of the habits of these marine borers, preservative treatments must be used at relatively high concentrations and may be supplemented with mechanical barriers, such as copper sheathing or floating collars.

Quarantine requirements

Under natural conditions the earth's creatures in each locality reach a balance. If this balance is destroyed by the introduction of new species, the result may be a rapid build-up in the population of the introduced species because of the absence from the area of natural predators, and harm may occur to crops, dwellings and even the human inhabitants.

The rapid and voluminous interchange of goods and people that is now occurring between the continents means a much greater risk of disturbance of the natural balance, so strict quarantine procedures at points of entry to Australia, although annoying to the traveller and importer, are of vital importance to the welfare of the country.

Anyone intending to import logs or sawn timber into Australia must follow the procedures laid down by the Commonwealth Department of Agriculture, Fisheries and Forestry's Australian Quarantine and Inspection Service (AQIS). The importer must also comply with all other regulatory and advisory bodies prior to and following importation (e.g. the Australian Customs Service, state Departments of Agriculture, Imported Foods Program, Therapeutic Goods Administration, and the Agricultural Pesticides and Veterinary Medicines Authority).

Intending importers should contact the Plant Quarantine Office in the relevant capital city and obtain an import permit. The permit calls for a description of the timber, the country of origin, the name of the craft by which it will be conveyed, and the approved place where it will be available for inspection by quarantine officers.

Inspection is made to see that the timber is not infested and that it is free of bark, soil, seeds or spillage that might create a possible hazard. In the case of logs a final clearance is withheld until sawing or veneering has been completed. If infestation is discovered, importers must treat the timber at their own expense. Fumigation with methyl bromide gas is very effective.

Most other countries have similar requirements for the inspection of timber imports. New Zealand prohibits the import of forest products with bark attached but exceptions can be made under some circumstances for veneer-producing logs and turpentine piles, which are subject to inspection before dispatch and possible retreatment on arrival.

In the case of goods imported within cargo containers, the timber component of the container—usually a thick plywood floor—must also be protected against pests and diseases that may inadvertently be harboured in the wooden component. The AQIS publication *Cargo Containers. Quarantine Aspects and Procedures* lists the chemicals approved for the preservation of such timber components. This publication is updated regularly to ensure only approved preservatives are used.

FURTHER READING

Referenced

Australian Standards. (2005). AS/NZS 1604 *Specification for Preservative Treatment* series.

Australian Standards. (1996). AS 2870 *Residential Slabs and Footings—Construction*.

Australian Standards. (2001). AS 3600 *Concrete Structures*.

Australian Standards. (2000). AS 3660.1 *Termite Management: New Building Work*.

Bootle, K. R. (1977). Ventilation under timber floors. Tech. pubn 11. Sydney: Forestry Commission of NSW.

Casimir, J. M. (1958). *Ernobius mollis*, an introduced bark beetle. Tech. notes 11(3). Sydney: Forestry Commission of NSW: 24–7.

Commonwealth Dept of Agriculture, Fisheries and Forestry (2004). *Cargo containers—quarantine aspects and procedures*. Canberra: Australian Quarantine Inspection Service.

Creffield, J. W. (1996). Wood destroying insects. Wood borers and termites. Melbourne: CSIRO Publications.

Edwards, D. W. (1982). *Anobium* attack and Australian-grown radiata pine. Internal report. Sydney: Forestry Commission of NSW.

Fairey, K. D. (1977). *Lyctus* susceptibility of the commercial timbers used in New South Wales. Tech. pubn 19. Sydney: Forestry Commission of NSW.

Forestry Commission of NSW. (1978). Timber borers of common occurrence. Tech. pubn 18.

Forestry Commission of NSW. (1978). Subterranean termites and their control in NSW. Tech. pubn 14.

French, J. R. J. (1968). The European house borer *Hylotrupes bajulus*. Tech. pubn 4. Sydney: Forestry Commission of NSW.

Keirle, R. M. (1974). Marine borers and the breakdown of timber in the sea. Wood tech. leaflet 9. Sydney: Forestry Commission of NSW.

Knudson, R. M. and Schniewind, A. P. (1975). Performance of structural wood members exposed to fire. *For Prod J* 25(2): 23–32.

Walsh, P. P. (1978). Concrete slabs for houses. Tech. paper (2nd series) 25. Melbourne: CSIRO Division of Building Research.

Walters, N. E. M. (1972). Case histories of the dry rot fungus *Serpula lacrymans*. *CSIRO For Prod Newsletter* 387: 4–7.

Websites

Australian Government, Forest and Wood Products Research and Development Corporation, viewed 4 March 2005, <http://www.timber.org.au>.

Chapter 16

Preservation methods

Wood is a complex organic polymer, and when used as a building material, like most other building materials, it may be subject to a number of degradative forces, including biological agencies, the weather and fire. In addition, Australia's size and diverse climate present some unique problems; there is a wide range of wood destroying fungi; and we have, in the hottest part of the country, one of the world's most voracious termites, *Mastotermes darwiniensis*, and elsewhere there are many other species of termites. Our timbers may also be attacked by marine borers and wood-boring insects, such as lyctids and anobiids. (Chapter 15 describes in more detail some of these agencies of timber degrade.)

The biodegradable feature is both a strength and a weakness of timber; it is good for natural recycling, but a disadvantage for a building material that is expected to provide a reliable service life. Clearly, using chemicals to impregnate the wood cells and make them resistant to decay, insects, weather and fire is essential to obtain adequate service life from low-durability timber species.

Some timber species are naturally durable and contain chemicals in their heartwood cells that repel or protect them from the various agents of degradation. In these cases, wood-preservation processes supplement this durability by protecting the sapwood of the naturally durable species.

Preservation is a technology to extend the service life of otherwise non-durable timber. As such, therefore, it can be looked upon as a means of conserving a natural resource. Treated timber will outperform untreated material, and since it is derived mainly from renewable forests, it has clear advantages over non-renewable alternative materials. In addition, the costs, both in energy and to the environment, for the production of timber (treated or otherwise) are far less than those for concrete, steel, aluminium, plastic, and so on.

Even the old bush 'remedy' of a coat of finely ground charcoal in raw or boiled linseed oil on the wood surface will give some short-term measure of protection to non-durable species that are in contact with the soil, but for long-term reliability deep penetration with fungicides and insecticides is needed.

Chemicals that are used in the preservation of wood are variable in effect because of the many kinds of degradative agencies and climatic variables referred to above. For example, a compound that is lethal to one type of fungus may have little effect on another; in addition, chemicals that are toxic to fungi may not be sufficiently toxic to termites and marine organisms, so the determination of effective preservative treatments can be complicated.

The main preservatives that are used in commercial treatment plants in Australia can be classified as:

- *water-borne formulations*—which are for heavy duty applications, such as poles, piles and bridges, and for lighter duty applications, such as domestic decking and fencing
- *light organic solvent-borne preservatives* (LOSPs), which are used for the treatment of relatively high-value products, such as joinery and house framing
- *oil-borne preservatives*—which are used for heavy duty applications, such as poles, piles and bridges, while high-temperature creosote (HTC) is mainly used for fence post treatments, where the quality of the finish is less critical than the overall cost of the commodity.

Apart from the marine environment, ground contact is the main hazard to timber and should be avoided unless the species used has a very high natural durability or has been adequately impregnated with non-leachable preservatives.

For timber that is not in ground contact, reduced loadings of preservative are appropriate. Then there are the special cases where only protection against borer attack is required. The AS/NZS 1604 2005 *Specification for Preservative Treatment* series lists the various degrees of hazard and gives requirements for the acceptable amounts of penetration and retention for the approved, commercially available preservatives in Australia.

Preservative treatments are undertaken by trained operators at licensed treatment plants (Plate 38). It is most important that treated off-cuts and wastes are disposed of by approved methods. They should never be burnt as fuel or in barbecues. In many cases, appropriate attention to building detail (e.g. shedding water or keeping it out altogether) can often provide sufficient protection to the timber component against decay to obviate the need for preservative treatment.

Relative durability of species

Natural durability refers to the inherent ability of the heartwood of a timber or tree species to resist decay and insect attack when it is used in ground contact; performance above ground will generally be better. As a rule, durable timbers can be used to build structures without the need for special techniques for their protection. These species will be resistant to fungal attack, wood borers and termites. However, they may not show this resistance to all of these biodeteriogens at the same time. For example, some timbers in Australia are resistant to decay but are attacked by termites.

Traditionally, in Australia, a durability rating has been assigned to the outer heartwood of trees; the sapwood, transition wood (if present) and core wood (inner heartwood and pith) are not considered to be durable. Durability can also vary both within and between trees of the same species and according to position along the length of a tree. Thus, natural durability ratings in Australia are deemed to be guides only in the selection of a timber to do a particular job.

Classification of the durability of a species is not something that can be done with great precision because of the variability of wood properties within species, even within the individual tree, and the variable nature of the hazard, but a classification that has been widely accepted as a general guide is that based on one developed many years ago by CSIRO. It was essentially a rating of the durability of the species' *heartwood* when used in ground contact and exposed to attack by decay and termites; because of this combined assessment the classification does not truly reflect the special qualities of species that are very resistant to termites but much less so to decay (e.g. brush box). A further complication is the size of the specimen at risk. As with exposure to fire, the section size has a significant effect on the rapidity of breakdown; the periods quoted below are relevant to 50 × 50 mm cross-section specimens for in-ground exposure under average Australian conditions and for 35 × 35 mm cross-section specimens exposed above the ground. The ratings should be considered merely as a guideline to *relative* durabilities. As already mentioned, the extent of decay and termite hazard varies greatly in a continent with such a wide range of climates.

The ratings were divided into four classes:

Class 1 Very durable. In excess of 25 years in the ground.
Class 2 Durable. Between 15 and 25 years in the ground.
Class 3 Moderately durable. Between 5 and 15 years in the ground.
Class 4 Non-durable. Between 1 and 5 years in the ground.

It will be appreciated that the classification was very broad and was of no assistance in evaluating the relative merits of species in the same classification. It is well-known that timber exposed fully to the weather but not in ground contact could be expected to have a very much longer service life than timber in ground contact.

In 2003 a new Australian Standard, AS 5604-2003 *Timber—Natural Durability Ratings*, was published to provide natural durability ratings for timber species for use by producers and users of timber product and to reduce the problems associated with different ratings in different Standards that did not always agree with each other. The new Standard was drafted to provide an authoritative source to which the other Standards would refer. The Standard was revised in 2005 to include marine borer resistance classes.

AS 5604 rates:

- the sapwood of a species as being either susceptible or non-susceptible to lyctid borers
- the heartwood of a species as being either resistant or non-resistant to termite attack (inside, above-ground applicable to an H2 situation in the AS/NZS 1604 series)
- the natural durability class of the heartwood when in ground contact
- the natural durability class of heartwood when outside above ground
- the natural durability class of heartwood when exposed to marine borers in southern waters (i.e. south of Perth in the west and south of Batemans Bay in the east).

There are four natural durability classes and Table 16.1 has been compiled from the information published in AS 5604-2003 *Timber—Natural Durability Ratings*.

Table 16.1 Natural durability—probable life expectancy

Class	Probable in-ground life expectancy (years)	Probable above-ground life expectancy (years)	Probable marine borer resistance life expectancy (years)
1	>25	>40	>60
2	15–25	15–40	41–60
3	5–15	7–15	21–40
4	0–5	0–7	0–20 (usually <5)

Again, the classification is very broad and is of no assistance in evaluating the relative merit of species in the same classification. Timber that is exposed fully to the weather but not in ground contact could be expected to have a very much longer service life than timber in ground contact. The above-ground column in Table 16.1 equates to outside above-ground exposure, which is subject to periodic moderate wetting when ventilation and drainage are adequate.

All sapwood has poor resistance to decay; resistance is determined largely by the extractives formed when sapwood changes into heartwood. Termites are less easily deterred by these extractives and will attack most species, although slowly in the case of the very durable species. They tend to avoid species that have a relatively high silica content (e.g. brush box, turpentine) because of their abrasive nature. Marine organisms, too, are deterred to some extent by a high silica content.

Since the fungi that are responsible for decay favour wood that is neither very dry nor very wet, the danger zone for timber members that are embedded in the ground is 200–300 mm above and below the ground line. This is where practically all posts and poles fail, so even with preservative-treated timber it is a desirable procedure to examine this zone at regular intervals for signs of decay.

Timber supplies from traditional native forest resources are being reduced, worldwide, as a result of environmental/sustainability arguments. At the same time, there is an increasing demand for timber and wood fibre (including pulp and paper), and tree plantations are increasingly being utilised to meet more and more of our consumption demand. Trees from plantations are usually young and relatively fast grown. Their wood properties, including durability and treatability, can be different from the wood of trees obtained from more slowly grown native forests. Clearly, this has important ramifications for timber users in their desire to extract maximum service life.

The sapwood of the majority of species is comparatively easily penetrated by preservatives, whereas most heartwood can be very difficult to treat because of the changes that occur to the wood cells at the time of heartwood formation. Most treatment methods for round timbers (e.g. posts, poles, piles) aim to provide a considerable loading of preservative in the ring of sapwood, which should be kept as intact as possible during the harvesting operations. The removal of bumps to improve the aesthetic appearance of round timber must be avoided if the underlying heartwood is not of high durability. Such removal also reduces the structural strength of round timber product.

Immunisation against borer attack

While other borers can sometimes have nuisance value, immunisation in Australia is essentially directed against the lyctid borers, which threaten the sapwood of many hardwood species, especially those of the rainforest with wide sapwoods.

The Australian Standard requires all sapwood to be fully treated for the control of lyctid beetles and so a spray treatment to the sapwood surface is unacceptable. Since lyctid-susceptible timber is often appropriate for use as internal components, it is usual to treat such material with preservatives such as boric acid, borax or other boron-based compounds. A minimum loading of 0.047% mass/mass (% m/m) elemental boron is specified in the Standard to prevent attack.

Copper–chrome–arsenic (CCA) preservatives can also be used, the necessary loading being the equivalent of 0.035% m/m elemental arsenic. There are numerous ways of carrying out the immunisation process and these are described later.

Detection of starch in sapwood

There is no point in immunisation treatment against lyctid borers if there is no starch-bearing sapwood present, so it is important to have a simple test for starch. An aqueous iodine solution that is applied to the suspect timber will rapidly develop a blue-black colour when starch is present. Appendix A of AS 1604.1-2005 *Specification for Preservative Treatment—Sawn and Round Timber* sets down the procedure for preparing the iodine test solution and for its application to the timber surfaces. The colour change will show up more readily on the exposed end-grain. Care must be taken to avoid contamination of the solution.

Methods of immunisation

Nowadays, lyctid-susceptible timber is more often than not treated in a commercial, vacuum pressure impregnation plant. For successful execution some preliminary drying of the timber is desirable. It is loaded into the cylinder (block stacking will enable more economic use of the cylinder) and a vacuum is held for about 30 minutes before the cylinder is flooded with the treatment solution, usually borax or CCA. A pressure of about 1400 kPa is applied for about 60 minutes, when the pressure is released and the solution is pumped out. This process is the one most commonly used for commercial operations as it permits a rapid throughput of timber.

A number of non-pressure processes may also be used and these are outlined below.

Dip diffusion

This method involves the dipping of the green timber, immediately after sawing, usually in a concentrated solution of borax and boric acid. After the excess liquid has drained off, the timber is stacked in a solid block and covered completely with, say, plastic sheeting to prevent drying and to facilitate the diffusion of the preservative throughout the sapwood. The period for which the timber is left in the stack before stripping it out to dry will depend on the thickness of the sawn timber but will usually be several weeks.

Cold soaking

In this method, the timber is stripped out with stickers, as for seasoning, so that the treatment solution can readily contact every surface, and it is then lifted into a tank containing the treatment solution, which is commonly borax. As the timber will tend to float in the solution, the stack needs to be weighted down in some way, otherwise the top boards are likely to be inadequately treated. This method may require a soaking time of up to 2 weeks for 25-mm thick timber, depending on the time of year and the species, so it is only suitable when a small throughput is required. Discolouration of the timber is sometimes a hazard. The process is seldom used commercially in Australia.

Hot and cold bath

As with the above method, after the timber is stripped out with stickers it is immersed in the treatment solution and weighted down to prevent flotation. The solution is then heated to about 85°C and maintained at that level for about 4 hours; it is allowed to cool to at least 60°C over a period of 16 hours before the timber is removed. Timber up to 50-mm thick can usually be treated satisfactorily in a 24-hour schedule. Since the timber will continue to undergo further useful diffusion of the preservative after removal from the solution, it should not be subjected to kiln drying for at least 5 days.

Steaming and cold quench

In this method, the partially seasoned timber is placed in the treatment vessel with restraints to prevent the stack from partially floating when the treatment solution flows in. The timber is first steamed for several hours with live or exhaust steam to raise its full cross-section to about 85°C, taking care to drain away the condensate. The steam is then cut off and the cold treatment solution is flooded in as quickly as possible, making sure that sufficient is added to keep the stack fully immersed at all times. After a soak of about 6 hours the solution is pumped out and the timber is removed to the drying area.

Spot test for immunised timber

The effective execution of the treatment process involves regular monitoring of the concentration of the treatment solution and analysis of treated wood to ensure the presence of the necessary amount and distribution of preservative. The details of the sampling procedures are given in AS/NZS 1605:2000 *Methods for Sampling and Analysing Timber Preservatives and Preservative-Treated Timber* and further details on the analysis of the treated wood and treatment solution may be sought from the forestry authorities in New South Wales and Queensland.

If it is important for timber users to have an immediate means of obtaining an indication of the presence of the treatment chemical, even if it does not reveal the actual concentration present, then a chemical spot test of freshly prepared and treated timber surfaces may be carried out in accordance with AS/NZS 1605:2000.

Preservative treatment against decay and termite attack

Preservative methods vary from simple brush treatments and momentary immersion through to those involving capital-intensive sophisticated treatment plants, typically employing pressures up to 1400 kPa and operating under strict licensing and guidelines, in accordance with Federal and state requirements.

It is common to apply a regular brushing treatment to the inside of boats, for example, with solutions of fungicides such as copper naphthenate and copper 8-quinolinolate in light mineral oil solvent as a deterrent to fungi, while dip treatments, usually with an immersion time of 3 minutes, may be used for windows and other joinery. By including waxes and resins as well as a fungicide, the end-grain is sealed to some extent against moisture entry (and exit) and the article is dimensionally stabilised as well as given a degree of protection against decay, provided it is then painted to ensure retention of the preservative. Such dip treatments are more accurately described as water-repellent treatments; they are not preservative treatments in the true sense of the word since they are unlikely to penetrate all sapwood that may be present or provide a skin of heartwood which has received a significant depth of penetration. A more complete degree of preservation for commodities such as windows and external joinery is achieved through LOSPs, which are delivered in double-vacuum or low-pressure treatment plants.

For commercial production it is usually desirable to have equipment that is capable of providing both vacuum and pressure to speed up the impregnation process, but dip diffusion and sap replacement are two methods involving little capital investment.

In the wet conditions found in tropical countries, such as Papua New Guinea, there is often a need for some preservative treatment of building components against decay and insect attack even when they are neither in ground contact nor fully exposed to the elements.

Methods involving a combination of vacuum and pressure

Full cell treatment

With this method, the wood cells remain full of the treatment solution at the end of the process and the method is used mostly for water-borne preservatives, such as CCA, where the recovery of solvent is not of economic importance and where there is no problem arising from the subsequent bleeding of preservative. After the timber is placed in the treatment cylinder a vacuum is applied to remove as much air as possible from the timber and so help to obtain the maximum absorption of the solution. The vacuum is maintained while the preservative is pumped into the cylinder. Then a pressure of about 1400 kPa is applied until the required uptake of solution has occurred. The term 'Bethell process' is sometimes applied to the full cell method.

Empty cell treatment

Empty cell treatment depends on the air trapped in the cells to expel surplus preservative and so avoids the risk of its subsequent bleeding from the timber, which can be a problem with creosote and furnace oil. The two main types of empty cell treatment are the Lowry process and the Rueping process.

In the Lowry process the solution is flooded in at normal atmospheric pressure and the displaced air escapes freely. The treatment pressure is then applied until the required uptake of solution is achieved. The pressure is released, the solution is pumped out of the cylinder and a short period of vacuum is applied, which causes the compressed air in the wood to expel much of the free liquid within the cells.

In the Rueping process additional air is placed in the wood cells by applying considerable air pressure before the solution is in the cylinder and maintaining it at that level until the timber is fully immersed, when the full treatment pressure is applied. When the final vacuum is applied the presence of the extra air results in a greater expulsion of the free liquid in the cells and so ensures less risk of bleeding of preservative when the treated article is in service.

Boultonising

Most pressure treatments involve preliminary air drying to remove some of the water present in the wood cells but this period of waiting is bypassed in the Boultonising process, which involves the immersion of the timber under vacuum in hot creosote or other oil. The heat drives out the water, which is replaced in the cell walls by the oil.

Temperatures above 120°C and treatment times of more than 12 hours can affect the strength of the timber and tend to increase the amount of surface checking but generally the weakening effect of Boultonising is only of significance with the lower density species, particularly softwoods. The aim of the method is to remove a measured amount of water by boiling the oil under vacuum and then applying a pressure of about 1400 kPa until the required retention is obtained. A final vacuum is usually applied to make the timber clean enough to handle comfortably.

Oscillating and alternating pressure

Timber that is difficult to impregnate can often be penetrated more deeply if it is first presteamed and then processed with oscillating periods of pressure and normal conditions, or alternating periods of vacuum and pressure.

Some common preservative chemicals

Today's preservatives have to be effective, long-lasting, economically feasible, and have minimum environmental impact. The preservatives used in Australia include:

- water-borne preservatives—CCA, ammoniacal copper quaternary (ACQ), copper azole (CuAz) and a number of boron-based compounds
- oil-borne preservatives—creosote and pigment-emulsified creosote (PEC)
- light organic solvent-borne preservatives (LOSPs)—tributyl tin naphthenate (TBTN), copper naphthenate, zinc naphthenate, azoles, plus a number of synthetic pyrethroids, such as permethrin and bifenthrin, and some resins and waxes to increase water repellency.

In addition to the above primary listing of preservatives, a number of remedial products are used in situ to reduce or eliminate existing decay and insect problems. These formulations include propriety products that come in many forms, such as gels, brush ons and insertable rods and tablets.

Methods for treating solid timber, both round and sawn, include full cell and empty cell processes, as described above, and, for value-added joinery, the LOSP process described below. In the cases of engineered wood products, such as plywood, laminated veneer lumber, glued laminated timber, the chemicals may be delivered by any of these processes but, in addition, the preservative may be added to the glue during manufacture of the product. For example, the application of preservative to plywood may be made to the veneers, the glue, a combination of both, or to the finished sheet using normal vacuum pressure treatment processes.

Treatment with LOSPs

LOSPs are preservatives that contain insecticides for internal use, and combinations of fungicides and insecticides for external use, and sometimes water repellents. LOSPs may also contain mouldicides. All of these preservative components are incorporated in a light organic solvent carrier, such as white spirit.

LOSPs are used to protect timber against insects, including termites, and decay, although they are not intended for use in ground-contact situations. In addition, LOSPs can provide a degree of weather protection when water repellents have been incorporated. The LOSP process leaves the treated timber dry after treatment, and does not cause it to swell and distort in any way.

This treatment method involves the use of low pressure, empty cell or double vacuum methods to give an uptake of preservative suitable for joinery, cladding and so on, but it is not suitable for timber in more hazardous situations or in ground contact. The timber is dried to equilibrium moisture content and all machining, drilling and so on is preferably done before treatment. The timber is block stacked with stickers at every third layer. After an initial vacuum the cylinder is flooded with solution and the vacuum maintained for 10 minutes; then pressure is returned to atmospheric level or, in resistant species, an elevated pressure may be applied for another 3 minutes. A final vacuum for 15 minutes removes most of the solvent. The Rueping process is also used with LOSPs.

Condition of timber before preservative treatment

Before timber is subjected to any of the preservative treatments outlined above, a few preliminary tasks are performed.

Bark must be removed from round timber not only to aid drying but, in the case of softwoods, to allow penetration of preservative through the rays. In hardwoods the presence of the bark is less critical since most penetration is along the vessels and the most essential feature is that the end-grain does not become clogged. Therefore, any end coatings that are used to inhibit splitting during the preliminary air drying must be cut off before the start of the preservation process.

If a pressure process is involved there is usually a need for the moisture content of the wood to be reduced, especially if oil-type preservatives are being used. With water-borne types it is usual to reduce the moisture content to the vicinity of the fibre saturation point (i.e. about 25–30 per cent), although plantation pines, if given a presteaming treatment, can be treated immediately after felling.

During the preliminary drying there is a risk of insect attack (e.g. from bostrychid borers) and bluestain, so care is needed in regard to proper stacking, yard hygiene, and spraying to control insect attack. Drying under cover is very desirable in the wetter climates. The development of severe bluestain can cause excessive absorption of chemicals.

In large sections of timber, such as railway sleepers, which are predominantly of difficult-to-treat heartwood, additional points of entry for preservative to assist in providing a skin of treated wood are obtained by *incising*, which involves the passage of the timber between rollers fitted with many short knife blades.

A variant of this is the process called *brucising*, a combination of bruising and incising, which is produced by fitting the rollers with blunt-toothed chain sprockets. Incising is usually carried out parallel to the grain, resulting in a parting rather than a severing of the vessels; a means of incising at a slight angle would be more effective.

Surface checking is also very helpful in increasing the points of preservative entry, and all bolt holes should be drilled before treatment to ensure a good skin of treated wood in their vicinity. Machining after treatment could remove much of the protective shell of preservative-treated wood.

Effective distribution of preservative

In addition to obtaining the desired loading of preservative in the timber it is important to get a relatively even distribution. Hardwoods are likely to cause more problems in this regard than softwoods; preservative enters along the hardwood vessels but the amount of penetration into the surrounding fibres depends on wood density, moisture content, temperature and pressure of the process, as well as the type of preservative used. This variable penetration has been a factor in the rapid entry of soft rot fungi into hardwood poles.

The problem of uneven penetration can be addressed by careful control of the treatment operation, ensuring that each load preferably contains only one size, one species group and one moisture content range. Some overtreatment may be necessary to ensure that all the treated wood reaches the minimum requirement. Inadequate predrying, with high moisture gradients, is a common cause of uneven penetration.

In areas where soft rot is a serious problem in poles, regular maintenance of the ground-line area of the pole is essential. One approach has been to present a physical barrier by encapsulating the butt of the pole in polyethylene sheeting and a bitumen coating, while another involves the provision of a bandage of polyurethane foam that is impregnated with fungicidal salts and backed by bitumen-lined polyethylene sheeting, which is heat-shrunk onto the pole. The bitumen tends to flow into the surface checks on the pole.

Preservative loadings

The Australian Standards series AS/NZS 1604 *Specification for Preservative Treatment* provides guidelines for the requirements for penetration and retention of the commercial preservatives used on a large scale in Australia in relation to various degrees of hazard and the end-use requirements.

In view of the likelihood of considerable alterations to the requirements of the AS/NZS 1604 series, no figures will be quoted here on the loadings required for the various degrees of hazard. The interested reader should refer to the current edition of that Standard series.

In New South Wales and Queensland the forestry authorities administer the *Timber Marketing Act 1977* and the *Timber Utilization and Marketing Act 1987*, respectively, and have the power to make their own requirements concerning approved chemicals, treatment methods and loadings, which are usually in line with those in AS/NZS 1604 series, although they do not have to be and so it is essential for commercial operators and purchasers of preservative-treated timber in those states to maintain a close liaison with the forestry authorities.

In general, it is necessary for all sapwood to be fully penetrated by preservative, but since heartwood is difficult to penetrate the requirement is usually for only a skin of, for example, 5–10 mm of heartwood to have the full loading of preservative, depending on the cross-section, end use and so on.

Marine piling is usually subject to particularly severe attack by marine organisms so a double treatment is often recommended, first with CCA and then with creosote.

Fire retardants

Some chemicals are able to give wood a considerable degree of protection against fire but most are water-soluble and thus are restricted mainly for internal use. The most effective of these are mono-ammonium phosphate, di-ammonium phosphate, borax and sodium fluoride. Commercial fire-retardant treatments are not widely offered in Australia and the preservation Standard, AS/NZS 1604 series, does not specify them.

Information on the use of fire-retardant treated timber can be found in Chapter 21.

Safety aspects of timber preservation

By definition, a preservative consists of chemicals that are toxic to some organisms. This does not mean that they are toxic to humans but, of course, the preservation industry is very conscious of the need to ensure that both the chemicals at the treatment plant and treated timber that leaves the plant are handled in appropriate ways.

The treatment industry provides point-of-sale literature that is designed to advise the user about sensible handling and disposal procedures. In addition, a Materials Safety Data Sheet (MSDS) is available for registered and approved wood preservatives and preservative-treated timber. The MSDS contains information on toxicity, chemical and physical properties of ingredients in the preservative, recommended handling requirements, transport and storage information, actions for spillages and instructions to deal with accidental poisoning. MSDS sheets can be obtained from the preservative manufacturers.

It is sound practice to handle preservative-treated timber with gloves and to wear protective equipment, such as dust masks and eye protection, when working with it (Plate 39). Also, it is recommended that preservative-treated timber wastes (e.g. off-cuts, building site debris) are not disposed of by burning, especially in open fires and on barbecues. These materials may be taken to approved landfill sites for disposal.

Australian Pesticides and Veterinary Medicines Authority

The Australian Pesticides and Veterinary Medicines Authority (APVMA) assesses and registers agricultural and veterinary chemicals, including wood preservatives. The APVMA is a statutory Commonwealth authority with Australia-wide responsibility for registration and control of the chemicals under a national scheme. It was established with agreement of the six states (Tasmania, Victoria, New South Wales, Queensland, South Australia and Western Australia) and the two territories (Australian Capital Territory and Northern Territory) that make up the Commonwealth of Australia. The legislation establishing the APVMA came into effect in June 1993 and is intended to assure the public that chemicals on the market are effective, suitably formulated and labelled, are safe when used as directed, and do not have adverse effects on the environment. In other words, the APVMA controls the use of chemicals up to the point of sale of the chemical. The states and territories control chemical application, and each has their own suite of legislation that governs preservative use and treatment plant operation, and, in New South Wales and Queensland, the sale of treated timber.

The APVMA administers the *Agricultural and Veterinary Chemicals Code Act 1994*, which is a package of legislation dealing with registration and registration fees and charges. This Act commenced in March 1995. The Act includes, as a schedule, the 'Agvet Code'. The Act is a law of the Commonwealth that only applies in the Australian Capital Territory but each of the six states and the Northern Territory have enacted complementary legislation that has the effect that the Agvet Code provisions may be applied as a law of each state and the Northern Territory. The Code itself determines the detailed operational provisions for registering chemical products, including wood preservatives, and provides the APVMA with its range of powers.

Under the Agvet Code the APVMA evaluates, registers and regulates preservative chemicals up to the point of sale.

FURTHER READING

Referenced

Anon. (2004). Treated timber in Australia: CCA and the alternatives. NTDP tech. report. Issue 5. May 2004. Canberra: Forest and Wood Products Research & Development Corporation.

Australian/New Zealand Standard. AS/NZS 1604 series. *Specification for preservative treatment.*

Australian Standard. (2005). AS 1604.1 *Specification for Preservative Treatment—Sawn and Round Timber.*

Australian/New Zealand Standard. (2000). AS/NZS 1605 *Methods for Sampling and Analysing Timber Preservatives and Preservative-Treated Timber.*

Australian Standard. (2003). AS 5604 *Timber—Natural Durability Ratings.*

Greaves, H. (2002). *Wood and wood preservation. A complete guide to the AS/NZS 1604 Standards series.* Canberra: Standards Australia Handbook HB 164-2002.

National Association of Forest Industries. (2003). Timber—design for durability. Timber datafile P4. Canberra: NAFI.

National Association of Forest Industries. (2004). Protecting buildings from subterranean termites. Timber datafile P5. Canberra: NAFI.

Richardson, B. A. (1993). *Wood preservation.* London: Construction Press.

Wilkinson, J. G. (1979). *Industrial timber preservation.* London: Associated Business Press.

Websites

Forest and Wood Products Research and Development Corporation, viewed 6 March 2005, <http://www.timber.org.au>.

Preservedwood, viewed 6 March 2005, <http://www.preservedwood.com.au>.

Timber Preservers Association of Australia, viewed 6 March 2005, <http://www.tpaa.com.au>.

Wood Preservative Science Council, viewed 6 March 2005, <http://www.woodpreservativescience.org>.

Chapter 17

Use of wood residues

In the conversion of natural round logs to timber and veneers, a range of residues are produced. Many of these are fully utilised as by-products in urban areas but not to the same extent in rural localities. Residues are generated from sawmills in both the softwood and hardwood sectors and can be broadly classified as sawdust, off-cuts, shavings, chip and bark. There are substantial gains in utilising these residues, providing both environmental and economic benefits. However, wherever possible sawmills will always attempt to recover more timber from the log, rather than generate residues, due to the much higher financial gains from timber production and the associated value adding. By-products are mainly used in the production of board materials, such as particleboard and medium-density fibreboard (MDF), landscape and horticulture markets and also for renewable energy production in the forms of both heat and electricity.

Of the residues produced in most softwood operations excluding cypress, approximately 40 per cent is bark, 30 per cent woodchip, 20 per cent sawdust, and 10 per cent shavings and dockings. The bark is usually sold to the landscape industry, where it is graded into various sizes, with the fines used for soil mixes and compost. The remainder (i.e. woodchip, sawdust and shavings) is usually destined for board production, with some utilised in the rural and horticultural sectors as well as for energy production (Plate 40).

Cypress residues consist mainly of sawdust and wings (the outer tapered portion of the tree containing the bark). However, more recently some mills are debarking their logs and this material is chipped for fibreboard production. Cypress contains natural extractives that make its heartwood resistant to termite activity. Consequently, wings are also chipped or hogged for use as garden mulch. The sawdust is not, however, fully utilised. In recent years there has been extensive research into utilising cypress residues because of its unique properties.

Hardwood sawmills produce residues in the form of sawdust, wings, shavings, chip and hearts (the central portion of the log that is often eaten out by termites). From sawmills, wings and hearts constitute much of the residues, followed by sawdust and lesser volumes of shavings and chip. Hearts are more often being split and after the mud from termite activity is removed they are chipped along with the wings. Because hardwood sawmills are often relatively small and located in rural areas, residues may not be fully utilised. Where utilised, they generally find application in the landscaping and horticulture industries and in some instances as boiler fuel. It should be noted that some states in Australia prohibit the export of chipped hardwood residues for potential use in pulp manufacture.

In addition to the residues that are produced from the conversion of logs into sawn timber, residues are now being recovered from forestry operations. This includes chipping of non-millable logs, branches and limbs. Any material remaining from these processes stays in the forest, where it naturally breaks down.

Uses of residues

Bark

Generally, the bark is separated from the log in most softwood production but, due to the different nature of the bark in hardwoods, it may not be removed prior to sawing.

Bark is a problem contaminant in the manufacture of board products, largely because of its dark colour. For this reason softwood sawmills debark the logs before processing, enabling the bark to be separated out. Bark that breaks up into chunks, as does that on the mature stems of the plantation pines, finds a ready market as a soil cover in landscaping. The stringy types of bark, such as from hoop pine, are generally processed into larger pieces and more generally used in non-residential applications.

Bark is usually richer in polyphenolic compounds than wood itself. The bark of radiata pine is rich in tannins, which can be used as a replacement for phenol and resorcinol in waterproof phenolic-type adhesives.

Soil improvers

Residues are utilised as soil improvers in the form of mulch, compost or peat substitute in potting mixes. Sawdust and shavings have the attraction of being low cost, free of weeds and easy to handle, but their very low nitrogen content demands a careful approach to their use. Residues with preservative treatment are not appropriate for this application.

Mulch

The provision of a layer of organic material on the surface of the soil is often described as mulching. A mulch has valuable growth-promoting properties in that it holds moisture in the soil, reduces run-off, minimises compaction of the soil, provides a more even temperature, reduces weed growth, encourages earthworms and produces humus.

Sawdust, shavings and bark can be used as a mulch provided they are not incorporated with the soil. The freshly produced material contains a lot of extractives of polyphenolic nature, which are leached out by water and may have a phytotoxic (plant-killing) effect, particularly on young seedlings. Weathering for a few months, preferably with the addition of some limestone to speed the leaching of any extractives, will overcome that problem but the weathered material requires a number of light applications of nitrogenous fertiliser prior to it being incorporated into soil. If it is used just as a surface mulch the microbiological activity involving nitrogen uptake will be confined to the surface layer of soil and there will be no harmful effect. If considerable mixing with the soil occurs there will be a great drain on the nitrogen in that soil, resulting in the yellowing of plant leaves in the vicinity and stunting of plant growth.

The addition of nitrogenous fertiliser has long-term value. A lot of it is incorporated in the bodies of the microorganisms and as they die it will be released slowly to the soil. The desirable depth of a mulch is about 75–100 mm. The mulch should not be too close to the stems of fruit trees and so on, whose growth it is intended to encourage, as otherwise collar rot could be promoted. Topping up may be desirable every couple of years.

Compost

Sawdust may be used in planting mixes when given a preliminary composting treatment that involves the incorporation of supplementary nitrogen (urea is a common source), limestone or dolomite, superphosphate and potash. Blood and bone and poultry manure may also be added. The moisture content of the mix is critical to success and should be within the range 80–120 per cent.

Animal litter

Sawdust and shavings provide a satisfactory deep litter for intensive poultry production, absorbing as much as 90 per cent of the nitrogen in the excreta. The addition of superphosphate before spreading spent litter will help to prevent rapid leaching of the nitrogen content. It is important to avoid the use of preservative-treated wood in litter or bedding for animals that seek out food within that material. The spent litter is used as a soil fertiliser.

Energy

Wood residues also provide a valuable fuel source, which is both renewable and sustainable. Many of the larger sawmills have boilers either to generate steam or to heat oil as the heat transfer medium for the kiln drying of timber. Many products, including those used internally, such as house framing and flooring, as well as many used externally, such as decking, benefit from kiln drying. Drying makes timber lighter, less susceptible to insect attack, more stable and stronger.

Biomass fuel, to which timber residues belong, is becoming increasingly important for use in co-generation plants that produce both heat for production use and electricity. In these plants the electricity generated is used by the plant, with the excess exported to the grid. One of the larger plants of this type is the 17 MW co-generation plant of Visy Industries in New South Wales. In other areas wood residues are increasingly being used as a supplement in bagasse (sugar cane fibre) fuelled co-generation plants in sugar mills. Wood residue fuelled co-generation plants represent only a small proportion of the installed biomass capacity, which in turn is very small in relation to the capacity of coal- and gas-fired power stations. Because biomass-generated energy is essentially carbon neutral, its use as an alternative to fossil fuels is being encouraged.

Research

In recent years alternative uses for residues and combined use with other industry sectors has been investigated. Research has included composting sawdust with cattle feedlot manure. The feedlot waste (manure) is high in nitrogen and, if allowed to decompose naturally, a significant proportion of the nitrogen would be lost to the atmosphere or could enter watercourses, rather than being locked into the compost in a form that could be utilised by plants. To retain the nitrogen it is necessary to add a material that has a high carbon-to-nitrogen ratio. Sawdust is an ideal material that is able to provide this.

The agricultural industry needs to control a variety of pests (e.g. nematodes) and fungi (e.g. *Pythium, Rhizoctonia*) to produce good crops and currently a range of pesticides and fungicides are used to maintain control. Research has indicated that soil to which sawdust has been added has consistently suppressed root-knot nematodes.

Research with cypress includes the separation of extractives from heartwood residues to assess insecticidal and fungicidal properties. Similarly, research is also being undertaken to determine whether a mix of pine and cypress in board products will show enhanced termite and decay resistance.

FURTHER READING

Department of Communications, Information Technology and the Arts. (2003). *Australian renewable energy*. Canberra: Commonwealth of Australia.

Ironside, G. E. (1976). Potting composts from eucalypt mill waste by accelerated maturation technique. Australian Institute of Horticulture 2(3). Reprint 3. Sydney: Forestry Commission of NSW.

Ironside, G. E. (1977). Some technological aspects of hardwood mill residues for horticultural usage. Reprint 10. Sydney: Forestry Commission of NSW.

Ironside, G. E. (1977). Are pine bark mulches advantageous under damp conditions? Australian Institute of Horticulture 2(7). Reprint 342. Sydney: Forestry Commission of NSW.

Ironside, G. E. (1979). Preservatives in sawmill residues. Reprint 107. Sydney: Forestry Commission of NSW.

Liversidge, R. M. (1973). Utilisation of sawmill residue. *Aust For Ind J* 38(12): 42–7.

Nichols, D. and Yasaki, Y. (1979). Phytotoxicity of *Eucalyptus camaldulensis* and *E. regnans* sawdusts. *Aust For Res* 9: 35–9.

Pittaway, P., Slizankiewicz, V., Spence, M. (2001). AGWISE Part B: Waste reuse strategies for rural development and sustainability. National Centre for Engineering in Agriculture. Publication 179714/1. Appendix E. Toowoomba: University of Southern Queensland.

Yasaki, Y. and Nichols, D. (1978). Phytotoxic components of *Pinus radiata* bark. *Aust For Res* 8: 185–98.

Chapter 18

Wood as fuel

Wood is unlikely to be a primary source of energy in industrialised countries where even forest planting, roading and logging are currently dependent on liquid fuels. Wood saves far more energy when substituted for metals and concrete as a construction material than is provided by burning it as a fuel.

It also competes in its requirements for land with other uses, such as food production, water catchment, national parks and wilderness areas, so that if there are other energy sources (such as coal) available these will be preferred. Wood has an energy content of about 9.5 GJ/tonne, at 50 per cent moisture content, compared with about 26 GJ/tonne for coal and 38 GJ/tonne for oil. Wood can be converted into liquid fuels, such as ethanol and methanol, but the processes are expensive. However, it may be worthwhile for the sawmilling industry to provide its own energy by returning to the use of mill waste, as it has done for a very long time. Unused forest residuals could provide a considerable amount of fuel but a better economic return might be obtained by converting them into chips for paper production.

Environmentally, wood is a relatively clean source of heat energy, with a very low sulfur emission and low ash residue, but for satisfactory combustion it is usually necessary first to dry out some of its large water content, otherwise about half of its heat value is devoted to this task. The denser species have the advantage of yielding a larger amount of heat per unit volume but this tends to be partly counterbalanced by their slower rate of drying. Generally, the lower the density, the lower the ignition temperature.

The temperature reached by burning wood depends on the rapidity of combustion, which varies considerably between species. Those that are high in water-soluble extractives often tend to smoulder and char and perform poorly in the domestic open fireplace. Such wood can give better heat if stacked vertically in the grate. Other species contain extractives (such as the resins in conifers), which may assist in speeding combustion, but those species are not favoured for fuel in open fireplaces because of greater sootiness and spark production. Species that are good sources of fuel include the wattles, casuarinas, ironbarks and eucalypt boxes.

The calorific value of oven-dry eucalypt hardwood is about 19 kJ/g and that of softwood is about 21 kJ/g. Values vary slightly between species but these figures reflect the practical situation. The calorific value of green timber varies with species and the actual moisture content present. However, as a rough guideline it would average about 60 per cent of that of the oven-dry figure.

The calorific value (HE) at a particular moisture content (MC) can be calculated from its oven-dry value (HO) by using this formula:

$$HE = HO \frac{(100 - \frac{MC}{8})}{100 + MC}$$

The ability to obtain a satisfactory amount of the heat that is potentially available depends on the efficiency of the burner, which is determined not only by its design and air supply but also by the size of the fuel supplied.

The ash content of wood is very low, often being well below 1 per cent; sapwood usually yields more than heartwood. Bark has a considerably higher ash content, sometimes as much as 10 per cent but more usually 2 or 3 per cent. With rough-barked trees the amount present in practice can vary considerably because of soil incorporation during felling and haulage. Humphreys and Ironside (1980) report analyses for a wide range of NSW species. Bark has a calorific value akin to that of wood.

Sawdust and shavings

The increasing cost of energy has directed attention to the need to make better use of residues. Sawdust may amount to as much as 20 per cent of the log and bark 10 per cent. Sawdust is relatively bulky, occupying about three times the volume of the equivalent solid timber, and is produced in a very wet condition. Its finely divided nature requires special equipment for its combustion, such as a Dutch oven with automatic feed, so in that state it is only suitable for industrial plants. For household use it is necessary to compact sawdust and shavings into 'logs', briquettes or pellets. To do so it is necessary for the wood to be dried down to the range 8–15 per cent moisture content (preferably 8–10 per cent) to secure a satisfactory product when compacted.

The compaction process involves the use of a high-pressure ram that is capable of perhaps 300 000 kPa, which forces the material through a die. The high pressure develops a temperature up to 180°C, which is sufficient to soften the lignin and make the wood self-bonding. Adhesives are not suitable, largely because their fumes would be unpleasant during combustion. The moisture content is critical because the steam that is generated tends to rupture the product; for this reason, pellets are easier to produce satisfactorily than the much larger 'logs'. Because of the high energy input required for the compaction, the net energy balance is not favourable and the operation only seems to be viable if there is plenty of the waste material available close to a market. Bark, too, can be used but its higher ash content makes it less attractive.

Preservative-treated sawdust and shavings are unacceptable. Boron compounds can damage grates while the volatilisation of the arsenic from wood containing copper–chrome–arsenic (CCA) would be a potential health hazard in domestic fuel.

In commercial environments, research is being undertaken to allow the burning of CCA-preservative treated timber safely, recovering both the energy from the burning wood and the basic elements of the preservative treatment chemical.

Slow combustion heaters

Slow combustion heaters are designed to operate on fuel that is high in carbon content but low in volatile matter.

Wood does not compare well with other fuels on this criterion of acceptance, as indicated by the generalised figures shown in Table 18.1.

Table 18.1 Fixed carbon and volatile content

Fuel	Volatile matter (%)	Fixed carbon (%)	Ash (%)
Wood	80	20	<1
Peat	65	30	5
Brown coal	50	45	5
Black coal	30	65	5
Anthracite	4	93	3
Coke	1	92	7

If only a very limited volume of air is admitted, as can be the case when such stoves are shut down overnight, the wood will be virtually distilled to produce a considerable amount of wood creosotes and tars, which condense in the flue and may eventually cause a blockage. In recent years there has been a real improvement in the design of slow combustion heaters. The passage of air inside the heaters is designed to ensure more efficient burning of wood. Some heaters have air inlets that adjust the rate of air intake when it falls below the desired level during those periods that the heater is shut down (as for overnight burning). If wood is used because of the lack of a more suitable fuel, the air supply should be plentiful and well-dried, non-resinous wood used.

Charcoal

Charcoal is a form of carbon obtained by the incomplete combustion of wood, which has a considerably higher calorific value than wood and is on a par with other high carbon fuels. Its calorific value is in the range 29–37 kJ/g, while coal is 28–33 kJ/g, coke 28–30 kJ/g and kerosene 46 kJ/g.

Charcoal is manufactured in large 'kilns' in which the wood is heated with a limited supply of air, sufficient to effect the removal of volatile gases and tars but not enough to oxidise much of the carbon. An exothermic reaction begins at about 270°C, after which no further external heat is required. The temperature may reach 400–500°C. The distilled products comprise methanol, acetic acid, acetone and phenols (given the collective title of 'pyroligneous acid'), wood tar (which contains the distillation products insoluble in water) and wood gas. For some industrial uses the charcoal may need further heating to remove tars with a higher boiling point. The ash content of the charcoal varies considerably between species, from 0.3–4 per cent with occasional instances of nearly 7 per cent. Figures for a number of species are given by Humphreys and Ironside (1980). The ash content has some effect on the absorbent properties of activated charcoal.

As well as being a valuable concentrated fuel, charcoal finds considerable use in metallurgy and as a filtering and decolouring agent. There was a considerable demand for it in the manufacture of carbon disulfide, a principal ingredient in the manufacture of rayon, but this fibre has since been displaced by other synthetics.

Research is being carried out by the CSIRO in the use of finely divided charcoal as a supplement to fuel oil.

FURTHER READING

Bridie, R. M. (1980). Utilisation of sawmill residues for steam generation. *Appita* 34(1): 47–53.

Harries, E. D. (1979). Wood for energy generation: an estimate of availability from Australian forests. 19th Forest Products Research Conference. Melbourne: CSIRO.

Houghton, J. E. and Johnson, L. R. (1976). Wood for energy. *For Prod J* 26(4): 15–18.

Humphreys, F. R. and Ironside, G. E. (1980). Charcoal from New South Wales species of timber. Research note 44. Sydney: Forestry Commission of NSW.

Ince, P. J. (1979). How to estimate recoverable heat energy in wood or bark fuels. General tech. report FPL 29. Washington, DC: USDA Forest Products Laboratory.

King, K. R. (1979). Wood residue: a technical appraisal of its production, disposal and use. *TRADA Information Bulletin* 1/79.

Seidl, R. J. (1980). Energy from wood: a new dimension in utilisation. *Tappi* 63(1): 26–9.

Soltes, E. J. (1980). Pyrolysis of wood residues. *Tappi* 63(7): 75–7.

Stewart, G. A., Gartside, G., Gifford, R. M., et al. (1979). *The potential for liquid fuels from agriculture and forestry in Australia*. Melbourne: CSIRO.

Weiss, D. E. (1979). Energy from biomass. *Appita* 33(2): 101–10.

Chapter 19

Health problems in wood processing

The preparation of the smooth surface that is desired for most furniture and other wood-based articles of decorative appearance usually involves the process of *sanding*, which creates a fine dust that is liable to cause some irritation, especially in summer, from its abrasive physical properties alone. Careful attention to dust extraction systems, good ventilation and personal hygiene normally keep the problem under control. However, some species require a much greater need for care as their fine dust may cause allergies among some workers who either have an innate sensitivity to them or develop it after a period of exposure. This sensitivity may be reflected in dermatitis, inflammation of the nasal membranes or irritation of the respiratory tract.

There are two types of dermatitis, *irritant dermatitis* and *sensitisation dermatitis*. The former is due to the presence of chemicals in handled materials, such as alkaloids and some tannins, and the localised irritation persists only while the worker is working with the material. In sensitisation dermatitis the worker develops an allergic reaction—eczema-like symptoms—that may extend to large areas of the body and which can be triggered off by exposure to small amounts of the dust which would have little effect on unsensitised skin.

The face, eyes, neck, nose and mouth are vulnerable areas, as are areas subject to considerable sweat production (e.g. armpits, groin). The skin irritants may also affect the mucous membranes of the nose and throat, but often this is a separate problem. As well as soreness, the nose and eyes may discharge copious quantities of fluid and become inflamed; asthmatic wheezing may follow.

Such problems arise more in furniture factories than in sawmills, where the wood particle size is generally much larger. Efficient dust extraction is the basic requirement; where this is not fully achievable the use of a face mask will protect the mouth and throat from irritation but these masks are uncomfortable to use for extended periods. Protective clothing and good personal hygiene are essential and showering facilities should be available to remove the dust at the end of the day's work. Barrier cream is of little help against dust irritation, although it may be useful where mere contact with the wood causes an adverse reaction.

Species that can produce nasal or skin irritants include black bean, various silky oaks, grey satinash, nyatoh, coachwood, western red cedar, cypress, iroko, guarea, African mahogany, makoré, Crow's ash, silky beech, blackwood, miva mahogany, teak, spotted gum, white birch, kwila, Australian red cedar and yellow carabeen. A comprehensive list is provided by Bolza (1976).

Preservative-treated timber needs care in its handling, particularly at the time when the treatment process is carried out. When handling freshly treated timber that is still wet from the treatment fluids used, impervious gloves and an apron should be worn and hands should be washed before eating, drinking or smoking. It is also important to avoid exposure to the fine mists that may be produced immediately upon opening the treatment vessel door after some treatment processes.

Creosote stains skin and may cause dermatitis, but when handled carefully in order to minimise contact it usually presents no problems. Some individuals may exhibit sensitisation to creosote, and working with creosote-treated wood, particularly in bright sunlight, may give rise to a sunburn-like skin condition. This can be avoided if gloves and protective clothing are used and care is taken to avoid liquid creosote directly contacting bare skin. The use of barrier creams is also good practice when working with creosote.

Potassium dichromate (used in copper–chrome–arsenic [CCA] salts) can cause dermatitis and even ulcers if it is allowed to penetrate cuts and abrasions, so these should be suitably covered. Today's CCA formulations are predominantly oxide-based, with a lower risk of dermatitis from handling.

Sodium pentachlorphenate can cause dermatitis when wet timber is handled but there is little risk when the wood is seasoned. This preservative is now little used in Australia but occasionally may be encountered as an anti-sap-stain treatment.

It is always advisable to handle any timber, including preservative-treated timber, with care by adopting good practices, such as wearing eye protection, gloves and dust masks when sawing and machining. In addition, after handling preservative-treated timber hands should be washed before eating, drinking or smoking.

All today's preservatives can be supplied with Material Safety Data Sheets or Safety Data Sheets and these can be obtained from the preservative manufacturer. The most at-risk members of the population are not the consumers of treated wood but the workers at the treatment plants, and today's treatment plant operations emphasise good practice to minimise worker exposure to the chemicals.

The thermosetting adhesives that incorporate formaldehyde need careful handling because of the susceptibility of some people to the formaldehyde. Barrier cream and gloves should be used. When urea formaldehyde is used in the manufacture of particleboard, it is difficult to avoid incorporating a small excess of formaldehyde. Sometimes the fumes build up to an irritant level in closed, freshly constructed cupboards incorporating particleboard. Good ventilation will often be sufficient to remedy the situation; alternatively, a coating with varnish or paint will reduce the emission of formaldehyde to an acceptable level. Modern manufacturing plants of wood-based composites aim to produce product with defined, extremely low levels of post-fabrication chemical emissions, including formaldehyde.

There is a widespread perception that the use of CCA preservative in the preservation of plantation pines may pose a health hazard because of the arsenic content. The round timbers commonly used for park fences and children's playgrounds, for example, present no hazard so long as the timber has been properly treated, the CCA chemicals have been fully reacted and the timber surfaces are free of deposits that may have arisen as a result of the treatment process. If the users of treated timber wish, CCA-treated timber surfaces may be washed/scrubbed before using the timber. Also, the surfaces may be coated with a protective layer, such as polyurethane, or paint. The instances where CCA-treated timber can present a health hazard are in sanding the wood and in burning the off-cuts and sawdust in confined spaces. The fine dust created by sanding could be inhaled into the lungs, so dust extractors should be working properly and a protective mask and gloves worn. When the treated wood is burnt some of the arsenic will volatilise, so such material is obviously unsuitable fuel for barbeque fires and in stoves. Generally speaking, CCA-treated timber off-cuts should never be burnt.

Small quantities of CCA-treated timber wastes resulting from domestic work projects may be disposed of with normal household wastes. Larger quantities, say from building sites, can be disposed of at approved landfills that are authorised by local authorities.

All treatment plants, and also sawmills carrying out even dip treatment to inhibit bluestain development need to ensure that the drainage from these processes does not contaminate water supplies or harm plant and animal life. Best practice for all preservative treatment plants is outlined in AS/NZS 2843:1 2000 *Timber Preservation Plant Safety Code—Plant Design* and AS/NZS 2843:2 2000 *Timber Preservation Plant Safety Code—Plant Operation*. These Standards set down the criteria for plant design and operation and emphasise working with minimal worker health and environmental impacts.

FURTHER READING

Referenced

Australian/New Zealand Standard. (2000). AS/NZS 2843:1 *Timber Preservation Plant Safety Code—Plant Design*.

Australian/New Zealand Standard. (2000). AS/NZS 2843:2 *Timber Preservation Plant Safety Code—Plant Operation*.

Bolza, E. (1976). Timber and health. Special report. Melbourne: CSIRO Division of Building Research.

Ostler, R. J. (1979). Health problems associated with wood processing. *BRE Information Paper* 13/79.

Woods, B. and Calnan, C. D. (1976). Toxic woods. *Br J Dermatol* 94(13).

Websites

Timber Preservers Association of Australia, viewed 6 March 2005, <http://www.tpaa.com.au>.

Chapter 20

Some wood utilisation aspects of tree breeding

It is not within the scope of this book to discuss the complex issues involved in seed selection and tree breeding but it is appropriate to mention here some aspects of these topics that the wood user would wish the plant physiologist and silviculturalist to consider in their aims. The comment made is concerned essentially with *radiata pine*, the main plantation species in Australia, and, because of its short rotation of the plantation cycle, one that is likely to show rapid benefit from careful selection of new growing stock. Selection of superior trees should not be based only on maximum wood production but should aim to restrict the extent of the juvenile core of inferior material.

Apart from healthy vigorous growth, other important considerations are stem straightness, small and uniform taper, relatively high density, well-scattered branches of small diameter emerging at right angles to the trunk and freedom from spiral grain and cone holes.

Density

Radiata pine usually has a core of low-density wood in perhaps the first ten growth rings. Density increases steadily until about 15 years of age and it then levels off; the increase is attributed to a greater proportion of latewood.

Since wood of uniform density is desirable, selection for high density in those first few years of growth is important, especially so in view of the trend to fell trees as early as possible, even for structural products.

The wood of radiata pine appears to have about the same density irrespective of ring width, if of the same age.

Density is related directly to the percentage of latewood, and, in young trees, the distance of the subject wood from the pith. The percentage of latewood is affected strongly by heredity. There is contradictory information on the effects of environmental factors on latewood production so further research is needed on these aspects. Environmental factors include rainfall intensity, altitude, latitude, rate of growth, soil fertility and presence of or lack of trace elements in the soil.

A high proportion of latewood tends to increase the difference between radial and tangential movement, which leads to a greater amount of seasoning degrade. The good machining properties desired by joinery manufacturers are enhanced by uniform ring width, relatively high density and a low percentage of latewood. The band of latewood is often associated with a large amount of resin, which may bleed through finishes, especially on surfaces that are exposed to hot sunlight.

Reduction of defects

The main defects requiring reduction in extent are knots, spiral grain, cone holes, compression wood, needle trace, resin content and pith.

Knots

Pines are not as self-pruning as hardwoods but trees having a tendency in this direction should be viewed very favourably in elite tree selection.

The presence of knots, especially if of larger diameter (say over 50 mm), has a major impact on strength properties because of their grain-distorting effect. Clusters of knots have a much greater weakening than indicated by the sum of their diameters because of the divergence of grain around the whole area. While knotty timber can be used decoratively to good effect for internal panelling, for all other purposes knots are undesirable due to other factors besides decreased strength, such as wood workability and serviceability of finishes. Not only is the size of the knot important but also the angle at which the branch that is responsible emerges from the trunk. For those branches that emerge from the trunk horizontally (or very close to horizontally) there is a lesser amount of the enclosing wood and they are easier to prune neatly. There is also a lesser risk of the inclusion of bark pockets, which may encourage invasion of the sawn timber by the bark beetle *Ernobius mollis*.

Branch diameter tends to be inversely related to the branch angle: the smaller the branch diameter, the more likely it is to be at the desirable 90° to the trunk.

Branches tend to be either in whorls at relatively even intervals or randomly scattered. If the intended market is for use as structural timber, then a scattered distribution would have merit, but for joinery purposes the clear material between the whorls will be more suitable, provided the whorls are well spaced. After a tree in a plantation has been pruned the new wood grown by the tree outside the end of the pruned branch is knot-free.

The development of more economical methods for early pruning is a further desirable approach to the knot problem, but the resin content of knots is increased by pruning.

Spiral grain

The large amount of sloping grain that spiral grain creates in sawn timber has a marked weakening effect on mechanical properties and can also cause a lot of twisting during drying. Radiata pine is more prone than most pine species to spiral grain in the first 15 years of growth, the angle of spirality reaching as high as 10°. By selective breeding this figure could be kept below 5°. Even at 5° the longitudinal shrinkage is about twice that of straight-grained wood. By careful selection of breeding stock it should be possible to bring radiata pine more into line with other pines in this respect.

The spirality of small-diameter poles cut from radiata pine can be a problem in areas of wide moisture content variation. Rotation of the top of the pole (after installation) causes a number of problems when the rotation exceeds acceptable limits. These problems include electrical conductor breakage because the cross-arm is no longer at 90° to the conductor. In areas subject to hot, dry summers, as much as 30° rotation at the top of the pole has occurred. Preservative treatment with an oil-borne preservative (creosote) rather than water-borne preservative may lessen the amount of rotation due to the oily nature of the preservative limiting the rate of moisture uptake or loss in the pole.

Cone holes

Some trees retain on their trunks a lot of old cones. When boards are sawn from the log, the stalks of the cones invariably fall out, resulting in numerous small holes in the sawn product. Although their small size usually makes their presence of little consequence, in structural timber they are unacceptable to buyers of board products, so there is a lot of wastage of otherwise good timber.

Compression wood

The juvenile wood of fast-growth pine has shorter fibres, higher hemicellulose and lower cellulose content than the mature wood and the cells of that juvenile wood have thinner walls, which are likely to produce paper with a lower tear strength. This reduction in tear strength is increased when compression wood is present because its fibres tend to shatter during the pulping process.

Since compression wood is more likely to occur in juvenile wood, every effort should be made to minimise its development as a result of trees that are not straight. Straightness is a factor that is susceptible to considerable improvement through selective breeding.

The higher lignin content of compression wood leads to a greater consumption of chemicals in both the separation of the fibres and their bleaching.

Compression wood is undesirable in structural and board products because of decreased strength and stability; the much greater longitudinal shrinkage is particularly significant.

Needle trace

This aberration of tissue formation is an undesirable feature in board products. Apart from its appearance there are often breaks in its surface, which can make it an unsuitable base for finishes. A high degree of heredity is involved so its incidence should be capable of considerable reduction through selective breeding.

Resin content

Lens-shaped pockets of resin are common in some pines, especially patula pine. These pockets are unacceptable in board and dressed products. Radiata pine is less affected in this regard but it can have a very high resin content in the latewood bands of the heartwood. The resin of the knots can also be very destructive to finishes.

Low-resin content is desirable in all board products for easier machining and finishing, and in paper pulp production, for which a latewood percentage of under 20 per cent is preferable.

Pith

Elite trees should have a narrow pith that does not wander erratically. Radiata pine sometimes has a wide pith, which can downgrade significant quantities of timber. If the tree trunk is of even diameter and straight, there is less chance of wandering pith. Very fertile sites seem to be more likely to produce trees with a wandering pith.

Drying degrade

Significant longitudinal shrinkage is a very undesirable feature in both structural and board products. It is related to cell length and the micellar angle in the S2 layer of the secondary wall, both of which are readily measurable under the microscope.

Excessive longitudinal shrinkage is also characteristic of the compression wood that is common in leaning stems, so the selection of seed from very straight trees may be helpful. Avoidance of plantation siting on steep or windswept land will also help to reduce the production of this undesirable feature.

Tracheids of above-average length in the early stages of pine tree growth are likely to be associated with less longitudinal shrinkage. Long tracheids are also desirable for good tear resistance in paper, for which the usual raw material is young plantation thinnings.

A minimal amount of heartwood will ensure less variability in moisture content in the timber during the drying process.

Durability

Radiata pine heartwood is relatively non-durable yet it is difficult to impregnate with preservatives so there is an obvious advantage in encouraging the production of a maximum amount of the easily treatable sapwood.

A counter argument would be the difficulty of protecting the sapwood against bluestain before and during seasoning, and the greater potential susceptibility of the sapwood to attack by the *Anobium* borer and such exotic borers as *Hylotrupes*, which might become established here in future years.

In the seasoned sapwood of radiata pine the latewood is more permeable than earlywood. This is due to the pits between the cells remaining open, whereas those in the earlywood have closed during seasoning.

In the initial green condition the reverse situation is likely to apply. However, in the heartwood the latewood is often saturated with resin, which blocks the entry of preservatives.

Bark

In view of the interest in radiata pine bark as a source of tannins for the manufacture of adhesives, the variability in bark properties should also be considered in selection procedures. Bark that is rich in tannins and free of a tendency for the extract to form insoluble compounds is desirable.

Species hybrids

In recent years, in addition to selective breeding within a species, selective breeding of appropriate species' hybrids has produced a number of 'new' species with desirable characteristics of the parent species. These characteristics include increased termite resistance as well as the better growth outcomes discussed above.

FURTHER READING

Hillis, W. E. (1980). Some basic characteristics affecting wood quality. *Appita* 35(5): 339–44.

Chapter 21

Timber use and performance in fire

Timber and its performance in fire

Unless highly resinous or in a form with a high ratio of surface area to section size, such as shavings, chips and twigs, wood does not readily ignite. In the section sizes that are typical of structural components, the insulating nature of wood slows down the rate of incineration considerably. Timber of large section size does not burn easily. Its low thermal conductivity means that the heat of combustion is slow to penetrate into the wood (in contrast with what happens with metals) and the average rate of penetration of charring is about 35 mm per hour under average fire conditions. Wood chars more rapidly when a fresh surface is exposed rather than when it is under a layer of charcoal, the rate being about 0.8 mm per minute in the initial 5 minutes of exposure, reducing to about 0.6 mm per minute after half an hour.

The temperature of the wood 6 mm in from the charring may be only 180°C. One advantage of the charcoal is that it absorbs water and so helps to speed the quenching of the flames during fire-fighting operations. Because of this slow penetration of fire, heavy timber construction using the denser hardwoods has always been considered favourably for warehouse construction, where fire fighters may have to penetrate deeply into a building to reach the source of a fire. It provides a much safer support than metal construction which, although not combustible, soon reaches a softening point when exposed to the heat of the fire and may suddenly suffer complete loss of ability to support the structure. Steel loses half its strength at 500°C, at which temperature concrete also will often start to disintegrate. As most fires that are likely to be a threat to a building will generate temperatures of 700–900°C, basing building design and regulations merely on theoretical considerations of combustibility is unwise.

Fire characteristics of wood

When wood is heated the temperature rises steadily to about 100°C, where it remains until the considerable amount of water vapour that it contains is evaporated. The temperature rise then continues without much further effect until, at about 200°C, flammable gases begin to form and by 250–300°C these will be enough to sustain ignition if sufficient oxygen is present. At 350–450°C, depending on the density of the wood, non-piloted ignition occurs.

Stages of fire development

Fire usually starts in the easily burnt contents, which are the real hazard, and most buildings will be seriously affected by the resulting heat.

Accurate measurements recorded during test fires in a furnished room indicate that a few minutes after the fire started the temperature reached 400°C due to the combustion of the gases from the ignited material. Then, for about 10 minutes, the temperature dropped back to about 100°C because the formation of char reduced the rate of gas formation and much of the heat energy was spent in evaporating the water vapour present. This was followed by a sudden rise in temperature to 250–300°C, resulting in the formation of combustible gases until a flash point was reached and widespread ignition occurred with the temperature at 700°C.

Walls may be able to resist fire penetration for hours but windows, doors and air-conditioning ducts are very vulnerable. Windows are likely to crack and fall out well before the glass melts. Flames may project several metres beyond and above the window opening, which can lead to the spread of fire in multi-storey construction despite concrete floor separations.

Fires spread not only from flying embers but also from heat radiation, an important factor in fires in closely settled urban areas.

Burning of a timber structure will often slow down very significantly once the contents have been destroyed because of a temperature drop below that necessary for the burning of the charcoal on the surface of the timber.

Building regulations

Fire and the safety of the occupants of the building are important concerns in all types of buildings. Building regulations that restrict construction materials are dominated by fire safety. Fire performance and occupant safety considerations restrict the use of timber and wood products more than many other materials within Australian building regulations. The restrictions limit the choice of material that can be used for certain types and parts of buildings, such as structural components, the surfaces of walls, ceiling and floor coverings, cladding on the exterior of the building and exterior material choices in bushfire-prone areas.

Fire-hazard properties

The Building Code of Australia (BCA) limits the choice of products that can be used within a building by requiring different performance criteria (when exposed to fire) for materials in various applications. The deemed-to-satisfy provisions require all materials or assemblies used in a building, except for housing, to have nominated fire-hazard properties.

Floor materials and covering

A minimum critical radiant flux is set for floor materials and coverings that is dependent upon the building occupation, the location of the material in the building and whether a sprinkler system is installed. Buildings that are used for the aged or for health care have greater requirements due to the limited mobility of the occupants.

A prescribed minimum critical radiant flux for various building uses is set out in the BCA. A material critical radiant flux is determined by AS ISO 9239.1-2003 *Reaction to Fire Tests for Floor Coverings—Determination of the Burning Behaviour using a Radiant Heat Source.*

Normally, timber used for flooring meets the general requirement of a critical radiant heat flux of 2.2 kW/m^2 or greater. Table 21.1 lists the common timbers that have been tested. All species tested exceed this requirement. Some high-density timber species meet the greatest requirement for floor covering control and therefore can be used in places where fire safety is paramount.

Table 21.1 Fire-hazard properties for floor materials and coverings

Critical radiant flux (kW/m^2)	
2.2 and less than 4.5	4.5 and greater
Alpine ash, blackbutt, brownbarrel, celery-top pine, manna gum, messmate, mountain ash, radiata pine, rose gum, shining gum, silvertop ash, Sydney blue gum, yellow stringybark	Beech myrtle, blackwood, brush box, cypress, grey box, grey ironbark, jarrah, karri, merbau, New England blackbutt, red bloodwood, red ironbark, red mahogany, red river gum, silver wattle, spotted gum, sugar gum, southern blue gum, Tasmanian blue gum, tallowwood, turpentine, yellow gum

Note: Data from Warrington Fire Research. (2005). *Assessment of timber floor, wall and ceiling linings to Specification C1.10a, SFR41117.2.*

Walls and ceilings

Timbers used for walls and ceilings must fall into one of three material groups. These material groups are tested in accordance with AS ISO 9705-2003 *Fire Tests—Full-Scale Room Test for Surface Products* or are predicted after testing in accordance with AS/NZS 3837:1998 *Method of Test for Heat and Smoke Release Rates for Materials and Products Using an Oxygen Consumption Calorimeter.*

AS ISO 9705 is a full-scale test where a room lined with the test sample is ignited and the time to flash over determines its material group.

AS/NZS 3837 is a bench test that measures heat release rates that are then correlated to the full-scale room tests mentioned above. The advantage of the latter method is that it is easy to do many samples, a bonus for timber that has many species and thicknesses needing consideration.

Group 1 material is the best and is generally considered to be for non-combustible materials or materials that are considered equivalent to non-combustible but show some signs of combusting during the test. Group 2 materials are generally for products such as fire-retardant treated timber and group 3 material generally relates to natural timber products. Table 21.2 contains a list of commercial timber species that pass. Some thin products, such as paper or loose wood fibres, may not.

Like floor materials, wall and ceiling materials are limited in certain areas due to various building occupations, the location of the material in the building or if a sprinkler system is installed.

Table 21.2 Fire-hazard properties group for timber wall and ceiling lining materials

Species	Material group
Alpine ash, Baltic pine, beech myrtle, blackbutt, blackwood, brownbarrel, brush box, coast grey box, cypress, grey box, grey ironbark, jarrah, karri, manna gum, marri, merbau, meranti, messmate, mountain ash, New England blackbutt, radiata pine, red bloodwood, red ironbark, red mahogany, red river gum, rose gum, shining gum, silvertop gum, silver wattle, Sydney blue gum, tallowwood, Tasmanian blue gum, turpentine, WA blackbutt, WA sheoak, western red cedar, yellow gum, yellow stringybark	3

Note: Data from Warrington Fire Research. (2005). *Assessment of timber floor, wall and ceiling linings to Specification C1.10a, SFR41117.2; and CSIRO. (2003). Assessment of the material group of various timber products using the cone calorimeter, 02/276.*

Data on manufactured products

Factory produced wood-based products, such as hardboard, medium-density fibreboard (MDF), particleboard and plywood, can also be assessed by the above test methods. However, since such products may vary widely in formulation from time to time and between manufacturers (raw materials plus additives) the confirmation of specific indices should be authenticated by the manufacturer of the particular named or branded products and/or a registered testing authority.

Non-combustibility

Where the deemed-to-satisfy provisions in the BCA require a material, construction or part of a building to be non-combustible when tested in accordance with AS 1530.1-1994 *Methods for Fire Tests on Building Materials, Components and Structures*, the use of timber or timber products is not permitted as a deemed-to-satisfy solution.

Non-combustibility requirements in the deemed-to-satisfy provisions do not, however, prevent or influence the processing of an alternative solution under the performance requirements.

Exempted building parts and materials

The requirements in the BCA for floors, walls and ceilings do not apply to timber-framed windows, solid timber handrails or skirtings, timber-faced solid-core fire doors, joinery units, cupboards, shelving and the like as they do not significantly increase the hazards of fire.

Charring and fire-resistance through charring

As explained above, wood that is exposed to high temperatures will decompose to provide an insulating layer of char that retards further degradation of the wood. Initially the wood rapidly chars but as the char increases the rate slows.

The rate of charring varies among timber species and predominately is dependent on its density and moisture content. Other factors are anatomy, chemical composition and permeability. Charring in the longitudinal grain direction is reportedly double that in the transverse direction and chemical composition affects the relative thickness of the char layer.

Since the moisture content of wood will come into balance or equilibrium with the environment that it is in, timber used inside will have a stabilised moisture content of about 12 per cent. When considering fire safety in building design, the moisture content is not considered in the design of fire-resistance for timber due to its low percentage. The density, on the other hand, is used to predict the fire-resistance of large-section timbers as a rate of charring is codified, allowing designers to design fire-rated timber elements. AS 1720.4 *Timber Structures—Fire-Resistance of Structural Timber Members* provides a method to calculate the fire-resistance level for solid timber.

The ability of the member to maintain the load-carrying capacity of a structural wood member depends upon its cross-sectional dimensions. This rate of charring, and hence the rate of reduction of load-carrying capacity that is caused by the loss of effective cross-section, is predictable.

The temperature at the innermost zone of the char layer is assumed to be 300°C. Because of the low thermal conductivity of wood the temperature inward from the base of the char layer is about 180°C. This steep temperature gradient means that the remaining uncharred cross-sectional area of a large wood member remains at a low temperature and can continue to carry a load.

By substituting appropriate values in the equations below, the residual cross-section can be calculated with sufficient accuracy for design of the element and consequent compliance with the requirements of the BCA.

Notional charring rate

$$C = 0.4 + \left(\frac{280}{D}\right)^2$$

where:
C = notional charring rate, in mm/min
D = timber density at a moisture content of 12 per cent in kg/m^3.

Effective depth of charring

$$dc = Ct + 7.5$$

where:
dc = calculated effective depth of charring in mm
C = notional charring rate in mm/min as calculated
t = period of time, in min.

Note that the net effect of charring/fire will depend on the number of faces of the member exposed to the fire—one, two, three or four.

Broadly, the charring rate (C) is inversely proportional to the density (in kg/m^3) of the timber element but the calculation of expected performance must allow for charring (and hence reduction in cross-section size and thus load-carrying capacity) on one, two, three or four sides as appropriate.

An example of calculating the fire-resistance level of a structural element follows.

If a blackbutt timber post is required to be 50 × 50 mm to carry load for structural reasons, then it needs additional timber to protect it if it is to survive fire conditions for 60 minutes. If the average density of blackbutt at 12 per cent moisture content is 900 kg/m^3, then the notional charring rate from the equations above would be 0.5 mm/min. This would result in a charring depth of 37.5 mm each side of the post.

The size of post required, assuming the fire will affect all four sides, would be 50 + 37.5 + 37.5 = 125 mm square. If this size is not available, then the next available size up should be used.

Fire-retardant treatments

In building design there is often a need to improve the fire performance of timber and wood products. Timber and plywood that have had their fire performance improved are often used for interior finishes, particularly in public entertainment areas (i.e. auditoriums) and corridors where building occupants may need to travel past to escape a fire. In general, the building regulations require an improvement in the surface flammability performance. In recent times there has also been a demand in bushfire-prone areas to minimise the ignition and reduce the flame spread across exterior elements of a building.

Fire-retardant treatments of timbers do not prevent the wood from charring under fire exposure. The rate of charring through fire-retardant treated timber is approximately the same rate as through untreated timber. Most of this improvement is associated with the decrease in surface flammability rather than with any changes in charring rates.

Fire-retardant treatment of wood generally improves the fire performance by reducing the amount of flammable volatiles that are released during fire exposure or by reducing the effective heat of combustion, or both. This results in reducing the rate of flame spread over the surface. The timber may self-extinguish when the fire source is removed.

The mode of action of fire-retardants is that when they are subject to considerable heat they do one of the following:

- melt and form a glaze over the surface and exclude oxygen
- decompose to form gases that do not support combustion
- vaporise and absorb sufficient of the heat to prevent the temperature of the wood reaching a destructive level
- promote the formation of an insulating layer of charcoal.

The two general application methods are pressure impregnation and surface coating.

Pressure-impregnated fire-retardant treated wood

Wood is pressure impregnated with chemicals using pressure processes that are similar to those used for chemical preservative treatments. Similar cylinders and processes are used. The main difference is that considerably heavier absorptions of chemicals are necessary. The amount of chemical needed is dependent on the application and whether the timber is to be used in interior or exterior environments.

The penetration of the chemicals into the wood depends on the species, wood structure and moisture content. Since some species are difficult to treat, the degree of impregnation that is needed to meet the performance requirements for fire-retardant treated wood may not be possible.

Inorganic salts are the most commonly used fire-retardants for interior wood products and their characteristics have been known for more than 50 years. The pressure-impregnated fire-retardant treatments are often formulations containing inorganic salts, such as phosphoric acid, boric acid, zinc chloride and ammonium phosphates and polyphosphates. These chemicals are often combined to develop various fire performances. Other aspects that need considering are the hygroscopicity of the treatment, any strength reduction, any corrosive effect on fasteners, the ability to machine the timber, what the finished product may look like, and its ability to accept paints and stains or be glued.

Fire-retardant coatings

Sometimes the fire-retardant is applied to the timber as a coating. The common types of coatings are intumescent. An intumescent coating upon exposure to fire expands and forms a low-density film. This film insulates the wood surface below from the effects of high temperatures.

Exterior applications of fire-retardants

Fire-retardant treatments are normally salts and therefore water soluble. They can leach out in exterior applications or with repeated washings. Water-insoluble organic fire-retardants have been developed to meet the need for leach-resistant systems.

When testing the performance of exterior fire-retardants, the fire-retardant treated timber should be first artificially weathered to simulate years of service in an exterior application. In addition it should be exposed to ultraviolet light as this may degrade the coating that is used to slow down leaching or affect the chemical treatment.

For interior fire-retardants some leaching of the chemical may occur from repeated washing of the surface. Again, a simulated washing down of the surface over time should be employed. This accelerated weathering of the fire-retardant treated timber prior to testing is slowly finding its way into building regulations as the demand for fire-retardants increases.

For applications where elevated temperatures and high humidity may be experienced, such as roof sheathings, there is the potential for loss in strength over time. For such applications in elevated temperatures and high humidity some modification to strength is required. For fire-retardant treatments containing inorganic salts, the type of metal and chemical in contact with each other greatly affects the rate of corrosion.

Natural fire resistance

Some high-density timber species exhibit low flame-spread performance and can be used in areas within a building or in bushfire-prone areas without the application of fire-retardants. These timbers have been tested and have shown to meet or are better than the performance required for that application.

Multi-residential timber-framed construction (MRTFC)

During the early 1990s the timber industry gained approval within the deemed-to-satisfy requirements in the BCA to allow the use of low-rise, fire-protected, timber-framed residential buildings. These building utilise fire-rated linings to compartmentalise units within these building so that occupants can escape in the event of a fire.

The successful introduction of this form of construction has seen a number of timber-framed, three-storey, walk-up apartment buildings being built across Australia and timber-framed construction becoming commonplace in townhouse development. Three-storey walk-up apartment buildings require fire- and sound-rated walls, floors and ceilings, while townhouses require fire- and sound-rated separating walls.

The common form of wall construction is a double stud wall with fire-rated linings on the outside. An acoustic batt is normally used in the centre to dampen noise transmission. Figure 21.1 illustrates a typical wall detail.

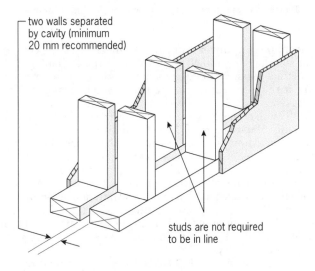

two walls separated by cavity (minimum 20 mm recommended)

studs are not required to be in line

Fig. 21.1 Double stud fire- and sound-rated wall

Sound transmission through floors is harder to resolve than sound transmission through walls due to the low frequency that footfall noise generates. Floor systems typically are a standard joist and sheet floor constructed with a plasterboard ceiling that is supported on resilient mounts and battens. The floor covering is normally a carpet or, if a hard surface is used, an acoustic mat is used between the hard floor surface and the structural floor. A typical floor/ceiling system is illustrated in Figure 21.2.

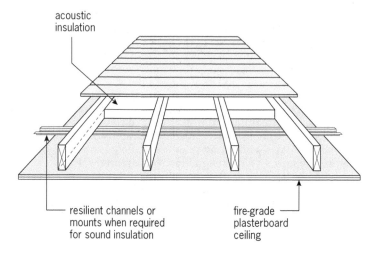

acoustic
insulation

resilient channels or
mounts when required
for sound insulation

fire-grade
plasterboard
ceiling

Fig. 21.2 Typical fire- and sound-rated timber floor/ceiling system

The adoption of a timber frame has been helped by the construction practices that have been developed to assist the technology. The key aspect that has assisted the take-up of this form of construction is the detailing at the intersection of non-fire-rated elements and fire-rated elements.

Normally where these two elements meet, there would be a break in the continuity of the fire rating, which is more often than not addressed by using fire-rated linings. A key recognition that timber itself can provide fire rating is utilised with timber blocks sealing up the breaks.

During the erection of the frame, it is normally undesirable to have the fire-rated lining installed to seal up breaks as this is out of sequence with when linings are generally installed. By introducing timber elements that take the place of the fire-rated linings (FRL; Fig. 21.3), a continuous fire rating can be maintained. This then allows the fire-rated linings to be installed during their correct construction sequence, thus preventing out-of-sequence activity.

Another key aspect of MRTFC is the acoustic treatment of the building. For a successful design it is necessary to ensure that acoustic separation is maintained. The main consideration in acoustic design in

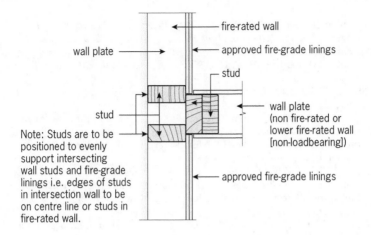

Fig. 21.3 Timber blocks are used to maintain fire resistance

timber-framed buildings is the separation of units so that noise is not transmitted into another unit. The greater the parting or path that noise has to travel, the better acoustic separation that is achieved.

Good acoustic design starts off with the building layout itself. Designing so that windows or entrance doors from different units do not face each other is a very good start. In addition, having rooms that are of like use adjoining each other is better than placing bathrooms against neighbouring bedrooms.

Timber-framed residential construction has also occurred in odd places, such as on the top of high-rise buildings, or in the conversion of other building types, such as offices to residential units. This can be achieved in building regulations through the alternative solution path of the BCA. An alternative solution uses a fire engineer to prove to the building authority that the design is as fire safe or safer than the deemed-to-satisfy solution, similar to how a structural engineer is used to design timber beams once they are outside typical span tables.

FURTHER READING

Australian Hardwood Network. (2003). *Australian hardwood and cypress manual.* Sydney: AHN.

Forest Products Laboratory, US Dept of Agriculture. (1974). *Wood handbook. Wood as an engineering material.* Agriculture handbook no. 72. Washington, DC: Govt Printing Office.

Australian Standard. (1994). AS 1530.1 *Methods for Fire Tests on Building Materials, Components and Structures.*

Australian Standard. (1990). AS 1720.4 *Timber Structures—Fire-Resistance of Structural Timber Members.*

Australian/New Zealand Standard. (1998). AS/NZS 3837 *Method of Test for Heat and Smoke Release Rates for Materials and Products Using an Oxygen Consumption Calorimeter.*

Australian Standard. (2003). AS ISO 9239.1 *Reaction to Fire Tests for Floor Coverings—Determination of the Burning Behaviour Using a Radiant Heat Source.*

Australian Standard. (2003). AS ISO 9705 *Fire Tests—Full-Scale Room Test for Surface Products.*

CSIRO. (2003). *Assessment of the material group of various timber products using the cone calorimeter, 02/276.*

National Timber Development Council. (2001). *Class 1a buildings, design and construction manuals—multi-residential timber-framed construction.* Melbourne: Forest and Wood Product Research and Development Corporation.

National Timber Development Council. (2001). *Class 2 & 3 buildings, design and construction manuals—multi-residential timber-framed construction.* Melbourne: Forest and Wood Product Research and Development Corporation.

National Timber Development Council. (2002). *Timber in buildings—internal fit-out.* Melbourne: Forest and Wood Product Research and Development Corporation.

Warrington Fire Research. (2005). *Assessment of timber floor, wall and ceiling linings to Specification C1.10a,* SFR41117.2.

Chapter 22

Australian Standards for the timber industry

The increasingly complex nature of our society requires a rationalisation of the ways of specifying and assessing the quality of products in order to give some measure of protection to the consumer who has no means of determining the merits of the claims made by the manufacturer's or retailer's salesperson. From the manufacturer's point of view, too, there is much to be gained from orderly production to an authoritative quality standard in that it puts some check on the unscrupulous competitor and the would-be buyer who demands the impossible.

In many countries there are now officially recognised standards organisations that have been set up to prepare rules that are acceptable to the majority of interested parties. Standards Australia was established in 1924. It is an independent, non-profit body, financed by membership fees (anyone can join and so obtain Standards at a discount, as well as receiving copies of a monthly bulletin listing new Standards and amendments to old ones) and the revenue received from the sale of the various Standards Australia publications or related activity. The organisation also carries stocks of many overseas standards of interest to importers and exporters.

Australian Standards are developed on the basis of cooperative effort and mutual agreement; the achievement of this agreement may involve long discussions, many meetings and often special technical investigations, but standards determined in this way usually have a better chance of success than those forced on an industry by government decree or bureaucratic authority. The membership of committees embraces all parties with an interest in the subject—producer, consumer, retailer, regulatory authority, technical and research bodies—so that all aspects of the subject have a chance to be discussed before the standard is published.

The use of standards is usually not mandatory (except in such fields as electric wiring rules, where it is obviously essential for public safety that everyone follows the same strict rules). A standard is not in itself compulsory and only becomes so when called up in legislation or in a contract; however, the presence of standards means that any specifier can call up the appropriate standards as a basis for contractual agreement in the supply of the material or goods.

Regulations governing the use of timber in buildings are tending more and more to require compliance with Australian Standards. In Australia, the Building Code of Australia, which regulates most housing that is constructed, regards the AS 1684-1999 *Residential Timber-Framed Construction* as being 'deemed to satisfy the requirements of the Building Code in regard to the use of timber in dwelling construction'. That Standard, in turn, calls up the various other Standards pertaining to the various components of the structure.

At the present time, Australian Standards cover virtually all sawn timber. There are standards for glued-laminated members, reconstituted wood products, such as plywood, particleboard and hardboard, railway sleepers, ladders, handles and windows—indeed most products involving a substantial timber component. AS 1720.1-1997 *Timber Structures—Design Methods* provides the basic information needed by engineers for calculating the special sizes required for large engineering structures. A list of the main Standards of importance appears below.

The decision as to what standards are to be prepared and who is to undertake the task is made by various industry boards or groups within Standards Australia. Where the standards relate to timber, the groups are made up of representative sawmillers, merchants, builders, architects, lending authorities, engineers, timber promotion organisations, forestry departments, public works departments and public utilities responsible for electricity, roads, railways, research agencies such as CSIRO and so on.

When Standards Australia agrees on the need for a new standard, or for the revision of an old one, it assigns the task to one of its technical committees. Standards are subject to change in the light of experience gained from their use and from new developments, so it is important to check with Standards Australia from time to time to make sure that your edition is up to date. For minor changes, amendment slips are produced by Standards Australia, obviating the need for the purchase of a completely new document.

The aim of each committee is to produce a standard based on a consensus of opinion. It is seldom possible to obtain a unanimous decision on all points so compromises have to be made; if there is a considerable body of opinion against a particular proposal, then there is no chance of it appearing in the final draft. Without such a general measure of agreement it is inevitable that contracting parties will tend to bypass the standard. Sometimes there are conflicts over a particular issue that is not vital to the main purpose of the standard and this may be referred by the drafting committee to the Standards Sector Board for a ruling.

Some timber producers brand their timber with the number of the appropriate standard and the relevant grading within that standard, such as 'F11–AS 2082'.

There have been many attempts to secure greater uniformity between the building regulations in the various states and between the rules of the various local government authorities but progress has been slow. The increasing acceptance of Australian Standards has been one way of gradually achieving this desired degree of uniformity.

Australian Standards referenced in this book

AS/NZS 1080.1: 1997 *Timber—Methods of test—Moisture content*

AS/NZS 1080.2.1: 1998 *Timber—Methods of test—Slope of grain by scribe*

AS/NZS 1080.2.2: 1998 *Timber—Methods of test—Slope of grain by reference to surface checks*

AS/NZS 1080.2.3: 1998 *Timber—Methods of test—Slope of grain by splintering*

AS/NZS 1080.2.4: 1998 *Timber—Methods of test—Compound slope of grain*

AS/NZS 1148: 2001 *Timber—Nomenclature—Australian, New Zealand and imported species*

AS/NZS 1328.1: 1998 *Glued laminated structural timber—Performance requirements and minimum production requirements*

AS 1530.1-1994 *Methods for fire tests on building materials, components and structures*

AS 1577-1993 *Scaffold planks*

AS 1604.1-2005 *Specification for preservative treatment—Sawn and round timber*

AS/NZS 1604.2: 2004 *Specification for preservative treatment—Reconstituted wood-based products*

AS/NZS 1604.3: 2004 *Specification for preservative treatment—Plywood*

AS/NZS 1604.4-2004 *Specification for preservative treatment—Laminated veneer lumber (LVL)*

AS/NZS 1604.5-2005 *Specification for preservative treatment—Glue laminated timber products*

AS/NZS 1605: 2000 *Methods for sampling and analysing timber preservatives and preservative-treated timber*

AS 1684-1999 *Residential timber-framed construction*

AS 1720.1: 1997 *Timber structures—Design methods*

AS 1720.2: 1990 *Timber structures—Timber properties*

AS 1720.4-1990 *Timber structures—Fire-resistance of structural timber members*

AS 1738-1975 *Timber for marine craft*

AS/NZS 1748: 1997 *Timber—Stress-graded—Product requirements for mechanically stress-graded timber*

AS/NZS 1859.1: 2004 *Reconstituted wood-based panels—Specifications—Particleboard*

AS/NZS 1859.2: 2004 *Reconstituted wood-based panels—Specifications—Dry-processed fibreboard*

AS/NZS 1859.4: 2004 *Reconstituted wood-based panels—Specifications—Wet-processed fibreboard*

AS 1860-1998 *Installation of particleboard flooring*

AS 1860.1: 2002 *Particleboard flooring specifications*

AS 1738-1975 *Timber for marine craft*

AS 2082: 2000 *Timber—Hardwood—Visually stress-graded for structural purposes*

AS/NZS 2098: 1996 *Methods of test for veneer and plywood*

AS 2209-1994 *Timber—Poles for overhead lines*

AS/NZS 2269: 2004 *Plywood—Structural*

AS/NZS 2270: 1999 *Plywood and blockboard for interior use*

AS/NZS 2271: 2004 *Plywood and blockboard for exterior use*

AS/NZS 2272: 1996 *Plywood—Marine*
AS/NZS 2311:2000 *Guide to the painting of buildings*
AS 2329-1999 *Mastic adhesives for fixing wallboards*
AS 2870-1996 *Residential slabs and footings—Construction*
AS/NZS 2843.1: 2000 *Timber preservation plant safety code—Plant design*
AS/NZS 2843.2: 2000 *Timber preservation plant safety code—Plant operation*
AS 2858: 2004 *Timber—Softwood—Visually graded for structural purposes*
AS/NZS 2878: 2000 *Timber—Classification into strength groups*
AS 3519: 1993 *Timber—Machine proof-grading*
AS 3600-2001 *Concrete structures*
AS 3660.1-2000 *Termite management—New building work*
AS 3818.1-2003 *Timber—Heavy structural products—Visually graded—General requirements*
AS 3818.2-2004 *Timber—Heavy structural products—Visually graded—Railway track timbers*
AS 3818.3-2001 *Timber—Heavy structural products—Visually graded—Piles*
AS 3818.4-2003 *Timber—Heavy structural products—Visually graded—Cross-arms for overhead lines*
AS/NZS 3837: 1998 *Method of test for heat and smoke release rates for materials and products using an oxygen consumption calorimeter*
AS/NZS 4063: 1992 *Timber—Stress-graded—In-grade strength and stiffness evaluation*
AS/NZS 4357: 1995 *Structural laminated veneer lumber*
AS 4440-2004 *Installation of nailplated timber roof trusses*
AS 4446-1999 *Manufacture of nailplate-joined timber products*
AS 4787: 2001 *Timber—Assessment of drying quality*
AS 5604-2003 *Timber—Natural durability ratings*
AS ISO 9239.1-2003 *Reaction to fire tests for floor coverings—Determination of the burning behaviour using a radiant heat source*
AS ISO 9705-2003 *Fire tests—Full-scale room test for surface products*

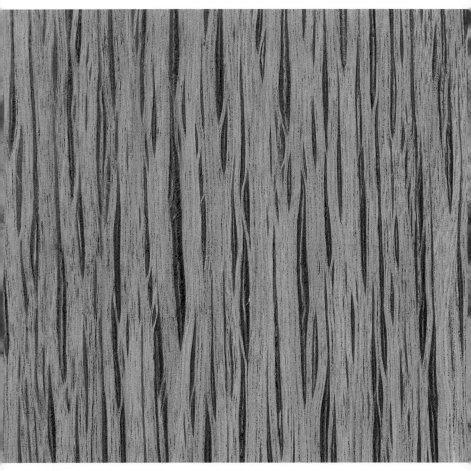

Plate 1 Rays, when large, produce a very distinctive appearance (see p. 6). This photograph of back-cut rose sheoak shows the multitude of lens-shaped rays

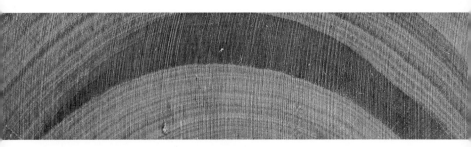

Plate 2 A band of compression wood showing on the end-grain (see p. 13). This example is of hoop pine

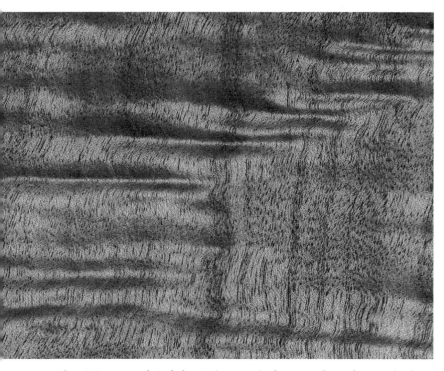

Plate 3 Top view of rippled grain (see p. 14). This example is of Queensland maple

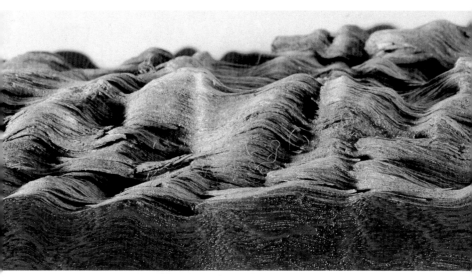

Plate 4 Side view of rippled grain (see p. 14)

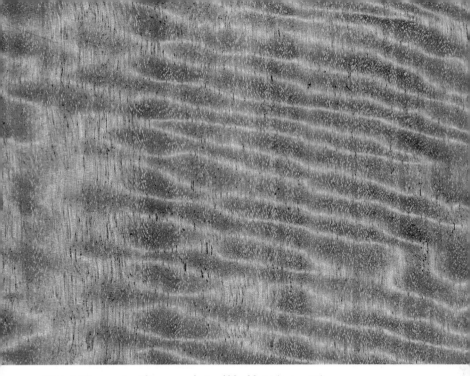

Plate 5 Wavy grain. This example is of blackbutt (see p. 14)

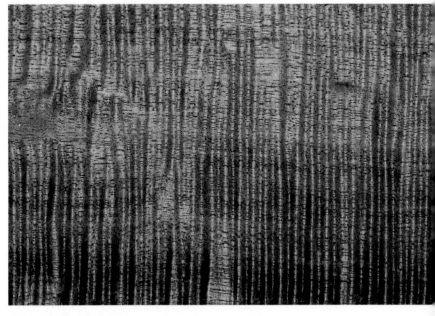

Plate 6 Fiddleback figure in an ash eucalypt (see p. 14)

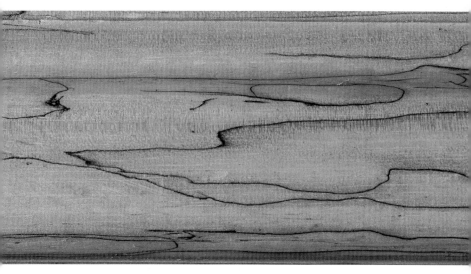

Plate 7 Fungal attack in a living tree (the example is ramin) producing a tracery of dark stain (see p. 19)

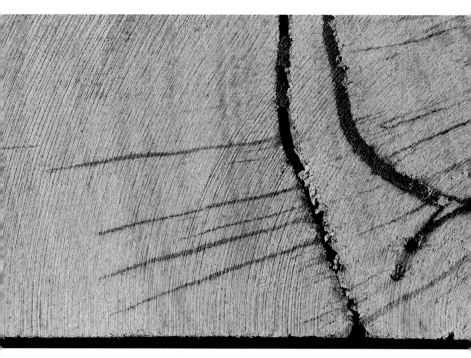

Plate 8 Lines of pencil streak arising from pin-hole borer tunnels in *Eucalyptus obliqua* (see p. 19)

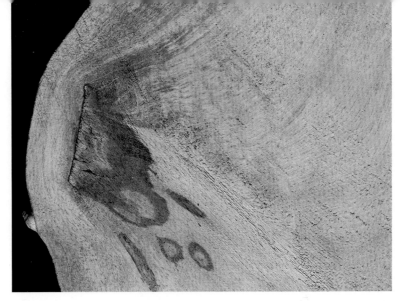

Plate 9 An illustration of a tree's capacity to grow over a pruned branch (see p. 27)

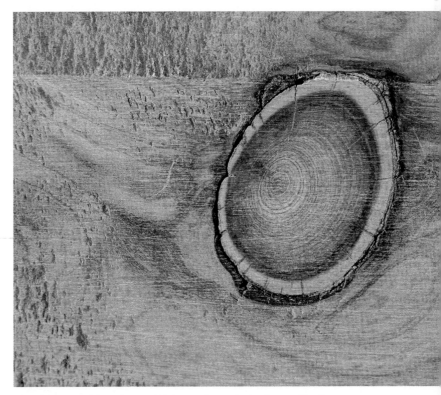

Plate 10 Encased knot (see p. 27). Note the enclosing layer of bark

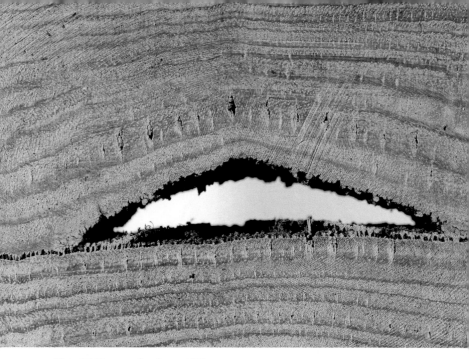

Plate 11 Gum pocket (see p. 29)

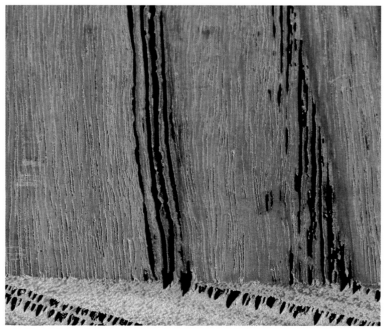

Plate 12 Gum veins (see p. 29)

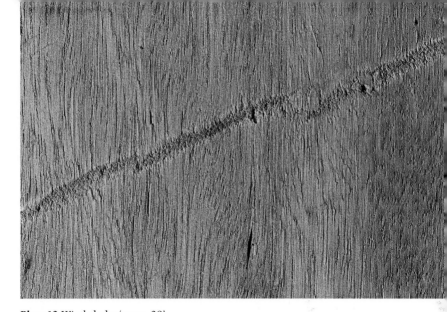

Plate 13 Wind shake (see p. 29)

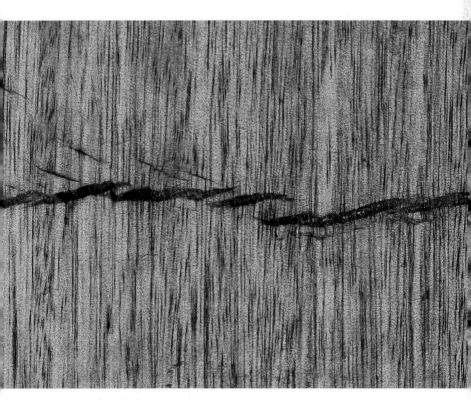

Plate 14 Felling shake (see p. 29)

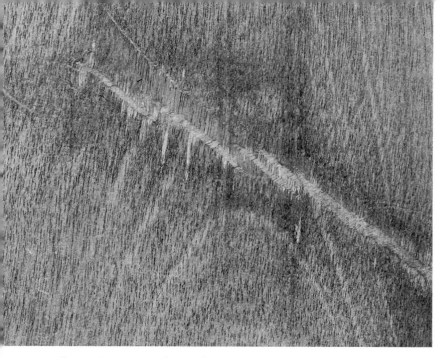

Plate 15 Compression fracture (see p. 31)

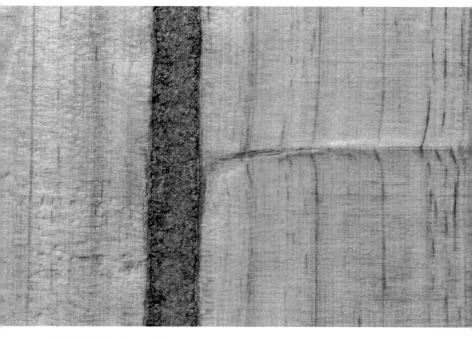

Plate 16 Pith (see p. 47)

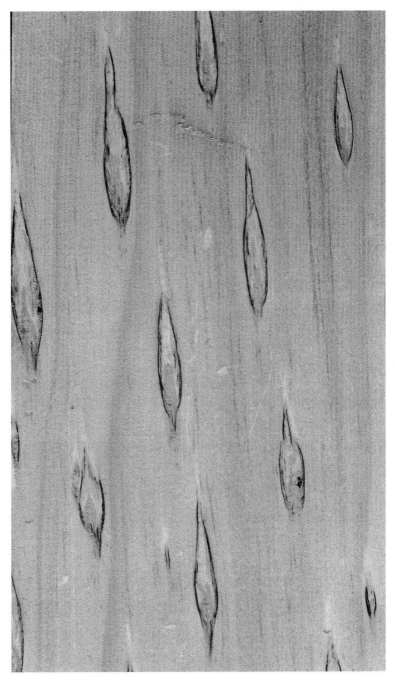

Plate 17 Needle trace (see p. 47)

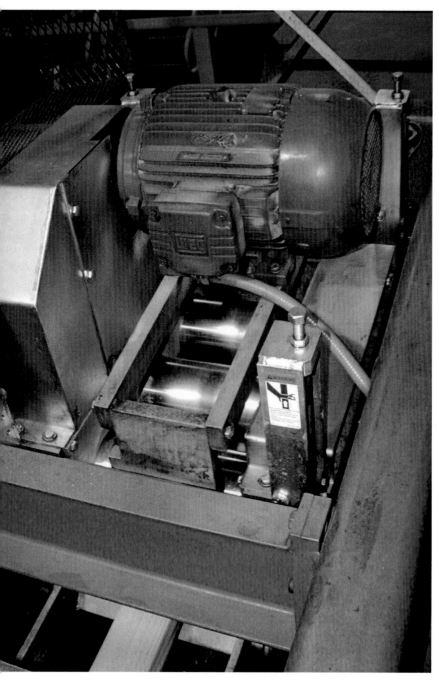

Plate 18 Metriguard machine for grading structural timber (see p. 48)

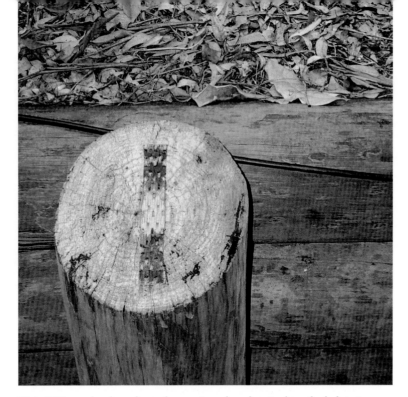

Plate 19 Example of accelerated corrosion of a galvanised toothed plate in contact with H5 CCA-treated pine (see p. 62). (Note the difference between the untreated centre of the log and the treated outer zone)

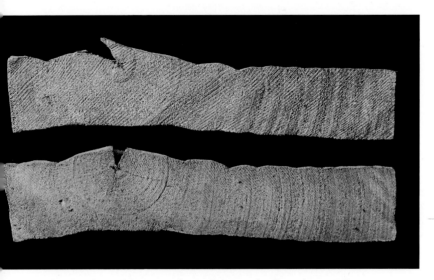

Plate 20 The undulating surface indicative of collapse (see p. 78)

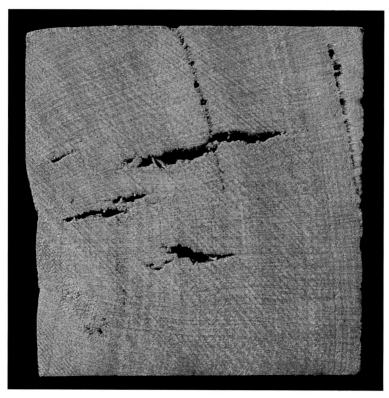

Plate 21 Internal checking, or honeycombing, often associated with collapse in cool-climate eucalypts (see p. 79)

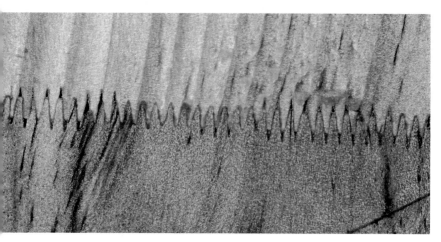

Plate 22 A finger-jointed lining board (see p. 97)

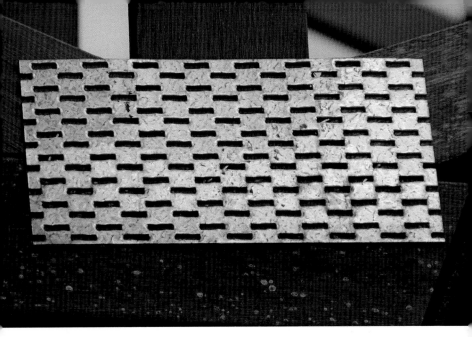

Plate 23 Nailplate connection (see p. 106)

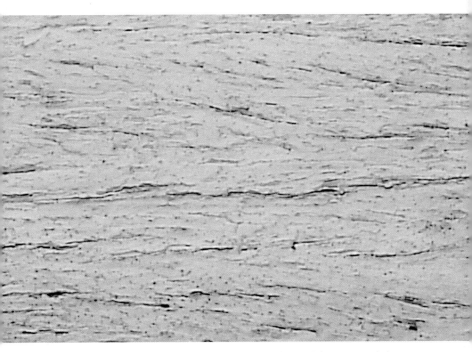

Plate 24 Hardwoods subject to surface checking often exhibit coating failure that is extensive (see p. 145)

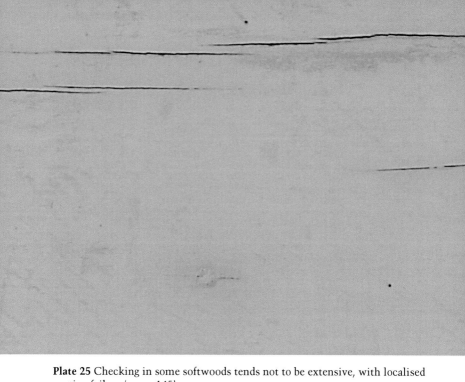

Plate 25 Checking in some softwoods tends not to be extensive, with localised coating failure (see p. 145)

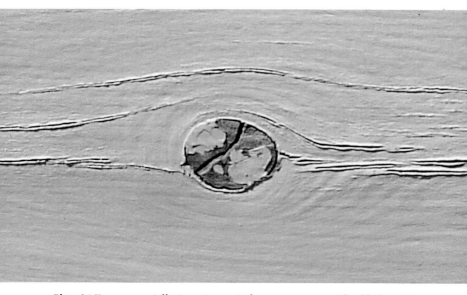

Plate 26 Knots, especially in resinous timber, present a considerable hazard to coatings (see p. 145)

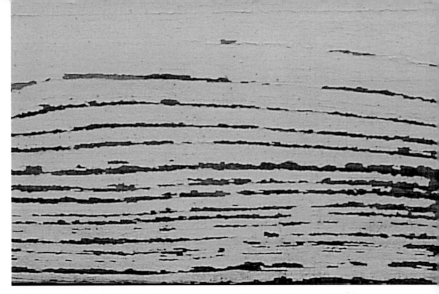

Plate 27 In softwoods with very pronounced growth rings coating systems usually fail more rapidly on the narrow bands of latewood (see p. 145)

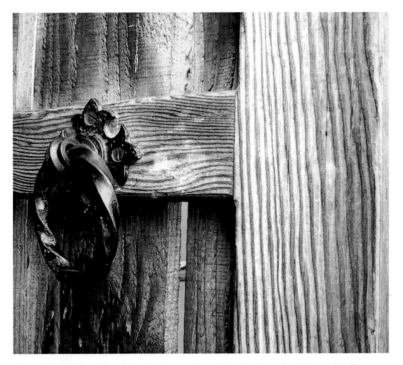

Plate 28 Weathered wood, showing surface degradation of earlywood cells, giving a washboard effect to this oregon gate, which has been exposed without the benefit of a surface coating (see p. 168) Source: courtesy Dr Harry Greaves

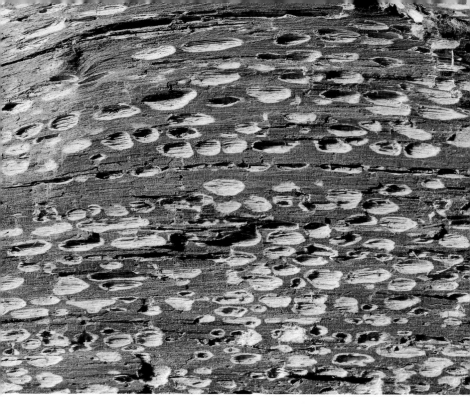

Plate 29 Decayed wood (see p. 169)

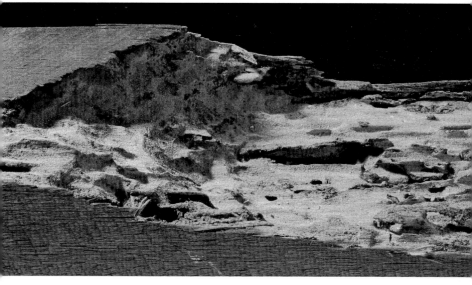

Plate 30 Wood partly destroyed by termites (see p. 173)

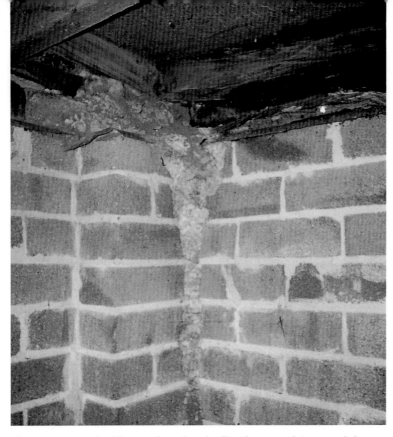

Plate 31 Termites build an earth-enclosed gallery between the nest and the timber being attacked, in this case bypassing the termite barrier (see p. 175)

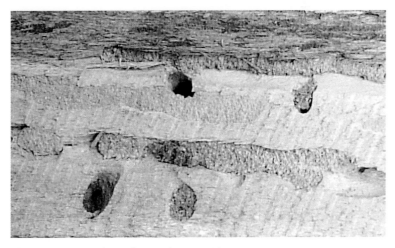

Plate 32 Longicorn borer damage (see p. 178)

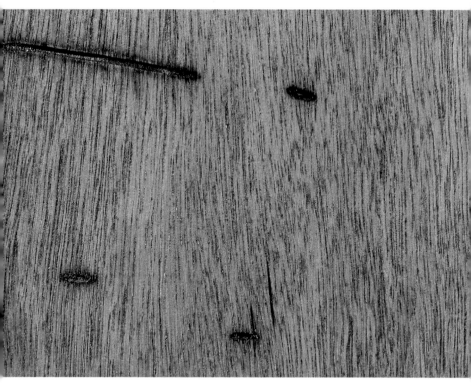

Plate 33 Pin-hole borer damage (see p. 179). Note the black stain within and surrounding the holes

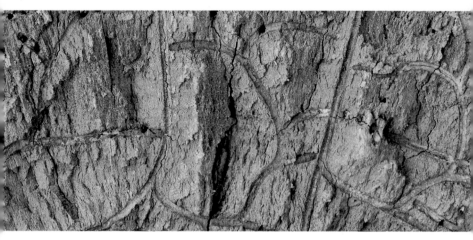

Plate 34 Instances of severe pin-hole damage can result in a brash fracture (see p. 179)

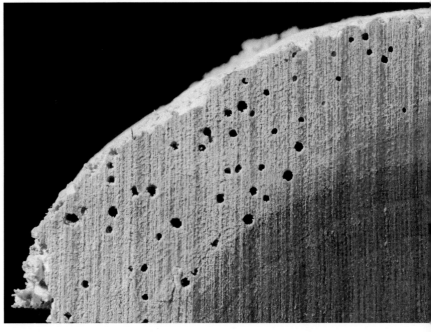

Plate 35 Hardwood sapwood riddled by the lyctid borer (see p. 179). There is no damage to the heartwood

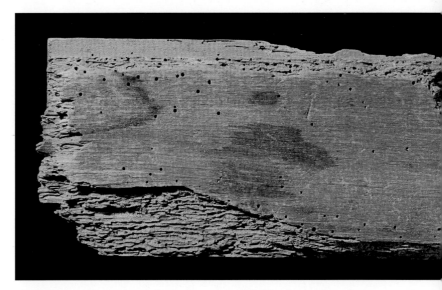

Plate 36 Sapwood of New Zealand white pine riddled by the *Anobium* borer (see p. 180)

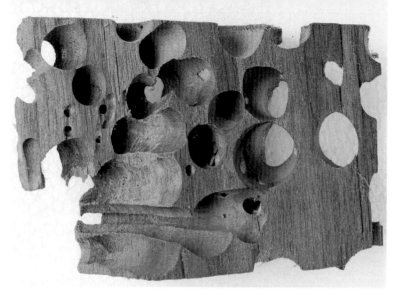

Plate 37 The typical network of tunnels formed by the *Teredo* borer (see p. 182)

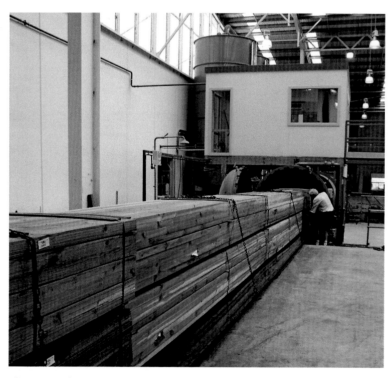

Plate 38 Modern preservative treatment plants in which the operations are under cover to minimise environmental impact (see p. 186) Source: courtesy Dr Harry Greaves

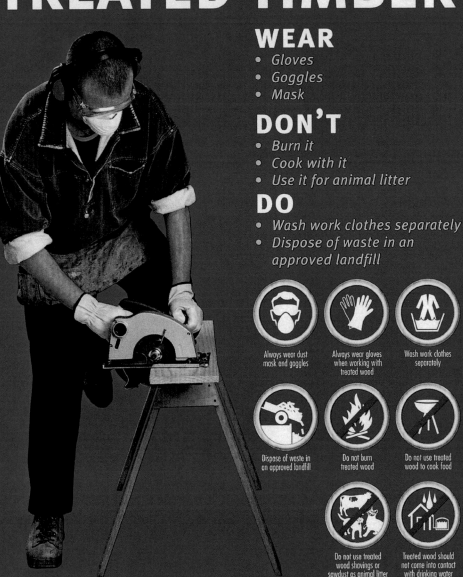

Plate 39 Point of sale safety information (see p. 196)

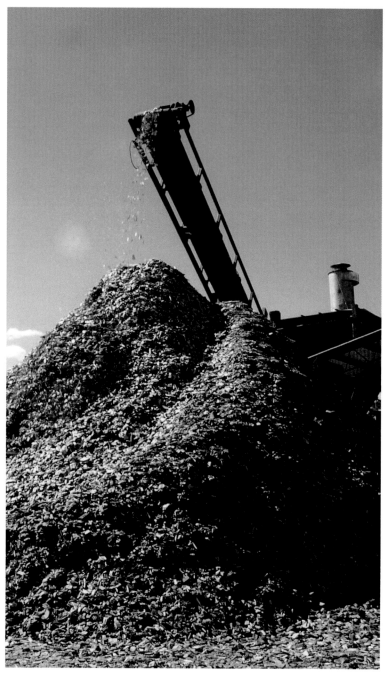

Plate 40 Cypress chip residue destined for 'green' power generation (see p. 198)

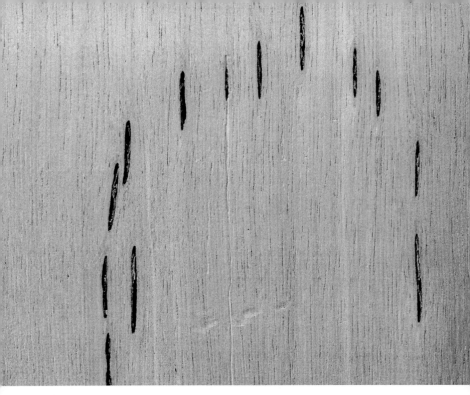

Plate 41 Latex canals in white cheesewood (see p. 266)

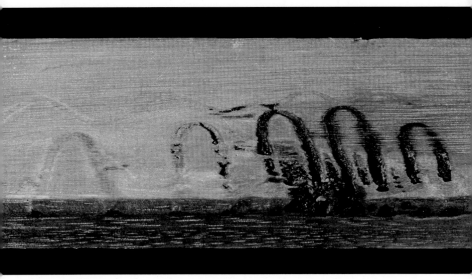

Plate 42 Scribbly borer marks in rose gum, producing hobnail on quarter-cut edge (see p. 281)

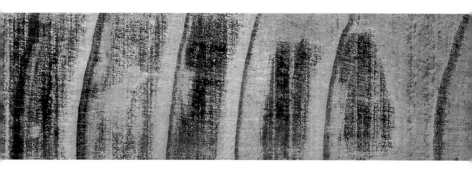

Plate 43 Areas of high resin content in radiata pine, indicated by the darker colour of the affected wood (see p. 327)

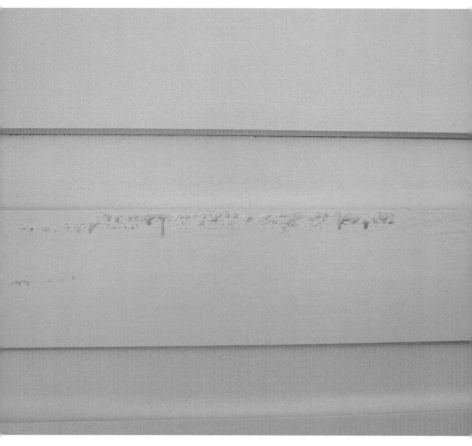

Plate 44 An example of the failure of an external stain finish on radiata pine with a high resin content (see p. 327). Note that the resin exudation is concentrated in the bands of latewood on this quarter-cut board

Properties of species and notes on uses

Species descriptions

Brief descriptions of the main features of the timber of the most commonly mentioned species have been provided in the section that follows. Selection of species was necessarily subjective, for the considerations of space prevent the inclusion of a large number of species of interest and an arbitrary choice has had to be made. For a guide to the classification of descriptions, see page 233.

Many Australian species, particularly those of rainforest origin, have had to be omitted when of little commercial availability, yet they are of potential importance in woodcraft work. Species in this category include:

- *Abarema hendersoni* (tulip siris)
- *Alangium villosum* (canary muskheart)
- *Bridelia exaltata* (scrub ironbark)
- *Daviesia arborea* (daviesia)
- *Drypetes australasica* (grey boxwood)
- *Endiandra compressa* (Queensland greenheart)
- *Guilfoylia monostylis* (scrub ooline)
- *Harpullia pendula* (tulipwood)
- *Olea paniculata* (native olive)
- *Pleiococca wilcoxiana* (silver aspen)
- *Rhodosphaera rhodanthema* (tulip satinwood)
- *Sarcopteryx stipitata* (corduroy)
- *Zanthoxylum brachyacanthum* (thorny yellowwood)

As well as the main Australian species of commercial importance, a large number of overseas timbers have been included, some because they are imported in considerable quantity, others because their names appear in overseas specifications and Australian species compete with them in world markets, and others because their names crop up in general literature on wood products, thus provoking local inquiry as to their properties.

A list of publications that have been of invaluable assistance in the assembly of this information is provided on page 363. Reference should be made to these publications for fuller accounts of the properties of the listed species and of others that it has not been possible to mention here.

Some explanatory notes on aspects of the summaries follow.

Naming of trees

Because of the many thousands of different species of tree their naming presents a complicated problem. Common names often change from state to state, even district to district. Over the years the 'standard trade name' proposed by Standards Australia in AS/NZS 1148 *Timber— Nomenclature—Australian, New Zealand and Imported Species* has had some effect among people closely involved in the timber industry but a lot of confusion remains. Because of this it is often advisable, when placing orders or writing about particular species, to include the botanical name as well.

However, botanical names are also still in a state of flux for many species. It is not uncommon for a botanical name, accepted for many years, to be changed because further investigation by botanical taxonomists (those concerned with the naming of plants) has led to the discovery that someone had given that particular species a different name at an earlier date and this different name then takes precedence. The situation is difficult for the wood technologist as well as the layperson and presents an unfortunate degree of confusion when one wishes to consult old sources of information in which different botanical names were used.

With the passage of time it is hoped that the position will become stabilised. In an endeavour to make the botanical names more useful to the reader, a number of earlier synonyms have been included in some of the species descriptions to assist in cross-references to other publications of previous decades. The names given in the current Australian Standards have been followed in the main but a few divergences in both common name and botanical name have been made where current practice in the industry runs contrary to the Standards.

The common names for Australian timbers are particularly confusing because the early European settlers applied Northern Hemisphere names, such as ash, beech, elm, hickory, oak and teak, to species that have nothing in common botanically with such species.

To enable botanical names to have an international basis, the early attempts in the 18th century to achieve standardisation were based on Latin and pseudo-Latin words. The Swedish botanist, Carl Linnaeus, did most to put the naming of plants in an organised basis; he elaborated a system by which each distinctive kind of plant was given a generic name indicative of its group, plus a specific name. Problems arose when botanists gave the same plant different names, or the same name to different plants, so it was necessary to develop the *International Code of Botanical Nomenclature*, which is reflected in the *Index Kewensis*, the standard world reference on plant names.

If one wishes to comply strictly with international rules of nomenclature, one has to provide the name of the author as well as the general and specific name, a ruling usually observed when writing for scientific journals but too cumbersome for everyday use. In the species descriptions the identity of the botanist who gave the name to the species is given in the abbreviated form accepted for scientific papers.

When one taxonomist makes a change to the name prescribed earlier, the name of that earlier author is often shown in brackets. For a comprehensive discussion of the complex problem of an international nomenclature, textbooks on botany should be consulted. A helpful introduction is given in *The Structure of Wood* by F. W. Jane, second edition by K. Wilson and D. J. B. White (1970).

Guide to classification of descriptions

The species descriptions that follow conform to the list of numbered subsections, which are explained below. For some species, there was no information available to the authors for a particular subsection and, in those instances, the numerical subsection has not been included. For example, Georgina gidgee only has numerical subsections for 1, 2 and 3.

1 *Size of tree and type of forest (location)*

The actual height and diameter of mature specimens are often quoted in reference books but are not necessarily a helpful guideline to the general appearance of the tree since the size of tree as felled for timber will depend largely on the age of the crop. Descriptions have been limited to small (up to 15 m average height), medium (to 30 m) and large (over 30 m), to give a broad indication of the nature of the tree.

Type of forest

As a result of differences in rainfall, soil quality and tree species, forests vary considerably in the nature of their growth. They may be classified into three main types, which are described below in very general terms.

Sclerophyll forest   In this forest there is a continuous canopy of the tree crowns. The length of the tree trunk is greater than the depth of the leafy crown and most of the trees have sclerophyllous leaves (i.e. they are of relatively hard and stiff texture). The main eucalypt forests are of this type.

Savannah   The savannah is open forest where the trees are of relatively scattered occurrence, the canopy is discontinuous, the length of the tree trunk is usually less than the depth of the leafy crown, and there is usually a ground cover of grass or small shrubs.

Rainforest   This forest requires a high level of soil moisture. The canopy is virtually continuous but may be arranged in several distinct layers. A prominent feature is the frequent presence of epiphytes and vines on the tree trunks. Because of the thick canopy of leaves, little sunlight penetrates to the forest floor, so there is an absence of grasses and herbage.

2 *Description of wood*

Describes the visual and physical characteristics of the wood, such as colour, smell, grain texture and extractives where present.

3 Density

'Green density' (GD) is the density of the wood at the time the living tree is felled. It varies considerably with the season, weather conditions, the age of the tree and so on; the quoted figures must therefore be accepted as a guideline only and when accurate green density figures are required for, say, assessment of transport costs, it is advisable to carry out accurate determinations on the material involved.

The air dry density (ADD) given is the average figure at 12 per cent moisture content. It can vary considerably with conditions of growth, climate and maturity of wood.

4 Drying and shrinkage characteristics

The figures given indicate the change in dimension in both the radial and tangential directions when the timber dries from the green, freshly felled condition down to 12 per cent moisture content. Some reference books give figures for shrinkage from green condition to 6 per cent, others to oven dry condition (0 per cent), so when making comparisons between species it is essential to check on the basis of the figures quoted.

Shrinkage varies very considerably within a species. Any attempt to give figures accurate to the decimal place is out of touch with reality; the average figures listed have been taken to the nearest half per cent.

5 Workability

Such characteristics as ease or difficulty of turning, ease or difficulty of nailing and bending and susceptibility to splitting.

6 Durability

It is difficult to determine a satisfactory classification in terms of durability because of the considerable within-species variability, as well as the wide range of climatic factors in Australia, which encourage widely differing hazards of decay and insect attack. The currently accepted Australian rating system is described on page 187 and in AS 5604 *Timber—Natural Durability Ratings*. The natural durability ratings are based on expert opinions and on the testing of stakes and poles embedded in the ground and represent a combined assessment of resistance to decay and termites. In particular end uses for a specific site, it is always worthwhile to seek local advice on species' suitability.

The sapwood of virtually all species has very poor durability in external locations, even when it is not susceptible to lyctid borer attack, so *all references to natural durability are concerned with the heartwood only.*

In considering the possibility of lyctid borer attack it is important to remember that only the sapwood of some hardwoods is susceptible and that *all softwoods are not susceptible to attack*.

In the species descriptions following, the ratings are set out thus:

- Lyctids 'S' or 'NS': where 'S' indicates that the sapwood is susceptible to the lyctid borer and 'NS' indicates that it is not.

- Termites 'R' or 'NR': where 'R' indicates that the heartwood is resistant to termite attack inside above ground—applicable to hazard class 2 (H2) in AS 1604 *Specification for Preservative Treatment* series—and 'NR' indicates that it is not.
- Durability 'IG', 'AG' and 'M': where 'IG' indicates in-ground, 'AG' indicates above-ground, and 'M' indicates exposure to marine borers, each followed by 1, 2, 3 or 4, where the number indicates the natural durability class of the heartwood in each situation. Marine borer resistance ratings apply to southern waters (i.e. south of Perth in the west and south of Batemans Bay in the east). Only class 1 timbers can be expected to to give a reasonable service life (12–30 years) in northern waters.

Where insufficient knowledge is available a rating is not included.

7 Strength grouping

The significance and method of allocation of strength groups is explained on page 37. Classification may change for some species through the influence of further test results.

8 Use

A selection of uses has been included as a guideline to the most suitable applications but omission of mention does not infer unacceptability for other purposes.

9 Availability

Availability has been mentioned in general terms and will be useful only as a very broad guideline. Most of the less common Australian species will be available only in the districts where they occur. The volume of production and importation of timber varies considerably from year to year.

Afrormosia *Pericopsis elata* (Harms) van Meeuwen
Synonym: *Afrormosia elata* Harms
Other common name: Kokrodua

1 A large hardwood of the west African rainforests. **2** Heartwood golden brown, often with dark streaks. Sapwood narrow (10–15 mm) and usually distinctly paler. Texture medium. Grain variable. Somewhat like teak in general appearance but lacks its oily nature. **3** GD about 1100 kg/m³; ADD about 700 kg/m³. **4** Easy to dry. Shrinkage about 3 per cent radial, 6 per cent tangential. **5** Easy to work. Turns satisfactorily. Care needed when nailing to avoid splitting. Not suitable for steam bending. Contains a lot of tannins so there is a risk of staining if wet wood comes in contact with ferrous fixings. Sanding dust can be irritating to eyes and skin. **6** Durability IG2; heartwood very difficult to impregnate with preservatives. **7** Probably S3, SD3. Some mechanical properties are listed on page 411. **8** Decorative veneer, furniture, high-quality joinery. **9** Seldom seen in Australia, mainly as veneer.

Aglaia *Aglaia* spp.

1 A hardwood of wide distribution in Papua New Guinea and the Solomon Islands but not a major species. **2** Heartwood pale brown to reddish brown. Sapwood straw to pink. Fragrant odour. **3** ADD varies with species, the range being 720–960 kg/m³. **4** Shrinkage about 2.5 per cent radial, 5.5 per cent tangential. **6** Lyctids probably S; durability IG3; heartwood difficult to impregnate with preservatives. **7** Because of the wide density range, strength may vary considerably; it is classified provisionally as S3, SD4. **8** Plywood, turnery, furniture, internal joinery. **9** Seldom seen in Australia.

Alder, blush *Sloanea australis* (Benth.) F. Muell.

1 A medium-sized hardwood of the coastal rainforests from the Illawarra district of New South Wales to north Queensland. **2** Heartwood pinkish brown, darkening on exposure. Sapwood whitish. Texture fine and even. Grain often rather interlocked. **3** GD about 900 kg/m³; ADD about 600 kg/m³. **4** Easy to dry but some collapse occurs. Shrinkage about 2.5 per cent radial, 5 per cent tangential; after reconditioning about 2 per cent radial, 4 per cent tangential. **5** Easy to work. Glues well. **6** Lyctids S; durability IG4, M4. **7** S5, SD6. Some mechanical properties are listed on page 411. **8** Internal joinery, plywood, turnery. **9** Seldom available commercially.

Alder, brown *Caldcluvia paniculosa* (F. Muell.) Hoogland
Synonyms: *Ackama paniculata* Engl.
Ackama muelleri Benth.
Other common name: corkwood (because of its bark)

1 A large hardwood of the coastal rainforests from the Hunter River in New South Wales to the Mackay district of Queensland. **2** Heartwood pale to dark pinkish brown, sometimes with a purple tint. Sapwood, about 25 mm wide, greyish brown, usually distinct from the heartwood. Texture fine and even. Grain usually straight. Very little figure. **3** GD about 900 kg/m³; ADD about 600 kg/m³.   **4** Slow in drying and liable to warp and twist if not carefully stacked with closely spaced stickers. Some collapse occurs and reconditioning is worthwhile. Shrinkage about 5 per cent radial, 9 per cent tangential; after reconditioning about 3.5 per cent radial, 6 per cent tangential.   **5** Relatively easy to work but inclined to brittleness so not suitable for steam bending. Glues well.   **6** Lyctids S; termites NR; durability IG4, M4; heartwood readily accepts impregnation with preservatives.   **7** S5, SD6. Some mechanical properties are listed on page 411.   **8** Plywood, furniture, internal joinery, turnery.   **9** Very limited.

Alder, hard *Pullea stutzeri* (F. Muell.) L. S. Gibbs

1 A small hardwood of the north Queensland rainforests.   **2** Heartwood greyish brown. Texture very fine and even. Grain straight. The rays are large enough to produce a considerable figure on the radial surface.   **3** ADD about 830 kg/m³.   **6** Durability IG4.   **7** Provisionally S4, SD4. Some mechanical properties are listed on page 411.   **8** Turnery.   **9** Of little significance commercially.

Alder, rose *Caldcluvia australiensis* (Schltr.) Hoogland
Synonyms: *Ackama australiensis* (Schltr.) C. T. White
Ackama quadrivalvis C. T. White et W. D. Francis

1 A large hardwood of the north Queensland rainforests between Innisfail and Cooktown.   **2** The wood is similar to that of brown alder. Heartwood pink to dark pinkish brown. Texture fine and even. Grain usually straight.   **3** ADD about 600 kg/m³.   **4** Slow in drying, with some collapse. The amount of shrinkage may be somewhat less than that of brown alder.   **6** Lyctids NS; termites NR; durability IG4, M4.   **7** S6, SD6.   **8** Plywood, interior joinery, turnery.   **9** A commercial species in north Queensland.

Alerce *Fitzroya cupressoides* (Mol.) Johnst.

1 A large softwood of southern Chile and Argentina.   **2** Heartwood reddish brown (very similar to Californian redwood), darkening on exposure; often has darker streaks. Sapwood narrow and whitish. Texture fine and uniform. Grain usually straight.   **3** ADD about 470 kg/m³.   **4** Easy to dry. Shrinkage about 2.5 per cent radial, 4 per cent tangential.   **5** Easy to work if tools are kept sharp.   **6** Lyctids NS; termites R; durability IG1, AG1; heartwood moderately resistant to impregnation with preservatives.   **7** S7, SD8.   **8** Outdoor furniture, cladding, joinery, roof shingles.   **9** Seldom seen in Australia.

Amberoi *Pterocymbium* spp., especially *Pterocymbium beccarii* K. Schum.

1 A hardwood widely distributed from Papua New Guinea to Sabah and the Philippines.   **2** Heartwood cream coloured. Sapwood whitish and not clearly distinguishable from the heartwood. Texture rather coarse. Grain straight.   **3** ADD about 370 kg/m³.   **4** Needs care in drying to avoid bluestain. Shrinkage about 2 per cent radial, 5 per cent tangential. **5** Easy to work. Glues satisfactorily. Unsuitable for turnery. **6** Lyctids S; termites NR; durability IG4, M4; heartwood easy to impregnate with preservatives. **7** SD8, below S7. Not a structural timber. Some mechanical properties are listed on page 411. **8** Plywood, interior joinery, packaging. **9** Occasionally imported in small quantities.

Amoora *Amoora cucullata* Roxb.

1 A hardwood widely distributed in Papua New Guinea but not of major commercial importance. Similar species occur in the Indian subcontinent and South-East Asia. **2** Heartwood red to reddish brown. Sapwood pale pink. **3** ADD about 540 kg/m³. **4** Shrinkage about 3 per cent radial, 7 per cent tangential. **6** Lyctids S, durability IG4, AG4; heartwood difficult to impregnate with preservatives. **7** S6, SD5. Some mechanical properties are listed on page 411. **8** Joinery, furniture, veneer, turnery. **9** Occasionally imported in small quantities.

Andiroba *Carapa guianensis* Aubl.
Other common names: Brazilian mahogany, crabwood

1 A large, fast-growing hardwood of the lowland forests of northern South America, Central America and the West Indies. **2** Heartwood pale pink to dark red when first cut, but changing to a dark reddish brown. Resembles the true mahogany (*Swietenia*) but likely to be somewhat darker and less lustrous. The sapwood can be up to 50 mm thick and is of a pale brown colour. Texture variable. Grain usually straight. **3** ADD about 650 kg/m³. **4** Slow in drying, with some risk of splitting. Shrinkage about 3.5 per cent radial, 7 per cent tangential. **5** Relatively easy to work. May need predrilling for nails. Glues well. Not suitable for steam bending. **6** Lyctids S; durability IG3. **7** Possibly S4, SD4. **8** Furniture. **9** Seldom imported.

Antiaris *Antiaris toxicaria* (Rumph. ex Pers.) Lesch.

1 A hardwood widely distributed through tropical Asia and Africa as well as New Guinea and occasionally in north Queensland. **2** Heartwood and sapwood both pale cream. Texture coarse. Grain wavy. The latex produced by the tree is poisonous (hence the botanical name of the tree). **3** ADD 400–470 kg/m³. **4** Needs care in drying to avoid bluestain. Shrinkage about 2 per cent radial, 4.5 per cent tangential. **5** Easy to work. Nails satisfactorily. **6** Lyctids S; durability IG4; heartwood is readily impregnated with preservatives. **7** S7, SD8. Not a structural timber. Some mechanical properties are listed on page 411. **8** Internal mouldings, packaging. **9** Small quantities occasionally imported.

Apple, black *Planchonella australis* (F. Muell.) Pierre
Synonym: *Sideroxylon oust rale* F. Muell.

1 A scarce hardwood of the coastal rainforests of New South Wales and Queensland. **2** Heartwood pale yellow with darker streaks. Sapwood may not be clearly distinguishable. Texture very fine and even.

Grain sometimes interlocked. **3** GD about 1130 kg/m³; ADD about 880 kg/m³. **4** Needs careful drying. Slight collapse occurs. Shrinkage about 4 per cent radial, 7.5 per cent tangential; after reconditioning 3 per cent radial, 5 per cent tangential. **6** Lyctids S. **7** S3, SD3. Some mechanical properties are listed on page 411. **8** Artificial limbs, carving, turnery, marquetry, bearings, fishing rods. **9** Not a commercial species.

Apple, broad-leaved *Angophora subvelutina* F. Muell.

1 A predominantly coastal hardwood extending from the central coast of New South Wales to south-east Queensland. It is not as widely distributed as rough-barked apple and is less likely to be found inland. **2** Heartwood pale reddish brown. Sapwood distinctly paler. Texture rather coarse but even. Grain often interlocked. **3** GD about 1160 kg/m³; ADD about 750 kg/m³. **4** Shrinkage about 3.5 per cent radial, 5.5 per cent tangential. **6** Lyctids S; durability IG3. **7** S4 and provisionally SD5. **8** Seldom milled because logs usually faulty but could be suitable for general construction as well as fencing and fuel. **9** Seldom offered commercially.

Apple, rough-barked *Angophora floribunda* (Sm.) Sweet
Synonym: *Angophora intermedia* DC.

1 A medium-sized hardwood common in New South Wales in coastal districts, western slopes and northern tablelands, and extending into Queensland as far north as Bundaberg. **2** Heartwood pink to reddish brown. Sapwood distinctly paler. Texture rather coarse. Grain sometimes interlocked. Gum veins common. **3** GD about 1180 kg/m³; ADD about 850 kg/m³. **4** Shrinkage about 3.5 per cent radial, 5.5 per cent tangential. **6** Lyctids S; durability IG3. **7** Provisionally S4 and SD5. Some mechanical properties are listed on page 411. **8** As the logs are usually faulty little is cut for construction purposes but it is commonly used for fence palings and fuel. **9** Mainly in fencing materials.

Apple, smooth-barked *Angophora costata* (Gaertn.) J. Britt.
Synonym: *Angophora lanceolata* Cav.

1 A medium-sized hardwood of the central coast and north-western slopes of New South Wales, and in eastern Queensland as far north as Rockhampton. **2** Heartwood pale brown. Sapwood wide and distinctly paler. Texture rather coarse. Grain often interlocked. Gum veins common. **3** GD about 1240 kg/m³; ADD about 990 kg/m³. **4** Shrinkage about 3 per cent radial, 6 per cent tangential. **6** Lyctids S; durability IG3, M4. **7** S3, SD3. Some mechanical properties are listed on page 411. **8** As the logs are usually faulty it is seldom cut for building framework. It is a good fuel. **9** Mainly in fencing materials.

Ash, alpine *Eucalyptus delegatensis* R. T. Bak.
Synonym: *Eucalyptus gigantea* Hook, f.

1 A large hardwood of the cold climate areas of Tasmania, eastern Victoria and south-eastern New South Wales. **2** Heartwood pale pink or pale yellowish brown. Sapwood not clearly distinguishable and about 25–50 mm wide. Texture moderately coarse. Grain usually straight but sometimes wavy, producing a fiddleback figure. Gum veins common. Growth rings made conspicuous by the darker latewood. Very similar in appearance to mountain ash. **3** GD about 1050 kg/m³; ADD about 620 kg/m³. **4** Needs much care in drying because of proneness to collapse and internal checking, as well as surface checking on the tangential surface. For good-quality boards it is usual practice to quarter cut the logs. Reconditioning is standard practice. Shrinkage about 4.5 per cent radial, 8 per cent tangential; after reconditioning 3.5 per cent radial, 6.5 per cent tangential. **5** Relatively easy to work. Satisfactory for steam bending. Glues well. A walnut colour is obtained when it is fumed with ammonia. **6** Lyctids of origin Victoria NS, origin elsewhere S; termites NR; durability IG4, AG3, M4. **7** S4, SD4. Some mechanical properties are listed on page 411. **8** Furniture, plywood, joinery, panelling, flooring, oars, skis, agricultural implements, handles, cooperage, general construction. **9** It is a major species in Tasmania and Victoria; the Tasmanian wood is often sold to other states mixed with mountain ash and messmate under the trade term Tasmanian oak. The relative proportions of each species can vary considerably.

Ash, Bennett's *Flindersia bennettiana* F. Muell. ex Benth.

1 A hardwood of the coastal rainforest between the Clarence River in New South Wales and the Maryborough district of Queensland. **2** Heartwood pale straw. Sapwood not easily distinguished. Texture medium and even. **3** ADD about 840 kg/m³. **4** Needs care in drying to avoid surface checks. **5** Relatively easy to work. As the surface is inclined to be greasy it can be difficult to glue. **6** Lyctids S; durability IG3. **7** Provisionally S4, SD4. **8** Joinery, furniture, veneer. **9** Seldom available.

Ash, Blue Mountains *Eucalyptus oreades* R. T. Bak.

1 A tall hardwood of the central tablelands of New South Wales. Also found in the MacPherson Ranges on the border of Queensland and New South Wales. **2** Heartwood pale brown. Sapwood not clearly distinguishable. Texture moderately coarse. Grain straight. Growth rings prominent. **3** GD about 1080 kg/m³; ADD about 700 kg/m³. **4** Needs care in drying because of collapse. Shrinkage about 5 per cent radial, 8.5 per cent tangential; after reconditioning about 3 per cent radial, 5.5 per cent tangential. **6** Lyctids NS; durability IG4, M4. **7** SD5 and provisionally S5. Some mechanical properties are listed on page 411. **8** General construction, joinery. **9** Seldom marketed.

Ash, Crow's *Flindersia australis* R. Br.
Other common name: Australian teak

1 A large hardwood of occasional occurrence in the coastal rainforests of northern New South Wales, and also in Queensland as far north as the Gladstone area. **2** Heartwood golden yellow.

Sapwood distinctively paler and 25–40 mm wide. Texture medium and even. Grain often interlocked. Has very greasy surface. **3** GD about 1050 kg/m³; ADD about 950 kg/m³. **4** Slow to dry and needs protection in the initial stages from too rapid a drying rate, which would cause surface checking. Negligible collapse. Shrinkage about 3 per cent radial, 4 per cent tangential. **5** Not easy to work. Hard to glue because of its greasiness; a swabbing with methylated spirits before use may be helpful. Does not hold nails very firmly, for the same reason. Only fair for steam bending. Wears very well. **6** Lyctids S; termites R; durability IG1, AG1. **7** S2, SD3. Some mechanical properties are listed on page 411. **8** Flooring (especially good for dance floors), decking, boat building, outdoor furniture. **9** Usually only in districts of occurrence.

Ash, European *Fraxinus excelsior* L.

1 A medium-sized hardwood widely distributed in Europe. **2** Heartwood pale straw to pale pinkish brown. Sapwood pale straw, wide and often hard to distinguish from the heartwood. Texture rather coarse. Grain usually straight. Growth rings give considerable figure to the tangential surface. **3** ADD about 700 kg/m³. **4** Seasons without much degrade if stacks are weighted to restrain warping. Protection needed against end splitting. Reconditioning worthwhile. Shrinkage about 3 per cent radial, 4.5 per cent tangential. **5** Easy to work and gives smooth finish. Glues well. Very suitable for steam bending. Good resistance to sudden impact. **6** Lyctids S; durability IG4; heartwood variable in ease of impregnation with preservatives. **7** S5, SD5. Some mechanical properties are listed on page 411. **8** A very popular species for sporting equipment because of its toughness and flexibility. Also valued for tool handles, furniture and light aircraft construction. **9** Small quantities are imported into Australia for specialised uses.

Ash, hickory *Flindersia ifflaiana* F. Muell.

1 A large hardwood of the rainforests of the Cairns district of north Queensland. Rather similar in appearance to Crow's ash but not as greasy. **2** Heartwood yellowish brown. Sapwood paler. Texture medium and even. Grain variable. **3** GD about 1200 kg/m³; ADD about 980 kg/m³. **4** Dries slowly. Needs care to prevent checking. Shrinkage about 3 per cent radial, 4.5 per cent tangential. Negligible collapse. **5** Not easy to work. Fair for steam bending. **6** Lyctids S; termites R; durability IG2; AG1. **7** SI and provisionally SD2. **8** Flooring, handles, decking, outdoor furniture, boat building. **9** Usually confined to districts of occurrence.

Ash, mountain *Eucalyptus regnans* F. Muell.

1 A very large hardwood of the mountain regions of Tasmania and eastern Victoria. It is the largest of the eucalypts; indeed, the world's tallest hardwood is a mountain ash of the Styx River area of Tasmania; it is about 350 years old, 98 m in height and 5.2 m in diameter at the ground.

It is not the world's tallest tree, which is a softwood, a Californian redwood, 112 m in height. **2** Heartwood pale pink or pale straw. Sapwood not always clearly differentiated. Texture rather coarse. Grain straight. Growth rings conspicuous. Gum veins common. **3** GD about 1030 kg/m³; ADD about 680 kg/m³. **4** Considerable collapse occurs during drying so reconditioning is standard practice for dressed products. For best results it is advisable to quarter cut the log. Shrinkage about 6.5 per cent radial, 13 per cent tangential; after reconditioning about 4 per cent radial, 7 per cent tangential. **5** Relatively easy to work. Good for steam bending. A pale walnut colour is obtained by fuming with ammonia. Glues satisfactorily. **6** Lyctids NS; termites NR; durability IG4, AG3, M4. **7** S4, SD3. Some mechanical properties are listed on page 411. **8** Furniture, joinery, plywood, handles, cooperage, wood wool, flooring, panelling, general construction. **9** A major species in Tasmania and Victoria. Often sold in other states, sometimes mixed with other species and marketed as Tasmanian oak.

Ash, red *Alphitonia excelsa* (Fenzl.) Reisseck ex Benth.
Other common name: red almond

1 A medium-sized hardwood of the drier types of coastal rainforest of New South Wales and Queensland; also found occasionally in inland districts. A closely allied species, *Alphitonia petrel* Braid et C. T. White (pink ash), is common in north Queensland. **2** Heartwood pink when freshly cut, darkening to a rich orange-red. Stripes of varying hue often occur. The sapwood is distinctively paler. Texture even and relatively fine. Grain straight. **3** GD about 1100 kg/m³; ADD about 740 kg/m³. **4** Needs careful drying to avoid surface checks. Shrinkage about 2 per cent radial, 6 per cent tangential. Only slight collapse. **5** Firm but not hard to work. **6** Lyctids NS; termites NR; durability IG2. **7** S3, SD3. Some mechanical properties are listed on page 411. Pink ash is very considerably weaker, provisionally S7, SD7. **8** Ornamental turnery, decorative veneer, panelling, joinery, flooring. **9** Not a commercial species.

Ash, silver *Flindersia bourjotiana* F. Muell.
Flindersia schottiana F. Muell.
Synonym: *F. pubescens* P. M. Bail.
Other common names: bumpy ash, cudgerie

1 A hardwood of the coastal rainforests from the Hastings River in New South Wales to north Queensland. **2** Heartwood very pale yellow and not distinct from the sapwood. Texture medium and even. Grain variable. **3** ADD averages about 670 kg/m³. **4** Rather slow to dry but with little degrade. Negligible collapse. Shrinkage about 3.5 per cent radial, 6 per cent tangential. **5** Easy to work. Good for steam bending. Glues well. **6** Lyctids S; termites NR; durability IG3, M4. **7** S4, SD5. Some mechanical properties are listed on page 412. **8** Furniture, panelling, decorative veneer, sporting equipment, handles, oars, cooperage, boat building. **9** Virtually limited to Queensland.

Ash, silvertop *Eucalyptus sieberi* L. Johnson
Synonym: *Eucalyptus sieberana* F. Muell.
Other common name: coast ash (NSW)

1 A large hardwood of the southern and central coast and tablelands of New South Wales, eastern Victoria and north-eastern Tasmania. **2** Heartwood pale brown, sometimes pinkish. Sapwood to 25 mm wide, not clearly distinguishable from the heartwood. Texture medium. Grain often interlocked. Growth rings noticeable but not prominent. Gum veins, pin-hole borer discolouration and 'pencil streak' are common. **3** GD about 1200 kg/m³; ADD about 820 kg/m³. **4** Slow in drying and prone to surface checking on the tangential surface. Collapse is significant and reconditioning is desirable. Shrinkage about 6 per cent radial, 10 per cent tangential; after reconditioning about 2.5 per cent radial, 5.5 per cent tangential. **5** Not difficult to work. Satisfactory for steam bending. Relatively easy to split along the rays and was therefore used by the pioneers for roof shakes. **6** Lyctids NS; termites NR; durability IG3, AG2, M4. **7** S3, SD3. Some mechanical properties are listed on page 412. **8** General construction, handles. It is one of the major species being converted into wood chips at Eden (NSW) for export for writing paper production. **9** Commonly used for building framework on the south coast and tablelands of New South Wales.

Ash, white *Eucalyptus fraxinoides* Deane et Maiden

1 A large hardwood of limited occurrence on the southern tablelands of New South Wales. **2** Heartwood almost white to pale brown. Sapwood not clearly distinguishable from the heartwood. Texture moderately coarse. Grain straight. Growth rings prominent. **3** GD about 950 kg/m³; ADD about 700 kg/m³. **4** Needs care in drying to avoid surface checking. Collapse occurs and reconditioning is desirable. Shrinkage about 5 per cent radial, 6.5 per cent tangential; after reconditioning about 4 per cent radial, 5.5 per cent tangential. **5** Relatively easy to work. Often has very good appearance but unfortunately is not plentiful. **6** Lyctids S; termites NR; durability IG4, M4. **7** S4, SD3. Some mechanical properties are listed on page 412. **8** Furniture, joinery, panelling, general construction. **9** Limited to districts of occurrence.

Backhousia, stony *Backhousia hughesii* C. I. White

1 A medium-to-large hardwood of the north Queensland rain-forests. **2** Heartwood greyish brown. Texture fine and uniform. Grain often interlocked. When damaged the tree produces a greyish exudate, which sets into a hard material of a stony nature and consists of calcium carbonate and magnesium carbonate. **3** ADD about 1000 kg/m³. **4** Seasons with little degrade. **5** Hard to work. **6** Lyctids NS; termites NR; durability IG2. **7** Provisionally S3, SD2. **8** Building framework. **9** Limited to north Queensland.

Balau *Shorea* spp., mainly *Shorea albida* Sym. (heavy variety)
Shorea glauca King
Shorea laevis Ridl.
Shorea maxwelliana King
Shorea seminis van Sloot.
Other common names: selangan batu no. 1 (Sabah); alan (Sarawak)

1 A group of the denser (above 900 kg/m³) *Shorea* hardwoods of Malaysia, Indonesia and the Philippines. **2** Heartwood yellow to brown, distinct from the paler sapwood, which can be up to 50 mm wide. Texture moderately fine and even. Grain interlocked, producing a stripe figure on the radial surface. Resin pockets sometimes present. Susceptible to pin-hole borer damage. **3** ADD varies with species, from 900 to 1100 kg/m³. **4** Care needed in drying to avoid surface checking and end splits. Rate of drying is slow. Shrinkage varies considerably with species, probably averages about 3.5 per cent radial, 7 per cent tangential. **5** In relation to its density it is not hard to work, although if resin is present is does tend to build up on cutting equipment. Silica absent. Predrilling advisable when nailing. Unsuitable for steam bending. **6** Lyctids S; termites NR; durability IG2, AG1, M4. **7** S2, SD3. **8** Heavy construction, wharfage, sleepers, shipbuilding. **9** Seldom seen in Australia.

Balsa *Ochroma pyramidale* (Cav.) Urban

1 Although the lightest and softest of commercial timbers, it is botanically a hardwood. It is native to tropical America, the main commercial source being Ecuador, but it is being grown in other tropical areas, including Papua New Guinea. **2** Sapwood very wide and greyish white or oatmeal in colour. Heartwood pinkish brown and said to be considerably weaker in strength than the sapwood. Texture rather coarse but even. Grain usually straight. Grows very rapidly, producing a large tree in 10 years. Logs have to be converted to sawn material immediately after felling to avoid pin-hole borer damage and bluestain. **3** ADD ranges from about 50 to 400 kg/m³ but the desired commercial product is usually confined to the range 110–170 kg/m³. **4** Dries very quickly but its very soft nature dictates careful handling. Shrinkage figures vary considerably because of the wide range of possible densities. Probably about 3 per cent radial and 6 per cent tangential would be a reasonable guide. **5** Easy to work if very sharp, thin-edged tools are used to avoid crushing of the wood. Glues satisfactorily. Unsuitable for steam bending because it buckles too easily. Too soft for the use of nails and screws. Has high insulating value against heat and sound transference. Impregnation with hot wax can be used to prevent the excessive absorption of water. **6** Lyctids S; durability IG4, AG4; heartwood has no resistance to decay and is variable in its acceptance of impregnation with preservatives. **7** It is not a structural wood. Some mechanical properties are listed on page 412. **8** Model-making, stage sets, insulation of refrigerated trucks, packing of fragile goods (where its strength gives it an advantage over polystyrene), floats, rafts, core stock, surgical splints, surfboards, hat blocks. It has been used extensively, in conjunction with fibreglass-reinforced plastics, for boat construction. **9** Small quantities are imported.

Baltic, red *Pinus sylvestris* L.
Other common names: Scots pine, red deal, Baltic pine

1 A medium-sized softwood widely distributed throughout Europe and northern Asia. **2** Sapwood creamy white or pale yellow, 50–100 mm wide, and easily distinguished from the yellow-brown to reddish brown heartwood. Growth rings prominently marked by the darker denser summerwood. Texture relatively fine. Grain usually straight. The knots are usually grouped, whereas in white Baltic they are much more randomly distributed. The wood is resinous. **3** GD about 830 kg/m³; ADD about 500 kg/m³. **4** Dries rapidly but is liable to bluestain. Shrinkage about 2 per cent radial, 4.5 per cent tangential. **5** Easy to work unless the small hard knots are numerous. Glues satisfactorily if very resinous material is excluded. Nails well. **6** Lyctids NS; durability IG4, M4. **7** S6, SD6. Some mechanical properties are listed on page 412. **8** General construction, flooring, panelling, interior joinery. Preservative-treated material has been used for poles, pit props, etc. **9** Not commercially available in Australia but may often be seen in the form of containers for imported goods.

Baltic, white *Picea abies* (L.) Karst.
Synonym: *Picea excelsa* Link
Other common names: Norway spruce, white deal

1 This medium-sized softwood is the traditional Christmas tree of northern Europe. **2** The sapwood is white to pale yellow and not clearly differentiated from the heartwood. The growth rings are less conspicuous than those of red Baltic and the wood is much less resinous. Texture medium. Grain usually straight but there is a tendency for spiral grain to be present. **3** ADD about 420 kg/m³. **4** Dries easily but there is a risk of bluestain and surface checking. Shrinkage about 1.5 per cent radial, 4 per cent tangential. **5** Easy to work, except for the small tight knots that soon dull tool edges. Glues satisfactorily. **6** Lyctids NS; durability IG4, M4. The sapwood is susceptible to the *Anobium* borer under favourable conditions; many floors laid in white Baltic in eastern Australia between 50 and 80 years ago are now showing considerable *Anobium* infestation in the sapwood. **7** S7, SD7. Some mechanical properties are listed on page 412. **8** General construction, flooring, cladding. Considerable quantities were imported into Australia in past years for the two latter purposes. **9** Occasionally imported, mainly in the form of cladding.

Bamboo Various species of *Arundinaria, Bambusa, Dendrocalamus, Pseudosasa, Phyllostachys* and *Schizostachyum*

1 Bamboo is not a tree but a very large grass so the felled material is not defined as timber. It is included here because of its common use in furniture and blinds. The material seen in Australia is mostly imported from South-East Asia but small quantities are grown in the more tropical coastal districts of eastern Australia.   **4** Needs care in drying to prevent splitting. Splits start at the nodes because the cross walls at these locations are not free to move inwards. Collapse can occur. Dried material is more yellow than that which is dried rapidly in a kiln.   **5** Relatively easy to work. Material for blinds is usually split by knife. It accepts most clear finishes satisfactorily if properly seasoned.   **6** Lyctids S; durability IG4, AG4. Its starch content and porous nature make it susceptible to bostrychid and lyctid borer attack. This can be prevented by soaking the freshly cut material in a 3 per cent solution of borax or sodium octaborate for 1–2 weeks. The split bamboo absorbs preservative much more rapidly than the round cane. Even soaking in water gives some measure of protection against borer attack. Resistance to decay is poor in exposed conditions or ground contact but pressure impregnation with non-leachable preservatives can be carried out successfully.   **8** Furniture, fishing rods. It gives a high yield of cellulose so is a source of paper pulp.   **9** Imported material is commonly used for furniture and blind manufacture.

Banksia *Banksia* spp.

1 There are a number of species of this small hardwood in coastal districts of eastern Australia.   **2** Heartwood reddish brown, sapwood distinctively paler. Conspicuous ray figure, somewhat like that of silky oak. The trees are usually small and gnarled so do not provide a millable log, but the decorative nature of the wood could attract the artisan turner.   **3** ADD of saw banksia (*Banksia serrata*) 720 kg/m³, wallum banksia (*Banksia serratifolia*) 650 kg/m³ and white banksia (*Banksia integrifolia*) 560 kg/m³.   **4** Shrinkage is likely to be high so careful and slow drying is needed.   **6** Lyctids probably S.   **7** Probably S7 and SD7. Some mechanical properties of wallum banksia are given on page 412.   **8** Decorative woodware.   **9** Not a commercial species.

Basswood, New Guinea *Endospermum* spp.
Other common names: white milkwood, sendok-sendok, kauvula (Fiji)

1 A large hardwood of common occurrence in Papua New Guinea. *Endospermum* species of similar properties occur from Malaysia through to Fiji.   **2** Sapwood and heartwood both pale yellow. Texture rather coarse but even. Grain straight or slightly interlocked. Some brittleheart and tension wood likely in the logs.   **3** ADD varies widely from about 360 to 600 kg/m³. The New Guinea material is at the lower end of this range, while Fijian wood averages about 480 kg/m³.   **4** Dries rapidly but care is needed to avoid bluestain. Shrinkage about 1.5 per cent radial, 3 per cent tangential, or slightly higher.   **5** Easy to saw but gives a rather 'woolly' surface. Glues well.   **6** Lyctids S; durability IG4; heartwood absorbs preservatives readily.   **7** S7, SD7 to S5, SD6 depending on species. Some mechanical properties are listed on page 412. **8** Internal joinery, plywood, pattern-making. **9** Not commonly seen in Australia.

Basswood, silver *Tieghemopanax elegans* (C. Moore et F. Muell.) Viguier
Synonyms: *Panax elegans* F. Muell.
Polyscias elegans (C. Moore et F. Muell.) Harms

1 A small hardwood of the coastal rainforests from the Illawarra district of New South Wales to north Queensland. **2** Heartwood and sapwood both white to very pale brown. Texture moderately fine and even. Grain straight. Small ray figure on the radial face. **3** GD about 670 kg/m³; ADD about 460 kg/m³. **4** Shrinkage about 2 per cent radial, 5 per cent tangential. Negligible collapse. Needs protection against bluestain and surface checking. **5** Easy to work. **6** Lyctids S; durability IG4. **7** Provisionally SD8 and below S7. **8** Internal joinery, veneer. **9** Scarce.

Basswood, white *Tieghemopanax murrayi* (F. Muell.) Viguier
Synonyms: *Panax murrayi* F. Muell.
Polyscias murrayi (F. Muell.) Harms

1 A small hardwood of the coastal rainforests of New South Wales and Queensland. **2** Very similar in appearance and properties to silver basswood, but less dense. **3** GD about 610 kg/m³; ADD about 400 kg/m³. **4** Shrinkage about 3 per cent radial, 6 per cent tangential. Negligible collapse. Needs protection against bluestain and surface checking. **5** Easy to work. **6** Lyctids S; durability IG4. **7** Below S7 and SD8. Not for structural purposes. **8** Internal joinery, veneer. **9** Scarce.

Bean, black *Castanospermum australe* A. Cunn. et Fraser ex Hook.

1 A large hardwood of the rainforests from northern New South Wales through to north Queensland. Very little is now available in New South Wales. **2** Heartwood dark brown to almost black, relieved by paler streaks of the soft tissue surrounding the pores. Sapwood to 75 mm wide and pale yellow. Texture moderately coarse. Grain usually straight. Greasy to the touch. Heart shakes are common in the logs. **3** GD about 1100 kg/m³; ADD about 770 kg/m³. **4** Slow drying needed in well-protected stacks to avoid checking and excessive collapse. Reconditioning desirable. Shrinkage about 2 per cent radial, 6 per cent tangential; after reconditioning about 1.5 per cent radial, 3.5 per cent tangential. **5** Needs care in working. Nails satisfactorily. Its greasy nature may interfere with adhesives. Unsuitable for steam bending. The sanding dust is very irritating to nose and skin so good ventilation of the workshop is essential. It has higher than usual electrical resistance. **6** Lyctids S; durability IG2. **7** S4 and provisionally SD5. Some mechanical properties are listed on page 412. **8** Furniture, decorative veneer, carving, panelling, fancy turnery. **9** Scarce.

Beech, canary *Polyalthia michaelii* C. T. White
Polyalthia nitidissima (Dunal) Benth.

1 A medium-sized hardwood of the Queensland rainforests. **2** Heartwood pale yellow. Fine texture. Straight grain. **3** ADD about 550 kg/m³. **4** Easy to dry but precautions are needed against bluestain. **5** Easy to work. Glues well. **6** Lyctids S; durability IG4. **7** Provisionally S6, SD7. Some mechanical properties are listed on page 412. **8** Internal joinery. **9** Confined largely to districts of occurrence.

Beech, European *Fagus sylvatica* L.

1 A hardwood common throughout Europe. A number of other *Fagus* species grow in Canada and eastern Asia and have rather similar properties. **2** Heartwood pale brown, sapwood creamy and not clearly distinguishable. The heat of kiln drying can change the colour of the heartwood to reddish brown. Texture fine and even. Grain usually straight. The ends of the large rays give a characteristic fleck to the tangential surface. **3** ADD about 700 kg/m³. Japanese beech is somewhat lighter, about 640 kg/m³. **4** Care is needed in drying to avoid bluestain, surface checks and end splits. Shrinkage is relatively high, exceeding 4 per cent radial and 6 per cent tangential. **5** Relatively easy to work. Turns well. Easy to glue. Predrilling may be needed when nailing. Gives a very smooth finish. Very suitable for steam bending. **6** Lyctids NS; durability IG4; heartwood usually readily penetrated by preservatives. Sapwood can be attacked by the *Anobium* borer. **7** Probably S5, SD4 but it tends to vary considerably in strength. Some mechanical properties are listed on page 412. **8** Furniture (especially bentwood chairs), veneer, flooring, joinery, tool handles, brush backs, handles, wrest planks for pianos, shoe heels, decorative turnery. **9** Very limited quantities are imported.

Beech, myrtle *Nothofagus cunninghamii* (Hook.) Oerst.
Other common name: Tasmanian myrtle

1 A medium-sized hardwood of the heavier rainfall areas of Tasmania and eastern Victoria. Most supplies come from Tasmania. **2** Heartwood pink to reddish brown. Sapwood almost white and narrow. Texture fine and even. Grain sometimes wavy. Growth rings visible but not prominent. Little figure. **3** ADD about 700 kg/m³. **4** Its behaviour during drying is variable for it often has an uneven distribution of moisture. Dark-coloured wood needs extra care to minimise surface checking on the tangential surface and internal honeycombing. Some collapse occurs and reconditioning is desirable. Shrinkage about 3 per cent radial, 6.5 per cent tangential; after reconditioning 2.5 per cent radial, 4.5 per cent tangential. **5** Moderate working properties. Dresses to a very smooth surface but needs very sharp cutters. Needs care in nailing to avoid splits. Glues satisfactorily. Good for steam bending, carving and turnery except for a tendency to bruise on the end grain. Fumes to brown colour with ammonia. **6** Lyctids S; termites NR; durability IG4, AG3, M4. There is often a zone of intermediate wood between the sapwood and heartwood, which is relatively easy to impregnate with preservative. **7** S4, SD5. Some mechanical properties are listed on page 412. **8** Furniture, veneer, joinery, turnery (e.g. shoe heels), carving, flooring, panelling, handles, piano bridges. **9** Mainly in Tasmania and Victoria.

Beech, negrohead *Nothofagus moorei* (F. Muell.) Krasser

1 A large hardwood of the moist tops of the coastal ranges northward from the Harrington Tops near Gloucester, New South Wales, to southern Queensland. **2** Heartwood pink to reddish brown. Sapwood usually distinctly paler, variable in width up to 40 mm wide. Texture fine and even. Grain straight. **3** GD about 1050 kg/m^3; ADD about 770 kg/m^3. **4** Slow in drying. Some collapse, so reconditioning may be worthwhile. Rate of drying varies considerably. Shrinkage about 3 per cent radial, 7 per cent tangential. **5** Rather hard to work. Needs care in nailing and gluing. Can be bonded successfully with tannin–formaldehyde. Not easy to peel. **6** Lyctids S; termites NR; durability IG4, M4. **7** S4, SD3. Some mechanical properties are listed on page 413. **8** Flooring, panelling, turnery, plywood. **9** Seldom milled.

Beech, New Guinea *Nothofagus* spp., principally
Nothofagus grandis Steen
Nothofagus perryi Steen

1 Important hardwood species in Papua New Guinea. **2** Heartwood pinkish brown to reddish brown. Sapwood cream to pale yellow. Texture fine and even. Grain usually straight. **3** ADD about 830 kg/m^3. **4** Slow to dry and inclined to surface and end split. Quarter sawing is desirable. Shrinkage about 3.5 per cent radial, 8 per cent tangential. **5** Finishes well, giving a very smooth surface. May need predrilling for nails. Glues well. **6** Lyctids S; durability IG3. **7** S3, SD3. Some mechanical properties are listed on page 413. **8** Furniture, flooring, joinery, handles, turnery, veneer. **9** Seldom seen in Australia.

Beech, silky *Citronella moorei* (F. Muell. ex Benth.) Howard
Synonym: *Villaresia moorei* F. Muell. ex Benth.

1 A large hardwood of occasional occurrence in coastal rainforests of New South Wales and Queensland. **2** Heartwood pale yellow, with a grey-green tinge. Sapwood not clearly differentiated. Texture moderately fine. Grain often interlocked. The rays are prominent, giving an attractive figure to the radial surface. **3** GD about 1030 kg/m^3; ADD about 720 kg/m^3. **4** Care needed in drying to avoid bluestain and distortion. Slight collapse. Shrinkage about 3 per cent radial, 7 per cent tangential. **5** Relatively easy to work but the sanding dust is very irritating to nose and eyes. Particularly good ventilation of the workshop is essential. Glues well; the alkaline constituents of casein will turn it blue-green but this can be counteracted by washing with dilute oxalic acid. **6** Lyctids S; durability IG4. **7** S4, SD4. Some mechanical properties are listed on page 413. **8** Furniture, turnery, decorative veneer. **9** Scarce.

Beech, silver *Nothofagus menziesii* Oerst.
Other common name: southland beech

1 A medium-sized hardwood growing on both islands of New Zealand in the heavier rainfall areas but especially on the west coast of the south island. **2** Heartwood pink to reddish brown. Sapwood pale greyish pink. Texture fine and even. Grain usually straight. Slight growth ring figure on the tangential surface. **3** GD about 900 kg/m³; ADD varies considerably. The southern material is about 550 kg/m³, ranging up to 700 kg/m³ for north island wood. The lighter wood is preferred for furniture manufacture. **4** The rate of drying should be slow initially to avoid the risk of end splits. Back-cut material should be segregated from the quarter cut because the former dries considerably faster. Shrinkage about 3 per cent radial, 6 per cent tangential. **5** Good for steam bending and turnery. **6** Lyctids NS; termites NR; durability IG4, M4. **7** S5, SD6. Some mechanical properties are listed on page 413. **8** Furniture, turnery, flooring. **9** Only occasionally seen in Australia.

Beech, wau *Elmerillia papuana* (Schlecht.) Dandy
Other common names: elmeril, hui

1 A widely distributed hardwood in the rainforests of Papua New Guinea. **2** Heartwood pale brown to golden brown. Sapwood creamy and to 50 mm wide. Texture moderately fine and even. Grain variable. Some stripe figure on radial surface. Spicy odour. **3** ADD about 480 kg/m³. **4** Easy to dry but care needed to avoid bluestain. **5** Easy to work. Glues and nails well. Satisfactory for steam bending. Free of silica. **6** Lyctids NS; durability IG3. **7** S6, SD6. Some mechanical properties are listed on page 413. **8** Furniture, veneer, joinery, boat building, turnery, carving. **9** Occasionally seen in small quantities.

Beech, white *Gmelina* spp., especially *Gmelina leichhardtii* (F. Muell.) F. Muell. ex Benth.

1 A large hardwood of scattered occurrence in the coastal rainforest from the Shoalhaven River in New South Wales to Queensland, and also in Papua New Guinea. **2** Heartwood pale brown, not clearly distinguishable from the sapwood. Texture medium and even. Grain often interlocked. **3** GD about 950 kg/m³; ADD about 500 kg/m³. **4** Extremely slow in drying but there is little degrade and negligible collapse. Shrinkage about 1.5 per cent radial, 3.5 per cent tangential. Once dry it remains very stable. **5** Easy to work. Sometimes difficult to glue so surface should be freshly prepared and not too smooth. **6** Lyctids S. The heartwood traditionally has had a reputation of very good external durability but recent references have been less favourable, possibly a reflection of less mature material. **7** S6, SD6. Some mechanical properties are listed on page 413. **8** Furniture, especially outdoor furniture, boat building, carving, turnery, pattern-making, shives for beer casks. **9** Scarce.

Belah *Casuarina cristata* Miq.
Synonym: *Casuarina lepidophloia* F. Muell.

1 A small-to-medium hardwood of the heavy soils of the inland plains in New South Wales and also in Victoria, Queensland, South Australia and Western Australia. **2** Heartwood dark chocolate brown. Sapwood creamy and narrow (10–15 mm). Texture very fine and even. Grain usually straight. In contrast with most casuarinas it has fine inconspicuous rays. **3** GD about 1250 kg/m^3; ADD about 1150 kg/m^3. **4** Shrinkage about 2.5 per cent radial, 5 per cent tangential. **5** Because of its very dense nature it is hard to work. **6** Lyctids NS; durability IG2. **7** Provisionally S2, SD2. Some mechanical properties are listed on page 413. **8** Because of its limited size and availability it is mainly used in areas of occurrence for fencing and fuel but it could be of interest to the artisan turner for decorative wood ware. **9** Not a commercial timber.

Belian *Eusideroxylon zwageri* Teysm. et Binn.

1 A large hardwood of Sabah, Indonesia and the Philippines. **2** Heartwood varies in colour from light brown to dark chocolate brown. Sapwood pale yellow and up to 50 mm wide. Texture medium and even. Grain usually straight or only slightly interlocked. Freshly cut wood has a lemony odour. **3** GD about 1300 kg/m^3; ADD about 1000 kg/m^3. **4** If dried slowly there is little degrade, otherwise there could be surface checking. Shrinkage about 2.5 per cent radial, 4.5 per cent tangential. **5** Considering its density it is relatively easy to work. Deposits may build up on saws but there is very little silica. Predrilling for nails may be needed, especially on radial surfaces. Rather difficult to glue. **6** Lyctids NS; durability IG1, AG1, M4; heartwood has good resistance to marine borers. **7** SI and provisionally SD1. Some mechanical properties are listed on page 413. **8** Marine piling, wharfage, shipbuilding, outdoor furniture. **9** Not seen in Australia but a rival to the durable eucalypts on overseas markets.

Birch In Europe: *Betula pubescens* Ehrh.
Betula verrucosa Ehrh.
In Japan: *Betula maximowicziana* Regel

1 These are the main species but there are numerous other birches, medium-sized hardwoods that are very hardy, growing further north than any other European tree. In very cold regions it may be little more than a shrub. Found from southern France to the Arctic in Europe, also in North America and Asia. **2** Heartwood cream to pale brown generally but the Japanese species is bright yellowish red. Sapwood may not be clearly differentiated. Texture fine and even. Grain straight. Little figure. **3** ADD about 670 kg/m^3. **4** Dries rapidly. Needs careful stacking to avoid warping. Susceptible to bluestain. Shrinkage about 3 per cent radial, 6 per cent tangential. **5** Easy to work, glue and finish. Turns and peels well. **6** Lyctids S; durability IG4; heartwood easy to impregnate with preservatives. Sapwood susceptible to attack by *Anobium* borers. **7** Probably S4, SD4. **8** Plywood, furniture, turnery. The bark is useful for tanning leather. **9** Usually only seen as imported furniture.

Birch, white *Schizomeria ovata* D. Don
Other common name: crabapple

1 A large hardwood of the coastal rainforests from the Shoalhaven River in New South Wales to the Mackay district of Queensland. **2** Heartwood variable in colour, from off-white to pale brown, often with pinkish or purplish streaks. The sapwood is not distinctly different in colour and may be up to 150 mm wide. Texture fine and even. Grain variable. **3** GD about 980 kg/m³; ADD about 640 kg/m³. **4** Relatively easy to dry except for dark heart material, which usually degrades very considerably. Collapse is slight. Precautions needed against bluestain. Shrinkage about 3 per cent radial, 6.5 per cent tangential. **5** Easy to work. Glues well. **6** Lyctids S; durability IG4, AG4, M4; heartwood relatively easy to impregnate with preservatives. **7** S5, SD5. Some mechanical properties are listed on page 413. **8** Plywood, furniture, turnery, internal joinery. **9** Mainly as plywood. Limited quantity.

Blackbutt *Eucalyptus pilularis* Sm.

1 A large hardwood growing in abundance in the coastal forests between Bega, New South Wales and Maryborough, Queensland. **2** Heartwood pale brown, but northern material may sometimes have a slight pinkish tinge. Sapwood distinctively paler. Texture medium and even. Grain usually straight. Gum veins common. **3** GD about 1100 kg/m³; ADD about 900 kg/m³. **4** Care needed in drying to inhibit tendency to surface check on the tangential surface. Regrowth logs are subject to much more spring and bow than the mature stems and their central core is likely to suffer considerable collapse. In the regrowth material it is preferable that the larger dimension of the sawn product be perpendicular to the rays so that the distortion due to growth stresses shall occur as bow rather than spring, since it is usually much easier to remedy bow when assembling timber components. Shrinkage about 4 per cent radial, 7 per cent tangential. Reconditioning is seldom advisable because of its effect in widening surface checks. **5** In dressing it the planer angle may need reducing to 15°. Only fair for steam bending. A poor base for paint because of its tendency to surface check but stain finishes can be used satisfactorily. The high extractives content of mature wood can cause some gluing problems, especially with phenolic adhesives, but young regrowth wood appears to be much less affected. **6** Lyctids NS; termites R; durability IG2, AG1, M3. **7** S2, SD2. Some mechanical properties are listed on page 413. **8** Poles, sleepers, flooring, building framework. The regrowth material has potential for structural plywood. **9** It is a major timber for building framework and poles in New South Wales and southern Queensland.

Blackbutt, New England *Eucalyptus andrewsii* Maiden
Eucalyptus campanulata R. T. Bak. et H. G. Sm.

1 A large hardwood of the coastal ranges and tablelands of northern New South Wales and southern Queensland. **2** Heartwood pale brown. Sapwood 25–75 mm wide and distinctly paler. Very similar in appearance to blackbutt. Texture medium and even. Grain usually straight. **3** GD about 1150 kg/m^3; ADD about 930 kg/m^3. **4** Slight collapse occurs in drying. Shrinkage about 5 per cent radial, 8.5 per cent tangential; after reconditioning about 4 per cent radial, 6 per cent tangential. **5** Similar to blackbutt in working properties. **6** Lyctids S; termites R; durability IG2, AG2, M2. **7** S3, SD3. Some mechanical properties are listed on page 417. **8** General construction. **9** A plentiful species in areas of occurrence.

Blackbutt, Western Australian *Eucalyptus patens* Benth.
Other common name: yarri

1 A large hardwood of occasional occurrence in the jarrah and karri forests of south-west Western Australia. **2** Heartwood pale yellowish brown. Texture medium to coarse and even. Grain commonly interlocked. **3** GD about 1120 kg/m^3; ADD about 850 kg/m^3. **4** Slow in drying. Risk of surface checking. Some collapse occurs. Shrinkage about 5 per cent radial, 10 per cent tangential; after reconditioning about 3.5 per cent radial, 7 per cent tangential. **6** Lyctids S; termites R; durability IG2, AG1, M3. **7** S4, SD5. Some mechanical properties are listed on page 413. **8** General construction, sleepers, flooring, panelling. **9** Limited.

Blackwood *Acacia melanoxylon* R. Br.

1 A medium-sized hardwood of occasional occurrence in tableland areas in South Australia and all the eastern states but the only areas of considerable commercial yield are the wetter districts of Tasmania. **2** Heartwood golden brown, often with narrow bands of darker colour indicative of the growth rings. Sometimes reddish streaks are also present. Sapwood distinctively paler and up to 50 mm wide. Texture medium and even. Grain usually straight but sometimes wavy, producing a fiddleback figure. **3** GD about 870 kg/m^3; ADD about 640 kg/m^3. **4** Easy to dry, with little checking and negligible collapse. Shrinkage about 1.5 per cent radial, 4 per cent tangential. **5** Easy to work but planer angle may need reducing for figured material. Good for steam bending. Nails and glues well. Polyester and other catalysed finishes are sometimes retarded in their curing. It can be bleached white with ammonia and hydrogen peroxide. The sanding dust is irritating to the skin and bronchial tubes of some people. Spots of a dark exudate may appear sometimes but readily sand off and do not appear to affect finishes. **6** Lyctids S; termites R; durability IG3, AG3, M4. **7** S4, SD4. Some mechanical properties are listed on page 413. **8** Furniture, decorative veneer, panelling, carving, turnery, flooring, boat building, gun stocks. **9** Confined to relatively small sizes. It is a species whose wider cultivation should be encouraged.

Blackwood, African *Dalbergia melanoxylon* Guill. et Perr.

1 A small hardwood of east and central Africa. **2** Heartwood very dark purplish brown with black streaks. Sapwood narrow and pale yellow. Texture very fine and even. Grain straight. Slightly oily nature. **3** ADD about 1200 kg/m^3. **4** Dries very slowly and needs a lot of care to prevent splitting. Very stable when seasoned. **5** Despite its very high density it is relatively easy to work and because of its very fine texture it gives an excellent finish. Needs predrilling for nails and screws. Excellent for turnery.   6 Lyctids NS; durability IG1, AG1.   7 Very strong, possibly S1.   8 Greatly favoured overseas for woodwind instruments, giving much volume of sound without losing tone quality; the favoured species for Scottish bagpipes. Also used for brush backs and knife handles.   9 Not seen in Australia.

Bloodwood, brown *Corymbia trachyphloia* F. Muell.

1 A small-to-medium sized hardwood of the northern inland slopes in New South Wales and in many parts of Queensland.   2 Heartwood pale yellowish brown. Less prone to gum veins than red bloodwood.   3 GD about 1250 kg/m³; ADD about 1050 kg/m³.   4 Shrinkage about 3.5 per cent radial, 4.5 per cent tangential.   6 Lyctids S; termites R; durability IG1, AG1.   7 S3, SD3. Some mechanical properties are listed on page 413.   8 Fencing.   9 Limited to areas of occurrence.

Bloodwood, pale *Corymbia terminalis* F. Muell.

1 A medium-sized hardwood of occasional occurrence in the dry inland areas of New South Wales, Queensland, Northern Territory and Western Australia.   2 Heartwood dark red.   3 GD about 1170 kg/m³; ADD about 980 kg/m³.   4 Shrinkage about 2.5 per cent radial, 3.5 per cent tangential.   6 Lyctids S; durability IG2.   7 Provisionally S3, SD3.   8 Fencing.   9 Limited to areas of occurrence.

Bloodwood, red *Corymbia gummifera* (Gaertn.) Hochr.
Synonym: *Eucalyptus corymbosa* Sm.

1 A large hardwood of the coastal districts of New South Wales and Queensland.   2 Heartwood dark pink to dark red. Texture coarse. Grain often interlocked. Its most characteristic feature is the abundance of concentric gum veins, which permeate the timber; because of their presence red bloodwood and other bloodwoods are usually utilised as round timber rather than sawn, yet they can give a very attractive appearance to the sawn material, which might be described as a representation of travertine stone in wood form, and which does have potential as a decorative panelling.   3 GD about 1150 kg/m³; ADD about 900 kg/m³.   4 Does not move much in drying but some opening up of the gum veins may occur. Shrinkage about 3 per cent radial, 4 per cent tangential.   6 Lyctids S; termites R; durability IG1, AG1, M3.   7 S3 and provisionally SD3. Some mechanical properties are listed on page 413.   8 Poles, piles, posts, decorative panelling.   9 A relatively common species in coastal New South Wales and Queensland.

Bollywood *Litsea* spp., especially *Litsea reticulata* (Meissn.) F. Muell.

1 A medium-sized hardwood of the rainforests from the central coast of New South Wales to north Queensland.   2 Heartwood usually pale brown but tones of yellow, pink and grey can also be present. Sapwood, to 20 mm wide, usually distinctly paler. Texture moderately coarse but even. Grain sometimes interlocked.   3 GD about 760 kg/m³; ADD

about 500 kg/m³. **4** Slow to dry but little degrade occurs. Collapse is slight. If thick material is being dried it can run the risk of severe moisture gradients, which may cause internal checking. Shrinkage about 2 per cent radial, 5 per cent tangential. **5** Soft. Easy to work. Glues well. Satisfactory for steam bending. **6** Lyctids S; termites NR; durability IG3, AG3, M4. **7** Provisionally S7, SD7. Some mechanical properties are listed on page 414. **8** Plywood, joinery, carving, boat building. **9** Scarce.

Bonewood *Emmenosperma alphitonioides* F. Muell.

1 A medium-to-large hardwood of occasional occurrence in the rainforests from the Illawarra district of New South Wales to southern Queensland. **2** Heartwood pale greyish yellow. Texture fine and even. Grain straight. Has a greasy nature. **3** GD about 1100 kg/m³; ADD about 860 kg/m³. **4** Dries quickly but care needed to avoid surface checking. Collapse is slight. Shrinkage about 4 per cent radial, 7 per cent tangential. **5** Because of its greasy nature extra care is needed in gluing. **6** Lyctids NS; durability IG3. **7** S3 and provisionally SD3. Some mechanical properties are listed on page 414. **8** Joinery, flooring, turnery, panelling. **9** Seldom milled.

Box, brush *Lophostemon confertus* R. Br.

1 A large hardwood that grows on the edge of the rainforests from the central coast of New South Wales to Bowen, Queensland. **2** Heartwood varies in colour from a pinkish grey to a rich reddish brown. Sapwood usually distinctively paler. Texture fine and even. Grain usually interlocked to varying degrees. Logs are usually sound right to the pith and are free of gum veins, but breaks known as 'water rings' are sometimes present. **3** GD about 1160 kg/m³; ADD about 900 kg/m³. **4** Material with considerably interlocked grain can distort severely in drying. Close spacing of the stack stickers, weighting down of the stack and restriction of the air circulation in the early stages of drying will help to minimise degrade. Provided the grain is relatively straight it has good resistance to surface checking. Shrinkage about 5 per cent radial, 10 per cent tangential; after reconditioning about 3.5 per cent radial, 7 per cent tangential. **5** Because of its density and interlocked grain, as well as its dulling effect on tool edges due to the presence of silica, it is not easy to work. Planer cutting angles need to be reduced. Unsuitable for steam bending. It is very resistant to wear and has good resistance to splintering. Its natural waxiness occasionally causes some adhesion problems with some highly solvent floor finishes but it is a very good base for paints and stains. The natural wax that it contains is called arjunolic acid and it may be present to the extent of 5–10 per cent w/w. Brush box is low in tannins and is much less inclined to stain than the eucalypts when leached by rain. **6** Lyctids NS; termites R; durability IG3, AG3, M2. Sapwood only occasionally attacked by lyctid borers. **7** S3, SD3. Some mechanical properties are listed on page 414. **8** Flooring, cladding, panelling, mallets, pulley blocks, bridge decking (in dry areas). **9** Moderate quantities in New South Wales and Queensland.

Box, grey *Eucalyptus microcarpa* Maiden
Eucalyptus moluccana Roxb.
Synonym: *Eucalyptus hemiphloia* F. Muell. ex Benth.

1 A medium-sized hardwood of the central and north coast districts of New South Wales and southern Queensland. Occasionally found in eastern Victoria. **2** Heartwood pale yellowish brown. Sapwood usually distinctly paler. Texture relatively fine and even. Grain usually interlocked. Seldom has gum veins. **3** GD about 1170 kg/m^3; ADD about 1120 kg/m^3. **4** Slow in drying but not prone to surface checking. Shrinkage about 3.5 per cent radial, 7.5 per cent tangential. **5** Because of its density it is rather difficult to work. **6** Lyctids S but only occasionally attacked by lyctid borers; termites R; durability IG1, AG1, M2. **7** S2, SD2. Some mechanical properties are listed on page 414. **8** Heavy engineering construction, bridges, wharves, shipbuilding, piles, poles, sleepers. An excellent fuel wood. **9** Mainly in districts of occurrence.

Box, grey, coast *Eucalyptus bosistoana* F. Muell.

1 A large hardwood of eastern Victoria, and the southern and central coasts of New South Wales. **2** Heartwood pale brown, sometimes with a tinge of pink. Sapwood distinctively paler. Texture relatively fine and even. Grain usually interlocked. A very similar wood to grey box. **3** GD about 1180 kg/m^3; ADD about 1100 kg/m^3. **4** Slow in drying. Shrinkage about 4 per cent radial, 7 per cent tangential. **5** Satisfactory for steam bending. **6** Lyctids S; termites R; durability IG1, AG1, M3. **7** SI, SD1. Some mechanical properties are listed on page 414. **8** Heavy engineering construction, piles, poles, sleepers. **9** Mainly in districts of occurrence.

Box, kanuka *Tristania laurina* (Sm.) R. Br.

1 A medium-sized hardwood of high rainfall coastal districts between Gippsland in Victoria and north Queensland. **2** Heartwood pinkish, darkening to red towards the centre of the tree. Sapwood distinctly paler. Texture fine and even. Grain often interlocked. **3** GD about 1160 kg/m^3; ADD can vary considerably from about 830 to 1000 kg/m^3, averaging about 900 kg/m^3. **4** Needs care in drying and should be handled similarly to brush box. Shrinkage about 6 per cent radial, 12 per cent tangential; after reconditioning about 4.5 per cent radial, 7 per cent tangential. **5** Similar to brush box in workability. **6** Lyctids NS; termites NR; durability IG3, M4. **7** S2, SD3. Some mechanical properties are listed on page 414. **8** Mallets, handles, flooring. **9** Seldom milled.

Box, steel *Eucalyptus rummeryi* Maiden
Other common name: steel butt

1 A large hardwood of occasional occurrence on the north coast of New South Wales, especially in the Richmond Range area west of Casino. **2** Heartwood pale brown. The wood bears a close resemblance to grey ironbark and has similar properties. **3** GD about 1300 kg/m^3;

ADD about 1130 kg/m³. **6** Lyctids NS; termites R; durability IG1, AG1. **7** Probably S2, SD2. Some mechanical properties are listed on page 414. **8** Girders, poles. **9** Scarce.

Box, swamp *Lophostemon suaveolens* (Sol. ex Gaertn.) Sm.

1 A medium-sized hardwood of low-lying ground from the north coast of New South Wales to north Queensland. **2** Heartwood dark reddish brown. Sapwood distinctly paler. Texture fine and even. Grain interlocked. **3** GD about 1040 kg/m³; ADD variable, averaging about 850 kg/m³. **4** Needs care in drying, behaving rather like brush box. Shrinkage about 4 per cent radial, 9 per cent tangential; after reconditioning about 3 per cent radial, 5 per cent tangential. **6** Lyctids NS; termites R; durability IG2, AG1, M2. **7** S6, SD6. Some mechanical properties are listed on page 414. **8** Piling, marine structures, mallets. **9** Seldom milled.

Box, white-topped *Eucalyptus quadrangulata* Deane et Maiden

1 A medium-to-large hardwood of the better soils of the coast and adjacent ranges in New South Wales and southern Queensland. **2** Heartwood pale yellow. Sapwood not distinct. Texture moderately fine. Grain sometimes interlocked. **3** GD about 1230 kg/m³; ADD about 1030 kg/m³. **4** Relatively easy to dry. Collapse slight. Shrinkage about 3 per cent radial, 7.5 per cent tangential. Tends to suffer considerable splitting when large dimension stock is dried; better when sawn free of heart. **5** Considering its density it is relatively easy to work. **6** Lyctids NS; termites R; durability IG2, AG2. **7** S2, SD2. Some mechanical properties are listed on page 414. **8** Heavy engineering construction, poles, piles, sleepers, flooring, cladding. **9** A common commercial species in areas of occurrence.

Box, yellow *Eucalyptus melliodora* A. Cunn. ex Schau.

1 A medium-sized hardwood growing on the better soils of the tablelands and inland slopes in New South Wales, also in Victoria and Queensland. It is the best Australian tree for honey production and should be reserved for this purpose. **2** Heartwood pale yellow-brown. Sapwood paler and usually distinguishable. Texture moderately fine and even. Grain usually interlocked. **3** GD about 1300 kg/m³; ADD about 1100 kg/m³. **4** Slow to dry but not much degrade. Shrinkage about 3 per cent radial, 6 per cent tangential. **5** The interlocked grain and high density make it difficult to work. **6** Lyctids NS; termites R; durability IG1, AG1. **7** S3, SD4. Some mechanical properties are listed on page 414. **8** Heavy engineering construction, bridges, posts, poles, sleepers. **9** Only in districts of occurrence.

Boxwood, European *Buxus sempervirens* L.
Other common name: Turkish boxwood

1 A hardwood shrub or small tree of southern Europe, Asia and northern Africa; the best quality material comes from the Caucasus region. **2** Heartwood pale yellow. Sapwood distinctly paler. Texture very fine and even. Grain variable.   3 ADD about 900 kg/m³.   4 Dries very slowly. Prone to surface checking and splitting. Shrinkage is high, in excess of 4 per cent radial, 6 per cent tangential.   5 Hard to work when dry but gives a very smooth finish. Excellent for turning and carving.   6 Lyctids NS, durability IG2, AG1.   7 SD3 and provisionally S2.   8 Draughting equipment, rulers, engraving blocks, textile rollers, musical instruments, chess pieces.   9 Usually only seen in Australia in manufactured articles.

Boxwood, Macintyre's *Xanthophyllum octandrum* (F. Muell.) Domin
Other common name: sovereign wood

1 A hardwood of occasional occurrence in the north Queensland rainforests.   2 Heartwood pale golden yellow. Sapwood not clearly distinguishable. Texture medium and even. Grain usually straight.   3 ADD about 800 kg/m³.   4 Easy to dry.   5 Firm but not difficult to work. Needs care in gluing.   6 Lyctids S; durability IG4.   7 Provisionally S4, SD5.   8 Joinery, furniture, panelling.   9 Very limited.

Boxwood, yellow *Planchonella pohlmaniana* (F. Muell.) Pierre ex Dubard
Synonym: *Sideroxylon pohlmanianum* (F. Muell.) Benth. et Hook.

1 A medium-sized hardwood of occasional occurrence in the coastal rainforests from northern New South Wales to the Atherton district of north Queensland.   2 Heartwood pale yellow brown, resembling European boxwood. Sapwood slightly paler. Texture very fine and even. Grain sometimes slightly interlocked. No odour or taste.   3 ADD about 960 kg/m³.   4 Easy to dry. Shrinkage about 3.5 per cent radial, 5.5 per cent tangential.   5 Firm but relatively easy to work. Glues well.   6 Lyctids S.   7 Provisionally S5, SD5.   8 Artificial limbs, drawing equipment, pivot laps for gyroscopes, fancy turnery, kitchen utensils.   9 Not commercially available.

Brigalow *Acacia harpophylla* F. Muell. ex Benth.

1 A small hardwood of inland Queensland and northern New South Wales. Very large areas of it have been cleared in recent times in Queensland to provide grazing country for sheep and cattle.   2 Heartwood dark reddish brown. Sapwood thin, yellow and quite distinct. Texture very fine and even. Grain relatively straight.   3 GD about 1100 kg/m³; ADD about 950 kg/m³.   4 Dries slowly and with little degrade. Shrinkage about 1.5 per cent radial, 3 per cent tangential.   5 Firm but not difficult to work. The sanding dust can be irritating to nose and eyes so good ventilation of the workplace is essential.   6 Lyctids S; termites R; durability IG1, AG1.   7 S1, SD1. Some mechanical properties are listed on page 414.   8 Fancy turnery, handles, fencing, survey pegs, walking sticks, brush backs. A substitute for mulga in fancy turnery. Good fuel.   9 Not commercially exploited but large quantities of small-diameter logs are potentially available in Queensland.

Brownbarrel *Eucalyptus fastigata* Deane et Maiden
Other common name: cuttail.

1 A large hardwood of the north-east corner of Victoria and the tableland districts and south coast in New South Wales. **2** Heartwood pale brown. Sapwood paler and usually easy to distinguish. Texture medium and even. Grain often interlocked. Growth rings visible but not prominent. Gum veins common. The wood is similar in appearance to messmate. **3** GD about 1140 kg/m^3; ADD about 750 kg/m^3. **4** Slow to dry. Considerable collapse can occur; the wood should be handled like that of the ash eucalypts. Shrinkage about 6 per cent radial, 9.5 per cent tangential; after reconditioning about 4 per cent radial, 7 per cent tangential. **6** Lyctids S; termites NR; durability IG4, AG3, M4. **7** S4, SD4. Some mechanical properties are listed on page 414. **8** General construction purposes not involving exposure to the weather. Not a good fuel as it tends to smoulder and char. **9** A common timber in the districts of occurrence.

Buchanania *Buchanania* spp., principally *Buchanania heterophylla* K. Schum., *Buchanania macrocarpa* Lauterb.
Other common name: pink satinwood

1 A rainforest hardwood of Papua New Guinea. Other species of *Buchanania* with slightly stronger wood occur to a limited extent in north Queensland. **2** Heartwood pinkish brown. Sapwood white or pale pink. Texture medium. Grain straight. Some tension wood. **3** ADD about 350 kg/m^3. **4** Easy to dry. Shrinkage about 3 per cent radial, 6 per cent tangential. **6** Lyctids S, durability IG4. **7** Provisionally S7, SD7, but some species might be weaker. **8** Internal joinery, veneer. **9** Seldom seen in Australia.

Butternut, rose *Blepharocarya involucrigera* F. Muell.

1 A medium-to-large hardwood of the north Queensland rainforests. **2** Heartwood pinkish brown (rather similar to Queensland maple). Texture relatively fine and even. Grain often wavy, producing an attractive figure. **3** ADD about 560 kg/m^3. **4** Easy to dry. **5** Firm but easy to work. Glues well. **6** Lyctids S; durability IG4. **7** S6, SD6. **8** Furniture, decorative veneer, joinery, panelling. **9** Mainly on Queensland markets.

Cadaga *Eucalyptus torelliana* F. Muell.

1 A medium-sized hardwood of north Queensland. One of the few eucalypts to grow in close association with rainforest species. **2** Heartwood pale brown to chocolate brown. Sapwood distinctly paler. Texture medium. Grain often interlocked, giving a striped figure to the radial cut. Gum veins common. **3** ADD about 920 kg/m^3. **5** Relatively easy to work but difficult to glue. **6** Lyctids S; termites NR; durability IG2. **7** S2 and provisionally SD3. **8** General construction. **9** Small quantities in north Queensland.

Calantas *Toona calantas* Merr. et Rolfe
Synonym: *Cedrela calantas* Burk.
Other common name: kalantas

1 A medium-to-large Philippine hardwood, also found in Indonesia and Malaysia. **2** Heartwood reddish brown. Sapwood narrow, pale red and distinctive. Texture moderately coarse. Grain often interlocked. Characteristic cedar odour. The wood is very similar to that of the Australian red cedar. **3** ADD about 480 kg/m³. **4** Dries rapidly with some risk of internal checking and collapse. Shrinkage about 4 per cent radial, 7 per cent tangential. **5** Easy to work if tools kept sharp, but can be 'woolly'. **6** Lyctids S; durability IG2, AG1. **7** Possibly S6, SD7. **8** Furniture, panelling, joinery, decorative veneer, boat building, carving. **9** Small quantities are imported.

Another species, *Azadirachta integrifolia* Merr., of very similar appearance but slightly harder and denser, is sold under the same name. It grows in the Philippines, where it is also called maranggo.

Callicoma *Callicoma serratifolia* Andr.

1 A small hardwood that is a common understorey tree in the coastal forests with high rainfall in New South Wales and southern Queensland. Not large enough to be of commercial interest but could be useful to artisans for turnery, etc. **2** Heartwood pinkish brown. Sapwood distinctively paler. Texture fine and even. Grain straight. **3** GD about 930 kg/m³; ADD about 560 kg/m³. **4** Shrinkage about 4 per cent radial, 8 per cent tangential; after reconditioning about 2.5 per cent radial, 6 per cent tangential. **6** Lyctids S; durability IG4. **7** S6, SD6. **8** Turnery. **9** Not a commercial timber.

Calophyllum *Calophyllum* spp.
Other common names: bintangor, damanu

1 A large hardwood whose area of occurrence extends from South-East Asia across to Papua New Guinea and Fiji. Small amounts occur in north Queensland rainforests. **2** Heartwood pinkish brown to reddish brown. Sapwood pale yellow or pink but not always distinct from the heartwood. Texture rather coarse but even. Grain usually interlocked, producing a ribbon figure on the radial face. **3** ADD varies considerably with species, from about 550 to 900 kg/m³. Papua New Guinea and Fijian material is usually about 600 kg/m³. **4** Careful drying is required to avoid warping and end splitting. Shrinkage is variable: for Papua New Guinea material it is about 2.5 per cent radial, 5.5 per cent tangential. **6** Susceptibility to lyctid borer attack varies with timber species, so caution is needed. The Papua New Guinea material is reported to be not susceptible, whereas the Fijian wood is susceptible. Termites NR; durability IG4, M4; heartwood resistant to impregnation with preservatives. **7** Variable because of density range. Most timber is likely to be S5, SD6. Some mechanical properties are listed on page 414. **8** General construction, flooring, joinery, veneer, turnery, furniture. **9** Seldom seen in Australia.

Camphorwood *Cinnamomum oliveri* F. M. Bail.
Cinnamomum virens R. T. Bak.
Other common name: black sassafras

1 A medium-sized hardwood of the coastal rainforests of northern New South Wales and southern Queensland. **2** Heartwood greyish yellow or pale brown. Sapwood not clearly distinguishable. Has a characteristic odour, as its name suggests. Texture medium and even. Grain usually straight. **3** GD about 840 kg/m³; ADD about 560 kg/m³. **4** Easy to dry but precautions against bluestain may be necessary. Shrinkage about 2 per cent radial, 5 per cent tangential. **5** Firm but easy to work. Glues well. **6** Lyctids S; durability IG4; heartwood relatively easy to impregnate with preservatives. **7** S5, SD5. Some mechanical properties are listed on page 414. **8** Plywood, joinery. **9** Scarce.

Candlebark *Eucalyptus rubida* Deane et Maiden

1 A medium-sized hardwood of the Great Dividing Range in Victoria. Occasionally found also in Tasmania and southern New South Wales. **2** Heartwood pale pink. Sapwood often indistinguishable and to 30 mm wide. Gum veins common. Texture medium and even. Grain straight. **3** ADD about 740 kg/m³. **4** Care needed in drying to avoid excessive degrade. Considerable collapse. Shrinkage about 5.5 per cent radial, 12 per cent tangential; after reconditioning about 3 per cent radial, 6 per cent tangential. **6** Lyctids S; termites NR; durability IG4, AG3, M4. **7** S5, SD5. Some mechanical properties are listed on page 414. **8** Building framework. **9** Limited quantities, virtually only in Victoria.

Candlenut *Aleurites moluccana* (L.) Willd.

1 A medium-sized hardwood of the rainforests of north Queensland. **2** Heartwood creamy white. Sapwood not clearly distinguishable. Texture coarse. Grain straight. **3** ADD about 450 kg/m³. **4** Easy to dry but there is a need to take precautions against bluestain. **5** Very soft. Easy to work. Glues satisfactorily. **6** Lyctids S; durability IG4; heartwood should be relatively easy to impregnate with preservatives. **7** Provisionally S7 and SD7; it is not really suited for structural purposes. **8** Interior joinery, plywood, kitchen utensils. **9** A commercial timber in north Queensland.

Carabeen, grey *Sloanea macbrydei* F. Muell.

1 A medium-sized hardwood of the Queensland rainforests. **2** Heartwood pale brown. Sapwood not clearly differentiated. Like yellow carabeen it is liable to considerable discolouration. Texture fine and even. Grain straight. **3** ADD about 570 kg/m³. **4** Easy to dry but precautions needed against bluestain. Shrinkage about 2 per cent radial, 4 per cent tangential. **5** Easy to work. Glues well. **6** Lyctids S, durability IG4. **7** Provisionally S6, SD6. **8** Plywood, joinery. **9** Limited to areas of occurrence.

Carabeen, white *Sloanea langii* F. Muell.

1 A medium-sized hardwood of the Queensland rainforests. **2** Heartwood pale creamy brown. Sapwood distinctively paler. Texture fine and even. Grain often interlocked. High sheen. **3** ADD about 570 kg/m³. **6** Lyctids S; durability IG4. **7** Provisionally S6, SD6. **8** Decorative veneer, panelling, joinery. **9** Limited to areas of occurrence.

Carabeen, yellow *Sloanea woollsii* F. Muell.

1 A large hardwood of the coastal rainforests of northern New South Wales and southern Queensland. **2** Heartwood pale yellow-brown. The inner heartwood can be a dark brown, commonly called 'black heart', which is very difficult to season without degrade. Sapwood can be very wide, of similar colour to the heartwood but it is often discoloured considerably by sapstain. Texture fine to medium and even. Grain straight. **3** GD about 880 kg/m³; ADD about 620 kg/m³. **4** Care needed when drying to avoid sapstain and surface checking. Some collapse occurs. Shrinkage about 2.5 per cent radial, 6 per cent tangential; after reconditioning about 2 per cent radial, 4 per cent tangential. **5** Firm but easy to work. Glues well. **6** Lyctids S; termites NR; durability IG4, M4; heartwood relatively easy to impregnate with preservatives. **7** S4, SD4. Some mechanical properties are listed on page 414. **8** Plywood, internal joinery, turnery. **9** Mainly as plywood.

Carbeen *Corymbia tessellaris*
Eucalyptus tessellaris F. Muell.

1 A medium-sized hardwood of eastern Queensland, extending down to the north-western plains of New South Wales. **2** Heartwood brown to chocolate brown. Sapwood distinctively paler. Texture relatively fine and even. Grain interlocked. Has a rather greasy nature. Attractive appearance. **3** GD about 1160 kg/m³; ADD about 1000 kg/m³. **5** Relatively easy to work, considering its density. **6** Lyctids S; termites R; durability IG1, AG1. **7** Provisionally SI, SD1. Some mechanical properties are listed on page 414. **8** Heavy engineering construction, handles. **9** Only in districts of occurrence.

Cedar, Alaska *Chamaecyparis nootkatensis* (D. Don) Spach
Other common name: yellow cedar

1 A medium-sized softwood of the Pacific coast of North America, from southern Alaska to Oregon. Not plentiful. **2** Heartwood pale yellow. Sapwood narrow and not clearly distinguished from the heartwood. Texture fine and even. Grain usually straight. Growth rings very close together and not prominent. **3** ADD about 500 kg/m³. **4** Easy to dry. Low shrinkage, probably about 1.5 per cent radial, 3 per cent tangential. **5** Easy to work. Good surface for coatings. Contact with iron when damp can result in brown staining of the wood surface. Careful control of conditions needed when gluing it; it bonds better with resin types than non-resins. **6** Lyctids NS; termites R, durability IG1, AG1. **7** Some mechanical properties are listed on page 415. **8** External joinery, boat building, battery separators, pattern-making, carving, wall panelling, vats. **9** Only occasionally seen in Australia.

Cedar, incense *Libocedrus decurrens* Torr.

1 A large softwood of Oregon and northern California. **2** Heartwood pale reddish brown (rather like that of western red cedar). Sapwood creamy. Texture fine and even. Grain usually straight. The logs often have pockets of decayed wood, hence the term 'pecky cedar'. **3** ADD about 400 kg/m³. **4** Easy to dry, with little degrade and low shrinkage. **5** Easy to work. A good base for coating systems. **6** Lyctids NS; durability IG2. **8** Pencil slats, venetian blinds. Not a structural timber. **9** Seldom seen in Australia.

Cedar, pencil *Palaquium* spp.

1 A widely distributed hardwood in Papua New Guinea. **2** Heartwood pinkish brown. Sapwood pale pink. Texture moderately fine and even. Grain variable. No odour. **3** ADD varies considerably, due to the large number of species included under this one name, from 540 to 720 kg/m³. **4** Easy to dry. Shrinkage about 1.5 per cent radial, 4 per cent tangential. **5** The ease of working varies because some species may contain a little silica. Glues and nails well. **6** Lyctids S; durability IG4; heartwood resistant to impregnation with preservatives. **7** Possibly S5 or S6, depending on density of species. **8** Internal joinery, veneer, carving, turnery. **9** Occasionally sold in Australia.

Other *Palaquium*, commonly called 'bauvudi' and native to Fiji, are also imported in small quantities. Little has been reported on their properties.

Cedar, pencil, Virginian *Juniperus virginiana* L.
Other common name: eastern red cedar (USA)

1 A small softwood of the eastern United States. **2** Heartwood reddish brown. Sapwood distinctly paler. Texture fine and even. Grain usually straight. Characteristic odour that repels moths. **3** ADD about 520 kg/m³. **4** Easy to dry. Low shrinkage, about 1.5 per cent radial, 2.5 per cent tangential. Stable in service. **5** Easy to work but needs care in nailing. **6** Lyctids NS; durability IG2. **7** S7, SD8. Some mechanical properties are listed on page 415. **8** The most outstanding wood for pencils but now in short supply. The cedar wood oil used in toilet preparations is obtained by distilling the sawdust and off-cuts. **9** Only seen in Australia as pencils.

Cedar, Port Orford *Chamaecyparis lawsoniana* (A. Murr.) Parl.

1 A large softwood native to south-west Oregon and northern California in the United States; it has been planted as a forest tree in many parts of the world, including New Zealand, but not in

Australia. **2** Heartwood pale yellow-brown. Sapwood slightly paler but not always distinctive. Spicy odour, somewhat like ginger, when freshly cut. Some resin exudation can occur. Texture medium. Grain usually straight. The wood repels moths. **3** ADD about 530 kg/m³. Plantation material may be considerably lower. **4** Easy to dry and very stable in service. Shrinkage about 2.5 per cent radial, 4 per cent tangential. **5** Easy to work. Good base for coatings. **6** Lyctids NS; durability IG2; heartwood moderately resistant to impregnation with preservatives. **7** S6, SD6. Some mechanical properties are listed on page 415. **8** Battery separators, vats for acids, clothes cupboards, blind slats, joinery, boat building. **9** Seldom imported to Australia.

Cedar, red *Toona australis* (F. Muell.) Harms
Synonym: *Cedrela toona* Roxb. var. *australis* (F. Muell.) C. DC.

1 A large hardwood of occasional occurrence in the coastal rainforests of eastern Australia, extending to Papua New Guinea, South-East Asia and as far as India. Now scarce in Australian forests and commercial supplies are frequently of imported timber. The tree is easy to grow but the growing tip is very susceptible to attack by a moth larva; this makes it very difficult to produce a straight stem for timber purposes. Red cedar is one of the few deciduous trees of the Australian forests. **2** Heartwood pale to dark red, depending largely on the maturity of the wood. Sapwood very pale pink or yellow and distinctive from the heartwood. Texture rather coarse and uneven due to the ring-porous nature of the wood. Grain straight or slightly interlocked. Distinctive odour, said to repel moths. **3** GD about 640 kg/m³; ADD about 420 kg/m³ for mature wood. **4** Easy to dry but needs careful stacking to avoid cupping. Some collapse can occur. Shrinkage about 2 per cent radial, 4 per cent tangential; after reconditioning about 1.5 per cent radial, 3 per cent tangential. **5** Soft and relatively easy to work but inclined to give a 'woolly' cut. Nails and glues well. **6** Lyctids S; durability IG2, M4 but this valuable timber is too scarce to be applied to external use. **7** SD8, and provisionally S7; some mechanical properties are listed on page 415. Fast-grown timber seems to have at least as good, probably better, mechanical properties than the average material from large logs. **8** Furniture, panelling, decorative veneer, boat building, carving. **9** Scarce in local forests but small quantities are being imported.

Cedar, red, western *Thuja plicata* D. Don

1 A large softwood, the largest of the North American cedars, occurring in British Columbia, Washington, Oregon, Idaho and Montana. **2** Heartwood variable, from pale brown to dark brown. Sapwood to 20 mm wide, is yellowish white. Texture fine but uneven due to the prominent growth rings. Grain straight. Not resinous. The degree of darkness of the wood is not indicative of the amount of extractives present. The extractives that are most helpful in providing resistance to decay are rather insoluble in water but are corrosive to metals such as copper and iron. **3** ADD about 350 kg/m³. **4** Easy to dry. Shrinkage about 1.5 per cent radial, 3 per cent tangential. **5** Easy to work but the sanding dust can be very irritating to the breathing passages, so a well-ventilated workshop is essential. It is rather brittle, so care is needed in working end grain. Since it is very soft there is a risk when dressing it that the cutters may compress the softer earlywood, which will later recover to produce a ridged surface. Glues well and is a good base for coatings. The damp wood is corrosive to iron, resulting in a black discolouration of the surrounding wood, so hot-dipped galvanised nails are commonly used in areas likely to experience any dampness. A yellowish colouring readily leaches from the wood, so white-painted woodwork at a lower level can be stained if storm rains penetrate, say, to the unprotected rear surface of cladding. **6** Lyctids NS; termites R; durability IG3, AG2; heartwood difficult to impregnate with preservatives. **7** S7, SD8. Not a structural timber. Some mechanical properties are listed on page 415. **8** Cladding, external joinery, garden furniture, window sashes and frames, greenhouses, roofing shingles and shakes. If the water run-off from a newly installed cedar roof is to be used for drinking purposes it should be boiled. Any brown scum should be removed before boiling. If damp conditions are common the shingles and shakes may be subject to soft rot attack and some form of fungicidal treatment may be needed. The use of a steep slope will be helpful by ensuring rapid drainage of rain and dew. **9** Considerable quantities are imported.

Cedar, South American *Cedrela* spp., including
Cedrela odorata L.
Cedrela mexicana M. Roem.
Other common names: Central American cedar, cigarbox cedar,
    Spanish cedar, West Indian cedar

1 A large hardwood of the rainforests from Mexico to Brazil and in the West Indies. **2** Heartwood pale red to a mid red-brown. Sapwood pinkish or pale brown, clearly distinguishable from the heartwood. Fragrant odour. Texture coarse. Grain usually straight. The presence of gum sometimes interferes with the drying of finishes. Logs need rapid processing to avoid pin-hole borer damage. Said to be a good deterrent to moths. **3** ADD varies considerably but is usually in the range 400–500 kg/m^3. **4** Easy to dry but end splits can be a problem. Shrinkage about 3 per cent radial, 6 per cent tangential. **5** Easy to work if tools are kept very sharp to counter the 'woolliness' of the wood. Some gummy exudations can build up on processing equipment. Nails and glues well. Suitable for steam bending. **6** Lyctids S; durability IG3. Sapwood susceptible to *Anobium* borer attack. **7** S6 and provisionally SD7, but it varies considerably in strength. Some mechanical properties are listed on page 415. **8** Its most famous use has been for cigar boxes. Furniture, clothes cupboards, boat building. **9** Occasional small shipments are received.

Cedar, white *Melia azedarach* L. var. *australasica* (A. Juss.) C. DC.

1 A medium-sized deciduous hardwood of occasional occurrence in the rainforests of New South Wales and Queensland. **2** Heartwood pale brown. Sapwood creamy and readily distinguishable from the heartwood. Texture very coarse and uneven due to the ring-porous nature of the wood. Grain straight. **3** GD about 640 kg/m³; ADD about 450 kg/m³. **4** Easy to dry. Collapse slight. Shrinkage about 2.5 per cent radial, 4.5 per cent tangential. **5** Easy to work. Because of its very coarse texture it is difficult to give it a high finish. **6** Lyctids S; durability IG4. **7** Provisionally SD8 and less than S7. Not a structural timber. Some mechanical properties are listed on page 415. **8** Internal joinery. **9** Rarely cut.

Cerejeira *Amburana cearensis* (Fr. Allem.) A. C. Sm.
Synonym: *Torresea cearensis* Fr. Allem.

1 A medium-sized hardwood of Brazil and Argentina. **2** Heartwood pale yellow to very pale brown with a slight tinge of orange. Sapwood greyish but not clearly delineated. Vessel lines very prominent. Oily or waxy appearance and an odour that is distinctive but not really pleasant. Texture coarse. Grain irregular. **3** ADD about 600 kg/m³. **4** Needs careful drying to avoid distortion. Shrinkage about 2 per cent radial, 4 per cent tangential. **5** Cuts woolly when green but dry material finishes very smoothly. Easy to work. Glues satisfactorily. **6** Lyctids probably S; durability IG3; heartwood moderately resistant to impregnation with preservatives. **7** Probably S5. **8** Furniture, veneer, joinery. **9** Small quantities occasionally imported.

Cheesewood, white *Alstonia scholaris* (L.) R. Br.
Other common name: milkwood

1 A medium-to-large hardwood of the north Queensland rainforests; also in Papua New Guinea and South-East Asia through to India. **2** Heartwood cream to pale yellow. Sapwood wide and visually indistinct from the heartwood. Texture medium to coarse. Grain straight. Latex canals, which are slits 6–50 mm long and up to 3 mm wide, are common (Plate 41). Often has strong odour and bitter taste. **3** ADD about 400 kg/m³. **4** Dries quickly with little degrade, except that it is very susceptible to bluestain. Shrinkage about 2.5 per cent radial, 4 per cent tangential. **5** Very soft but easy to work. Glues well. **6** Lyctids S; durability IG4, M4; heartwood readily impregnated with preservatives. **7** S7, SD8. Not a structural timber. If so used, extra nailing would be necessary. Some mechanical properties are listed on page 415. **8** Pattern-making, core stock, plywood, carving, mouldings. It should not be used in contact with food because of the risk of tainting. **9** Small quantities in east coast markets.

Chengal *Balanocarpus heimii* King

1 A large Malaysian hardwood, now scarce. **2** Heartwood yellow to dark brown. Sapwood paler and clearly defined, 20–40 mm wide. Texture moderately coarse. Grain slightly interlocked, producing some ripple figuring. **3** ADD about 850 kg/m³. **4** Slow in drying but little degrade. Shrinkage about 1 per cent radial, 2.5 per cent tangential. **5** Relatively easy to work but gum builds up on the saws. **6** Lyctids NS; termites R; durability IG1, AG1. **7** S1, SD2. **8** Structural members requiring high strength and durability, shipbuilding, sleepers. **9** Not seen in Australia but often quoted by overseas buyers as a yardstick of excellence.

Coachwood *Ceratopetalum apetalum* D. Don

1 A medium-sized hardwood of the central and north coastal rainforests of New South Wales and, occasionally, southern Queensland. **2** Heartwood pale pinkish brown. Sapwood, to 25 mm wide, not always clearly distinguishable. Characteristic odour variously described as 'caramel' or 'new mown hay'. Texture fine and even. Grain usually straight. The numerous bands of soft tissue produce a lot of figure on the tangential surface. **3** GD about 850 kg/m^3; ADD about 620 kg/m^3. **4** Relatively easy to dry but there is some risk of internal checking. Collapse slight and reconditioning not necessary. Shrinkage about 4 per cent radial, 8 per cent tangential. **5** Firm but not difficult to work. Turns well except for a tendency to bruise on the end grain. Glues satisfactorily. Unsuitable for steam bending. Tends to split in nailing. Takes water and spirit stains much better than oil stains. **6** Lyctids NS; termites NR; durability IG4, M4; heartwood not difficult to impregnate with preservatives. **7** S5, SD4. Some mechanical properties are listed on page 415. **8** Decorative veneer, plywood, turnery, carving, gun stocks, shoe heels, furniture, handles. **9** Becoming scarce.

Coconut wood *Cocos nucifera* L.

1 While Australia has only very limited stands of coconut palm, confined to tropical areas, it is a very important feature of the islands of the Pacific, as well as Papua New Guinea, the Philippines and South-East Asia. In the past the fruit has been the basis of economic interest but the large percentage of over-mature stands has created an interest in the wood and small quantities of it are reaching the Australian market. **2** The wood is very different in structure to that of the usual hardwoods and softwoods, which belong to the dicotyledon group of plants, whereas the coconut palm is one of the monocotyledons, most of which are grasses and herbs. A very important feature is that the palm soon reaches a fixed diameter (about 300 mm). Taper is very slight (about 5 mm/m of height) and the mature palm is usually not much more than 20 m in height. There are no annual rings, no rays, no heartwood, no branches, no knots. The bark is not clearly differentiated and is very hard to remove, although this is necessary for the predrying of pole and round-post material, which require preservative treatment. The mature wood is reddish brown, with white flecks from the vessels. **3** There is a very considerable density gradient between the very hard material on the outside (basic density 600–1100 kg/m^3) and the soft material in the centre (200–600 kg/m^3); the higher the location in the tree the lower the density. The higher density on the outside is associated with a much greater abundance of fibre bundles. **4** It is easy to dry material up to 25 mm thick without degrade, but precautions are necessary against bluestain. Thicker sections are liable to surface checking. Material with a basic density below 350 kg/m³ suffers severe collapse, which is difficult to recondition. Because of the absence of grain differentiation lateral shrinkage is uniform and less than 3 per cent, other than that due to collapse. **5** Difficult to cut because of the hard nature of the thick-walled fibre bundles in the outer layers and the abrasive nature of the parenchyma cells, which disintegrate during the milling operation and cause a lot of frictional heat. This problem is accentuated in dry wood, so it is preferable to do most cutting in the green material. Takes adhesives satisfactorily. **6** Lyctids NS; durability IG4. The freshly felled stems are very susceptible to staining fungi and pin-hole borer attack. Takes pressure impregnation with copper–chrome–arsenic salts satisfactorily but uneven distribution of the preservative occurs and soft rot attack can occur. **7** Strength is related closely to density; only the outer third of the diameter is suited for structural members but it is virtually free of defects. Green material is almost as strong as the seasoned product. **8** The denser material is suitable for general structural purposes, flooring, window frames, tool handles, furniture, carving, turnery. The softer material is suitable for wall panelling and internal trim. Very soft material and off-cuts are used as charcoal. Pole and post material requires impregnation with preservatives. **9** Small quantities are likely to be introduced in the future.

Further reading

Philippine Coconut Authority (1979). *Coconut wood—proceedings.*

Cooba *Acacia salicina* Lindl.

1 A small hardwood of wide but scattered distribution through the dry inland areas of eastern Australia. **2** Heartwood dark reddish brown. Sapwood much paler. **3** ADD about 700 kg/m³. **7** Provisionally S6, SD6. **8** Decorative turnery. **9** Not a commercial timber.

Cooba, river *Acacia stenophylla* A. Cunn. ex Benth.
Other common name: eumung

1 Very similar to cooba but often grows to quite a large tree on river banks in inland areas of heavy soil, producing a very attractive, easily worked furniture wood.

Cottonwood, eastern *Populus deltoides* Bartr. ex Marsh., especially varieties *angutata* and *monilifera*
Other common name: poplar

1 A medium-to-large hardwood of eastern North America. Hybrids of this species have been used in plantation forestry in eastern Australia in recent years but growth rates have been seriously affected by the arrival of a fungal rust, *Melampsora*, which destroys the leaves. **2** Heartwood greyish white to pale brown. Sapwood whitish but not clearly distinguishable from the heartwood. Texture fine and even. Grain usually straight. Free from gum and resin. When seasoned it is odourless and non-tainting to food. **3** GD about 750 kg/m³; ADD about 450 kg/m³. **4** Dries quickly but care is needed to avoid cupping and surface checking. Shrinkage about 2 per cent radial, 5 per cent tangential. **5** Rather 'woolly' to work because of the frequent presence of tension wood. Peels well. **6** Lyctids S; durability IG4. **7** S7, SD8 but it tends to vary considerably in strength. Some mechanical properties are listed on page 415. **8** Match splints and boxes, plywood, wood wool, furniture, general construction. **9** If leaf rust problems can be overcome, increasing quantities of small-diameter logs should become available. Information on this rust is given in the paper by Heather, W. A., Chandrashekar, M., Sharma, J. K. (1980). Forms and degrees of resistance in *Populus* spp. to the *Melampsora* leaf rusts occurring in Australasia. *Aust For* 43(1): 52–7.

Cudgerie, brown *Canarium australasicum* (F. M. Bail.) Leenh.
Synonyms: *Protium australasicum* (F. M. Bail.) T. A. Sprague
Bursera australasica F. M. Bail.

1 A medium-sized hardwood of the rainforests from northern New South Wales to north Queensland. **2** Heartwood pale brown. Sapwood wide and not clearly distinguished. Texture moderately fine and even. Grain variable. **3** ADD about 580 kg/m³. **4** Easy to dry. Shrinkage about 2 per cent radial, 4 per cent tangential. Protection against bluestain desirable. **5** Easy to work. Glues well. **6** Lyctids S; durability IG4. **7** Provisionally S6, SD6. **8** Joinery, plywood. **9** Seldom marketed.

Curracabah *Acacia concurrens* Pedley
Acacia leiocalyx (Domin) Pedley

1 A small hardwood native to northern New South Wales and inland parts of Queensland. **2** Heartwood dark brown. Sapwood distinctively paler. **3** ADD 800–900 kg/m³. **7** Provisionally S4, SD4. **8** Decorative turnery. **9** Not a commercial timber.

Cypress, black *Callitris endlicheri* (Parl.) F. M. Bail.
Synonym: *Callitris calcarata* (A. Cunn. ex Mirb.) F. Muell.

1 A small-to-medium softwood, sometimes growing in association with white cypress, but often in pure stands in hilly country and on stony ridges, in inland areas of New South Wales and Queensland, and occasionally in Victoria. **2** Heartwood may have many shades of brown. Sapwood pale yellow. Texture fine and even. Grain straight except around the many knots. Odour not as strong as that of white cypress. The bark has a high tannin content. **3** GD about 780 kg/m³; ADD about 710 kg/m³. **4** Needs slow initial drying to avoid surface checking. Shrinkage about 3.5 per cent radial, 4 per cent tangential. **5** Not hard to work but splits very readily so some predrilling for nails is required. **6** Lyctids NS; termites R; durability IG2, AG1, M3. Both sapwood and heartwood are very difficult to impregnate with preservatives. The cypress jewel beetle will attack the sapwood of trees weakened by bushfire or drought and its larval tunnels may appear sometimes in the sawn timber.   **7** Provisionally S5 and SD6. Some mechanical properties are listed on page 415.   **8** Flooring, panelling, posts, poles, general construction.   **9** Much less common than white cypress.

Cypress, northern *Callitris intratropica* R. T. Bak. et H. G. Sm.
Callitris columellaris F. Muell. sens. lat. has also been applied to it

1 A small-to-medium softwood of the Northern Territory north of 14°S, extending westward into the Kimberley region of Western Australia. There are also some stands on Cape York Peninsula in Queensland. The amount available has been much reduced by uncontrolled fires, to which the tree is very sensitive. Regeneration occurs quite well when fire is excluded. It is the most valued timber of local occurrence in the Northern Territory because of its termite resistance.   **2** The appearance and properties of the wood are very similar to those of white cypress but it is appreciably stronger.   **3** ADD about 670 kg/m³.   **6** Lyctids NS; termites R; durability IG2.   **7** Provisionally S4, SD5.   **8** General construction, flooring.   **9** Limited to areas of occurrence.

Cypress, white *Callitris glauca* R. Br. ex R. T. Bak. et H. G. Sm.
Callitris columellaris F. Muell. sens. lat. has also been applied to it
Other common name: *Murray pine*

1 A small-to-medium softwood widely distributed in inland areas of Australia with moderate rainfall. Much of the country in New South Wales and Queensland now devoted to wheat growing was originally covered with forests of cypress. The bark often produces a saleable resin called sandarac, but its collection is very labour-intensive. It cannot be recovered by extracting the bark with solvents because this would result in an unacceptable adulterated product. An increased flow of resin is often seen on the stumps of recently felled trees. Sandarac is used in confectionery and pharmaceuticals.   **2** Heartwood variegated browns. Sapwood pale yellow. Texture very fine and even. Grain straight. Distinctive and strongly persistent odour. Knots very common. A splinter burns to a white ash while that of black cypress burns to a dark grey or black ash.   **3** GD about 800 kg/m³; ADD about 680 kg/m³.   **4** Dries quickly but is prone to fine surface checking so reduction of the initial drying rate is necessary for dressed products in warm weather. Shrinkage about 2.5 per cent radial, 3 per cent tangential.   **5** Needs care in working because of its brittle nature. Accepts nail plate connectors without splitting. Inadvisable to dress it at low moisture content levels because of its brittleness. The sanding dust of most cypress is irritating to the mucous membranes of some people. Because of its susceptibility to fine surface checking cypress is one timber that gives a better painting performance when coated in the unseasoned condition; by slowing down the initial drying rate the coating inhibits the formation of checks.   **6** Lyctids NS; termites R; durability IG2, AG1, M2. The sapwood of cypress is unusual in that it, as well as the heartwood, is very difficult to impregnate with preservatives, even when high pressures are involved. Sap-replacement methods involving the steeping of the end grain of freshly felled material in the treatment solution gives some degree of penetration but it is a slow process suitable only for small-scale operations (e.g. for butt treatment of fence posts). 7 S5, SD6. Some mechanical properties are listed on page 416. 8 Flooring, panelling, building framework, posts, small poles. Because of its frequent knots and high extractives content cypress is not favoured for paper pulp production. The yield and strength of the pulp is relatively low and there is a high consumption of processing chemicals. 9 Plentiful in New South Wales and Queensland.

There are a number of other cypress of limited occurrence but of generally similar behaviour to white cypress. They include:

- brush cypress—*Callitris macleayana* (F. Muell.) F. Muell.
- coast cypress—*Callitris columellaris* F. Muell. sens. lat.
- dune cypress—*Callitris rhomboidea* R. Br. ex L. C. Rich.

These species are found in coastal areas of eastern Australia and usually have knots of smaller diameter than white cypress. The strength grouping is provisionally S6, SD7, except for dune cypress, which is provisionally S7, SD7. Some mechanical properties of coast cypress are listed on page 415.

Dakua salusalu *Decussocarpus vitiensis* (Seem.) de Laubenfels
Synonym: *Podocarpus vitiensis* Seem.
Other common name: red podocarp

1 A medium-to-large softwood of Fiji. 2 Heartwood pale golden brown. Sapwood not readily distinguishable. Texture fine and even. Grain straight. Compression wood may be present occasionally. 3 ADD about 450 kg/m³. 4 Relatively easy to season. Shrinkage about 2 per cent radial, 3 per cent tangential. 5 Easy to work. Nail-holding capacity rather poor. 6 Lyctids NS; durability IG4; heartwood not easy to impregnate with preservatives. 7 Possibly S7, SD7. 8 Internal joinery, furniture. 9 Small quantities occasionally imported.

Damson *Terminalia sericocarpa* F. Muell.

1 A medium-sized hardwood of the Queensland rainforests. 2 Heartwood pale brown. Sapwood yellow. Medium and even texture. Grain sometimes interlocked. 3 ADD about 640 kg/m³. 4 Easy to dry. 5 Relatively easy to work. Glues well. 6 Lyctids S; durability IG4. 7 Provisionally S5, SD6. 8 Joinery. 9 Limited mainly to areas of occurrence.

Doughwood *Melicope octandra* (F. Muell.) Druce
Synonym: *Melicope australasica* F. Muell.

1 A small-to-medium hardwood of limited occurrence in the rainforests of the upper north coast of New South Wales and of southern Queensland. 2 Heartwood cream. Sapwood not easily distinguishable from the heartwood. Distinctive odour when freshly cut, hence the common name. Texture fine and even. Grain straight. 3 GD about 770 kg/m³; ADD about 530 kg/m³. 4 Easy to dry but precautions

necessary against bluestain. Shrinkage about 2.5 per cent radial, 5 per cent tangential. **5** Easy to work. **6** Lyctids S; durability IG4. **7** S6, SD6. Some mechanical properties are listed on page 416. **8** Furniture, interior joinery. **9** Scarce.

Duboisia *Duboisia myoporoides* R. Br.
Duboisia leichhardtii F. Muell.
Other common name: corkwood

1 A small hardwood of frost-free areas of high rainfall in northern New South Wales and Queensland. **2** Heartwood pale yellow. Sapwood not visibly different. Texture fine and even. Grain slightly interlocked. Silky sheen. **3** ADD about 450 kg/m³. **7** Provisionally S7, SD8. **8** Although the wood is attractive, the tree is too small for commercial interest in the wood. However, the leaves are a valuable source of the alkaloids hyoscine (used for preventing travel sickness and as a depressant of the central nervous system) and hyoscyamine (which can be readily converted to atropine, used in ophthalmology as an eye pupil dilator). The leaves of *D. myoporoides* yield mainly hyoscine, while those of *D. leichhardtii* yield hyoscyamine. The dried leaves are exported to Europe for extraction of the alkaloids.

Ebony *Diospyros* spp.

1 There are a number of *Diospyros* hardwood species in west Africa and South-East Asia, which are variously called African ebony, Ceylon ebony and Macassar ebony. **2** Heartwood black or black streaked with brown. Sapwood usually distinctly paler. Grain often interlocked. Fine texture yields a very smooth finish. **3** ADD varies with species but is usually in the range 900–1100 kg/m³. **4** Drying should be done slowly to prevent checking. Shrinkage varies with species but is probably in the vicinity of 2.5 per cent radial, 5 per cent tangential. **5** Difficult to work because of its hardness and dulling effect on tool edges. Turns well. Glues satisfactorily. Needs predrilling for nails. The sanding dust can be very irritating to some people. **6** Lyctids NS; durability variable. **7** S5, SD6 but strength properties vary considerably with species. Some mechanical properties are listed on page 416. **8** Piano keys, fingerboards for violins and cellos, billiard cue butts, inlay, carving, cutlery handles. **9** Not commercially available in Australia.

Elm *Ulmus* spp.

1 A medium-to-large deciduous hardwood of Europe, Asia and North America. **2** Heartwood pale brown to pale reddish brown. Sapwood often wide and usually distinctively paler. Texture rather coarse because of the large pores, which are unevenly distributed. Grain variable; often interlocked in the European species. **3** ADD variable with species, from about 550 to 650 kg/m³. **4** Seasons without much difficulty. **5** The European material is more difficult to work than that from the other continents because of wilder grain. Inclined to cut somewhat 'woolly'. Nails, screws and glues well. Good for steam bending. **6** Lyctids S;

durability IG4; heartwood moderately resistant to impregnation with preservatives. **8** Furniture (traditionally favoured for Windsor chair seats), decorative veneer, turnery, tool handles, cooperage. **9** Usually seen only in made-up furniture, etc. in Australia.

Erima *Octomeles sumatrana* Miq.
Other common names: binuang, ilimo

1 A large hardwood whose range extends from Sumatra and Sabah across to the Philippines and Papua New Guinea. **2** Heartwood pale brown, sometimes with a slightly purplish tinge. Sapwood almost white but can have a greyish yellow tinge, to 150 mm wide, and usually distinguishable from the heartwood. Texture moderately coarse. Grain interlocked, producing a stripe figure on the radial face. Logs may contain brittleheart and pin-hole borer damage. Unpleasant odour when green. **3** ADD about 370 kg/m^3. **4** Easy to dry but susceptible to bluestain damage. Shrinkage varies considerably with origin, up to about 3 per cent radial, 7 per cent tangential. **5** Easy to work but 'woolly', needing sharp tools. No silica present. End grain tends to crumble because of the wood's softness. Peels easily. Unsuitable for steam bending because it buckles severely. **6** Lyctids S; durability IG4; heartwood moderately resistant to impregnation with preservatives. **7** S7, SD8. Not a structural timber. Some mechanical properties are listed on page 416. **8** Plywood, core stock, internal mouldings. **9** Sometimes imported, mainly for plywood manufacture.

Evodia *Euodia elleryana* F. Muell.
Synonym: *Evodia elleryana* F. Muell.

1 A small hardwood of the Queensland rainforests. **2** Heartwood cream colour. Sapwood not clearly defined. Texture medium and even. Grain straight. **3** ADD about 600 kg/m^3. **4** Easy to dry. Protection needed against bluestain fungi. **5** Easy to work. Glues well. **6** Lyctids S; durability IG4. **7** Provisionally S6, SD6. **8** Internal joinery. **9** Limited mainly to districts of occurrence.

Evodia, northern *Euodia vitiflora* F. Muell.
Synonym: *Evodia vitiflora* F. Muell.

1 A medium-sized hardwood of the Queensland rainforests. **2** Heartwood pale yellow. Sapwood not clearly defined. Moderately fine and even texture. Grain usually straight. Freshly cut wood has an unpleasant odour. **3** ADD about 630 kg/m^3. **4** Easy to dry but precautions needed against bluestain. **5** Easy to work. Glues well. **6** Lyctids S; durability IG4. **7** Provisionally S6, SD6. **8** Plywood, joinery. **9** Limited mainly to districts of occurrence.

Fir, amabilis *Abies amabilis* Dougl. ex Forbes
Other common name: silver fir

1 A large softwood of western North America, mainly in British Columbia and Washington state. **2** Heartwood pale brown. Sapwood visually indistinguishable from the heartwood. Texture medium. Grain straight. It is rather similar to Sitka spruce but of a coarser texture and more brittle. Not quite as strong as western hemlock. **3** ADD about 420 kg/m³. **5** Holds nails well. **6** Lyctids NS; durability IG4, M4. **7** S7, SD6. Some mechanical properties are listed on page 416. **8** General construction purposes. **9** Considerable quantities are included with western hemlock under the trade term Canada pine, a common import.

Fir, Douglas *Pseudotsuga menziesii* (Mirb.) Franco
Synonym: *Pseudotsuga taxifolia* (Lamb.) Britt.
Other common name: Oregon

1 Probably the most important softwood of North America, growing on the western fringe from Mexico to British Columbia. It is being used as a plantation species in other countries, including New Zealand, but there are only small areas of it in Australian plantations. **2** Heartwood yellow-brown to pale reddish brown. Sapwood distinctly paler, varying in width from about 50 mm in mature trees to 75 mm in fast-growing plantation stems. Regrowth wood varies considerably in density and strength and it may be necessary to consider the percentage of latewood and the spacing of the growth rings in assessing quality. Growth rings are very prominent because of the considerable difference in density and colour between earlywood and latewood; this also leads to a coarse and uneven texture. Grain generally straight. Resin content can be high, causing occasional bleed-through of paint films: the temperature of kiln drying helps to drive off the volatile fraction and makes the resin less mobile. The presence of the resin gives a distinctive odour to the freshly cut surface. Does not have the spiral grain problems of radiata pine and compression wood is relatively uncommon. The wood near the pith is of good quality, in contrast to that of radiata pine. **3** GD about 650 kg/m³; ADD about 530 kg/m³, for mature wood. **4** Relatively easy to dry but the tangential face is prone to surface checking, so a mild schedule is needed when kiln drying. End splitting is also likely if drying is too rapid. Shrinkage about 2.5 per cent radial, 4 per cent tangential. **5** As it is one of the hardest softwoods it is only moderately easy to work. Care is needed in dressing for the softer earlywood may be compressed and later, on recovery, produce a ridged surface. This characteristic makes it unsuitable for turnery. The strong contrast in hardness between earlywood and latewood makes it liable to wear unevenly. Not suitable for steam bending. Not a good base for paint because of the uneven nature of the wood and, in external applications, early failure is sometimes experienced on the latewood of tangential-cut material. Inclined to split when nailed near ends of piece. Differential glue absorption can occur. **6** Lyctids NS; termites NR; durability IG4, AG4, M4. Has been used in Australia for many years as a satisfactory window joinery timber when free of sapwood. The heartwood is difficult to impregnate with preservatives and even the sapwood is not readily penetrated, especially in the case of copper–chrome–arsenic salts. **7** S5, SD5. Some mechanical properties of material from a variety of sources are listed on pages

416 and 417. **8** Its availability in large sections and long lengths has made it a highly favoured import to Australia for many years for applications such as structural framing, joinery, vats, boat building. In North America it is the most important plywood species but it is seldom used for that purpose in Australia.

Gaboon *Aucoumea klaineana* Pierre
Other common name: okoume

1 A large hardwood of west Africa. **2** Heartwood salmon pink, darkening to pinkish brown. It has some resemblance to African mahogany. Sapwood of variable width, up to 75 mm. Texture medium. Grain usually straight but occasionally interlocked. No odour. **3** ADD about 430 kg/m³. **4** Easy to dry, with little degrade. Some risk of bluestain. Shrinkage about 3.5 per cent radial, 5 per cent tangential. **5** Works rather 'woolly' and has a blunting effect on cutting edges when dry but peels and slices well. Nails well. Glues satisfactorily. **6** Lyctids NS; termites NR; durability IG4; heartwood difficult to impregnate with preservatives. **7** Possibly S7, SD8. **8** Plywood, joinery, furniture. **9** Occasionally seen in Australia in the form of veneer.

Geronggang *Cratoxylon arborescens* Bl.

1 A large hardwood of Malaysia, Indonesia and the Philippines. **2** Heartwood pale red when freshly cut, darkening on exposure. Sapwood pale yellow, sometimes with a pink or orange tinge, 25–50 mm wide and usually easy to distinguish from the heartwood. Texture coarse and even. Grain often interlocked. Logs sometimes subject to brittleheart. **3** GD about 800 kg/m³; ADD about 500 kg/m³. **4** Easy to dry. Shrinkage about 2.5 per cent radial, 4.5 per cent tangential. **5** Easy to work even though some silica is likely to be present in the rays. Peels well. Too soft for turnery. Nails satisfactorily without risk of splitting. **6** Lyctids NS; termites NR; durability IG4, M4; heartwood is easily impregnated with preservatives. **7** S7, SD7. **8** Plywood, internal joinery, shelving. **9** Seldom seen in Australia.

Giam *Hopea* spp.
Other common name: heavy hopea (not to be confused with
    merawan, light hopea)

1 The numerous species of *Hopea* hardwood collectively known as 'giam' vary considerably in size; they occur throughout South-East Asia and extend as far east as Papua New Guinea. **2** Heartwood yellow, often with a greenish tinge when freshly cut, but becoming reddish brown on exposure. The sapwood, when first cut, is virtually indistinguishable from the heartwood but it remains yellow and does not darken appreciably. Texture fine and even. Grain slightly interlocked, giving some ribbon figure on the radial face. Resin canals are indicated by fine white lines visible on both radial and tangential surfaces. No taste or odour in the dry wood. **3** ADD about 1000 kg/m³. **4** Slow to dry but little degrade occurs if mild conditions are provided. Because of the variety of species involved shrinkage varies considerably, up to about 2.5 per cent radial, 5.5 per cent tangential.   **5** As it is very hard and horny it is not easy to work and difficult to produce a smooth surface. No silica is present but some gum build-up on saw teeth is likely.   **6** Lyctids S; termites NR; durability IG2.   **7** SI, SD1. Some mechanical properties are listed on page 417.   **8** Heavy structural members, boat keels, poles, piles, cross-arms, sleepers.   **9** Seldom seen in Australia.

Gidgee *Acacia cambagei* R. T. Bak.

1 A small hardwood of the dry inland plains of New South Wales and Queensland, and occasionally in South Australia and the Northern Territory.   **2** Heartwood dark chocolate brown. Sapwood pale yellow. Texture very fine. Grain variable; some trees produce wood with a very wavy figure, commonly described as 'ringed gidgee', which is much sought after for walking sticks and fancy turnery. Strong characteristic odour when freshly cut.   **3** GD about 1330 kg/m³; ADD about 1250 kg/m³.   **4** Slow in drying but little degrade if dried under cover. Shrinkage about 2 per cent radial, 3 per cent tangential.   **5** Hard to work.   **6** Lyctids NS; termites NR; durability IG1, AG1.   **7** Provisionally S1, SD1. Some mechanical properties are listed on page 417.   **8** Fancy turnery, decorative woodware.   **9** Not a commercial timber.

Gidgee, Georgina *Acacia georginae* F. M. Bail.

1 A small hardwood widely distributed in the dry interior of Queensland, South Australia and the Northern Territory. Very like gidgee.   **2** Heartwood coffee brown.   **3** ADD about 1330 kg/m³.

Gmelina *Gmelina arborea* Roxb.
Other common names: gamari, yemane

1 A medium-sized hardwood native to India and Burma but now being planted on a considerable scale in other tropical areas because of its rapid rate of growth. The stem may be inclined to develop in a crooked fashion so careful silvicultural practices are required. The tree is deciduous. It is said to coppice very satisfactorily.   **2** Heartwood pale yellowish white. Sapwood not readily distinguishable. Texture moderately coarse. Grain inclined to be interlocked, often producing a decorative appearance. Silvery sheen.   **3** ADD about 510 kg/m³.   **4** Dries without appreciable degrade. The quarter-sawn material dries much more slowly than back-sawn stock. Shrinkage is usually less than 2 per cent radial, 4 per cent tangential, and the timber has a good reputation for stability in service.   **5** Easy to work. Good base for coatings. Suitable for steam bending.   **6** Durability IG2.   **7** Not known, but in general the timber has about 60 per cent of the strength of teak.   **8** Furniture, carving, decking, boat building, plywood, paper pulp, matches, musical instruments.   **9** Not seen in Australia.

Grapia *Apuleia praecox* Mart.
Other common names: garapa, muirajuba

1 A medium-sized hardwood of South America, especially Brazil.
2 Heartwood lustrous golden yellow, developing a reddish hue on
exposure. Sapwood narrow and of distinctively paler colour. Slightly
rancid odour sometimes present. Texture fine and even. Grain usually
interlocked, producing a stripe figure on the radial surface. **3** ADD
900–1000 kg/m³. **4** Shrinkage about 3.5 per cent radial, 6.5 per cent
tangential. **5** Easy to work; can yield a very smooth surface. **6** Lyctids
probably S; durability IG2. **7** Possibly S2. **8** Furniture, joinery,
panelling. **9** Small quantities occasionally imported.

Greenheart *Ocotea rodiaei* (Schomb.) Mez

1 A large hardwood native to northern South America, especially
Guyana. **2** Heartwood pale to dark olive green, sometimes with
dark brown streaks. Sapwood pale yellow or greenish, to 50 mm
wide and often not clearly distinguishable from the heartwood.
Texture moderately fine and even. Grain variable. **3** ADD about
1000 kg/m³. **4** Very slow to dry and needs careful handling to avoid
checks and end splits. Shrinkage about 3.5 per cent radial, 5 per cent
tangential. **5** Difficult to fix without risk of splitting, so predrilling
is needed. Glues satisfactorily. Can be steam bent if given firm
support on the outer face. Rather hard to work. The sanding dust
can be very irritating and embedded splinters can cause considerable
infection. **6** Lyctids NS; durability IG1, AG1. One of the most
resistant species against marine borers. **7** S1, SD1. Some mechanical
properties are listed on page 417. **8** Marine structures, shipbuilding,
fishing rods (its great elastic strength makes it very suitable for this
purpose), vats for chemicals. **9** Rarely seen in Australia.

Guarea *Guarea thompsonii* Sprague et Hutch.
Guarea cedrata Pellegr. (scented guarea)

1 A large hardwood of the west African rainforests. *G. cedrata* extends
as far east as Uganda. **2** Heartwood pinkish brown. Sapwood narrow
and almost white. Texture medium and even. Grain variable. Slight
cedar-like odour. Some logs, especially of *G. cedrata*, contain gummy
material, which can be a problem when applying finishes. **3** GD
about 930 kg/m³; ADD about 600 kg/m³. **4** Dries easily but there
is some risk of surface checking. Shrinkage about 2 per cent radial,
4 per cent tangential. **5** Relatively easy to work but there is some
tendency to woolliness. The sanding dust can be irritating to both
skin and mucous membranes so good dust extraction is needed.
Nails and glues satisfactorily. Only just acceptable for steam bending.
If gummy material occurs, it may benefit from a rub down with
methylated spirits before the application of finishes. **6** Lyctids S;
durability IG2. **7** S4, SD5. Some mechanical properties are listed
on page 417. **8** Decorative veneer, joinery, furniture, boat building,
turnery. **9** Sometimes seen in Australia as veneer.

Gum, blue, southern
- (a) *Eucalyptus globulus* Labill. subsp. *bicostata* (Maid, et al.) Kirkp.
- (b) *Eucalyptus globulus* Labill. subsp. *globulus*
- (c) *Eucalyptus globulus* Labill. subsp. *maidenii* (F. Muell.) Kirkp.
- (d) *Eucalyptus globulus* Labill. subsp. *pseudoglobulus* (Naud. ex Maid.) Kirkp.
- (e) *Eucalyptus globulus* Labill. var. *st johnii* R. T. Bak., formerly *Eucalyptus stjohnii* (R. T. Bak.) (R. T. Bak.) syn. *Eucalyptus bicostata* Maid. et. al.

Other common names: (a) is also known as eurabbie and (b) as Tasmanian blue gum

1 A large hardwood of the cooler districts of south-eastern Australia, mainly in Victoria and Tasmania. The southern blue gum has been planted in many overseas countries; for example, it is a common feature of the Californian countryside. The leaves are usually rich in eucalyptus oil of cineole type. **2** Heartwood pale brown, sometimes with a pinkish tinge. Sapwood to 50 mm wide, paler but not always sharply distinguished from the heartwood. Texture medium and relatively even. Grain often interlocked. Growth rings prominent on end-section. **3** GD between 1100 and 1200 kg/m³; ADD about 900 kg/m³. **4** Needs care in drying to minimise checking of the tangential surface. Quarter cutting is desirable. Considerable collapse can occur. Shrinkage about 6 per cent radial, 12 per cent tangential; after reconditioning about 4 per cent radial, 7 per cent tangential. **5** Satisfactory for steam bending if carefully selected for straightness of grain. **6** Lyctids S; termites NR; durability IG3, AG2, M4. **7** S3, SD2. Some mechanical properties are listed on page 417. **8** General building purposes. **9** Confined to districts of occurrence.

Gum, blue, Sydney *Eucalyptus saligna* Sm.

1 A large, commonly occurring hardwood of the east coast of Australia from Batemans Bay, New South Wales to southern Queensland. **2** Heartwood dark pink to red-brown. Sapwood usually sufficiently paler to be readily distinguished. Texture moderately coarse and even. Grain straight or slightly interlocked. Gum veins common. **3** GD about 1070 kg/m³; ADD about 850 kg/m³. This species has been grown extensively in plantations in South Africa but the density of such rapidly grown wood is much less than that of mature Australian material, being in the range of 500–600 kg/m³. **4** Easy to dry but tangential surfaces are susceptible to surface checking. Collapse is very slight. Shrinkage about 5 per cent radial, 9 per cent tangential. Heart-centre material is inclined to split quite severely, so it is not recommended for large girders. **5** Relatively easy to work. **6** Lyctids S; termites NR; durability IG3, AG2, M3. **7** S3, SD3. Some mechanical properties are listed on page 417. **8** General building purposes, cladding, flooring, panelling, boat building. Has potential as a heavy furniture timber and for structural plywood. **9** Very common in coastal New South Wales.

Gum, grey *Eucalyptus propinqua* Deane et Maiden
Eucalyptus punctata DC.

1 Large hardwoods of the coastal districts between the Hawkesbury River in New South Wales and Maryborough in Queensland. **2** Heartwood red. Sapwood, to 30 mm wide, distinctively paler. Texture moderately coarse and even. Grain usually interlocked. Similar in general appearance to the ironbarks but often marked by characteristic grub holes. The end checking on grey gum logs is star-shaped from the heart, whereas ironbarks tend to check in small squares. **3** GD about 1240 kg/m^3; ADD about 1080 kg/m^3. **4** Slow in drying but little degrade occurs. Shrinkage about 7 per cent radial, 4.5 per cent tangential. **5** Because of its density and interlocked grain it is difficult to work when dry. **6** Lyctids NS; termites R; durability IG1, AG1, M2. **7** S1, provisionally SD2. Some mechanical properties are listed on page 417. **8** Heavy engineering construction, poles, sleepers. **9** A commercial species in New South Wales and Queensland.

Gum, grey, mountain *Eucalyptus cypellocarpa* L. Johnson, formerly *Eucalyptus goniocalyx* auctt. austral.
Other common name: monkey gum (NSW)

1 A large hardwood common in Victoria south of the alps, in the Grampian Ranges, and near Cape Otway; and in New South Wales mainly on the coastal fall of the southern tablelands. **2** Heartwood pinkish brown. Sapwood sometimes sufficiently paler to be distinctive. Texture moderately coarse and even. Grain sometimes interlocked. It can be so attractive as to qualify as a furniture wood but many logs contain an excessive amount of gum veins. **3** GD about 1100 kg/m^3; ADD about 880 kg/m^3. **4** Some collapse does occur in drying. To avoid surface checking it is advisable to quarter-cut material that is to be seasoned for boards etc. Shrinkage about 5 per cent radial, 10 per cent tangential; after reconditioning about 3.5 per cent radial, 7 per cent tangential. **6** Lyctids S; termites NR; durability IG3, AG2, M2. **7** S3, SD2. Some mechanical properties are listed on page 417. **8** General construction purposes. The attractive appearance of the timber suggests its potential for decorative veneer and heavy furniture, panelling, flooring and joinery. **9** Relatively common on the south coast of New South Wales.

Gum, Maiden's *Eucalyptus maidenii* F. Muell.

1 A large hardwood of occasional occurrence in eastern Victoria and southern New South Wales. **2** Heartwood pale brown. Sapwood not clearly differentiated. Texture medium and even. Grain often interlocked. **3** GD about 1100 kg/m^3; ADD about 950 kg/m^3. **4** Tends to check in drying and some collapse occurs. Shrinkage about 5 per cent radial, 10 per cent tangential; after reconditioning about 4 per cent radial, 6 per cent tangential. **6** Lyctids S; termites NR; durability IG3, AG2, M4. **7** S3, SD2. Some mechanical properties are listed on page 417. **8** General building purposes. **9** Generally limited to districts of occurrence.

Gum, manna *Eucalyptus viminalis* Labill.
Other common name: ribbon gum

1 A large hardwood of wide distribution in the cooler areas of Australia, from the Mount Lofty Ranges in South Australia through Tasmania and Victoria to all the tableland districts of New South Wales. Frost resistant. Coppices well from the stump. Has potential as a fast-growing source of pulp. **2** Heartwood pale pink or pale pinkish brown. Sapwood, to 35 mm wide, but not visually distinct. Texture medium and even. Grain variable. Growth rings prominent. **3** GD about 1100 kg/m³; ADD about 750 kg/m³. **4** Difficult to dry without considerable degrade from internal honeycombing, surface checking and collapse. Reconditioning usually desirable for dressed lines. Quarter sawing is recommended, followed by a slow initial rate of drying. Shrinkage about 6 per cent radial, 12 per cent tangential; after reconditioning about 3 per cent radial, 6 per cent tangential. **5** Not difficult to work. Glues satisfactorily. May need predrilling when nailed near ends of boards. **6** Lyctids S; termites NR; durability IG4, AG3, M4. **7** S4, SD4. Some mechanical properties are listed on page 417. **8** Internal joinery, furniture, panelling, flooring, handles. Potentially of interest for plywood manufacture. **9** Although a common eucalypt, the wood is of limited commercial availability because of seasoning problems.

Gum, mountain *Eucalyptus dalrympleana* Maiden

1 A large hardwood of the more alpine regions of south-eastern Australia, in Victoria, New South Wales and Tasmania. **2** Heartwood pale pink or pinkish brown. Sapwood of similar colour and not easily distinguishable. Growth rings prominent because of the darker latewood. Texture medium: fine in latewood but relatively coarse in earlywood. Grain usually straight. **3** GD about 1100 kg/m³; ADD about 700 kg/m³. **4** Some collapse occurs during drying but it is less than that suffered by mountain ash. It is advisable to quarter saw the log to lessen the effect of collapse and reduce the amount of surface checking. Shrinkage about 5 per cent radial, 9 per cent tangential; after reconditioning about 3 per cent radial, 5 per cent tangential. **6** Lyctids S; termites NR; durability IG4, AG3, M4. **7** S4, SD5. Some mechanical properties are listed on page 417. **8** Joinery, flooring, handles, general construction. Could be considered for furniture because of good appearance. **9** Seldom available commercially.

Gum, red, forest *Eucalyptus tereticornis* Sm.

1 A large hardwood of the coastal districts from Warragul in Victoria to the Cairns district of north Queensland, sometimes extending onto the adjacent tablelands. **2** Heartwood red. Sapwood distinctly paler. Texture moderately coarse and even. Grain often interlocked. **3** GD about 1200 kg/m³; ADD about 1050 kg/m³. **4** Not hard to dry. Shrinkage about 5 per cent radial, 8 per cent tangential. **5** The interlocked grain often makes it difficult to dress cleanly on the radial surface. **6** Lyctids NS; termites R; durability IG1, AG1, M2. **7** S3,

SD3. Some mechanical properties are listed on page 417. **8** Heavy engineering construction, machinery bearings, poles. **9** Mainly in districts of occurrence.

Gum, red, river *Eucalyptus camaldulensis* Dehnh.
Synonym: *Eucalyptus rostrata* Schlecht.

1 A medium-to-large hardwood found adjacent to most of the inland rivers of mainland Australia. It is a unique eucalypt in that it can stand quite long periods of flooding, and indeed such inundations play a very important role in the maintenance of river red gum forests. Because of its occurrence as an open woodland stand, trees tend to spread rather than form a long trunk so the length of millable log is usually small. **2** Heartwood red to reddish brown. Sapwood to 40 mm wide, distinctly paler. Texture relatively fine and even. Grain usually interlocked, often producing an attractive ripple or fiddleback figure. Gum veins common. The kino found in pockets in the wood has been used pharmaceutically in styptics and astringent gargles. **3** GD about 1130 kg/m³; ADD about 900 kg/m³. **4** Needs close stickering and weighted stacks when drying to minimise warping. Some collapse occurs. Shrinkage about 4 per cent radial, 8 per cent tangential; after reconditioning about 2.5 per cent radial, 4.5 per cent tangential. **5** Because of the interlocked grain it is necessary to adjust the cutting angle when dressing it. Unsuitable for steam bending because of the difficulty of obtaining the necessary straight-grained timber. Provided the grain is relatively straight it has good resistance to surface checking when exposed to the weather. **6** Lyctids S; termites R; durability IG2, AG1, M2. **7** S5, SD5. The classification is low because bending strength is affected considerably by the very interlocked grain. Some mechanical properties are listed on page 418. **8** Flooring, sleepers, heavy furniture, decorative turnery, panelling, sills, posts. **9** Mainly in Victoria and south-western New South Wales.

Gum, rose *Eucalyptus grandis* W. Hill ex Maiden
Other common name: flooded gum

1 A large, fast-growing hardwood of the east coast from the Hunter River in New South Wales to north Queensland. **2** Heartwood pink to pale red-brown. Sapwood not always clearly differentiated. Texture moderately coarse but even. Grain straight. The activity of a borer that makes 'scribbles' in the wood (Plate 42), and grub holes made by a large wood moth which lead to staining, often mar the appearance of the timber, which otherwise would be considered favourably for furniture. **3** GD about 950 kg/m³; ADD varies considerably with the maturity of the wood, with an average figure of about 620 kg/m³, although ranging up to about 750 kg/m³ for old growth. **4** Easy to dry. Shrinkage about 4 per cent radial, 7 per cent tangential. Inclined to surface check. **5** Relatively easy to work. Has possibilities for veneer, which glues well but is prone to end splits. **6** Lyctids NS; termites NR; durability IG3, AG2, M4. **7** S3, SD4. Some mechanical properties are listed on page 418. **8** Panelling, joinery, furniture, general construction. It is very good for fruit cases since the shooks can be stored for some time before use, even though in the green condition, without risk of serious fungal staining, which can happen with softwoods. **9** Plentiful in northern New South Wales and southern Queensland.

A hybrid of rose gum with *Eucalyptus urophylla* has shown a very rapid growth rate, as well as superior disease resistance, in Brazil where eucalypts are being planted on a very large scale. *Eucalyptus urophylla* is native to the Sunda Islands, located between Timor and Java.

Gum, round-leaved *Eucalyptus deanei* Maiden

1 A medium-to-large hardwood of the central and north coast of New South Wales and southern Queensland, at times extending to the tablelands. **2** Heartwood pinkish brown to reddish brown. Sapwood slightly paler and 50–75 mm wide. Texture rather coarse. Grain sometimes interlocked. Growth rings prominent on end-section. The quarter-cut material is of attractive appearance. **3** GD about 1220 kg/m³; ADD about 960 kg/m³. **4** Liable to considerable distortion in drying because of its very high shrinkage. Shrinkage about 8 per cent radial, 13 per cent tangential; after reconditioning about 5 per cent radial, 8 per cent tangential. **5** Not difficult to work. Finishes well. **6** Lyctids S; durability IG3. **7** S3 and provisionally SD4. Some mechanical properties are listed on page 418. **8** Because of its high shrinkage it is generally only used for lower quality framing. When carefully seasoned it could be used for flooring, panelling, etc. **9** Only in districts of occurrence.

Gum, salmon *Eucalyptus salmonophloia* F. Muell.

1 A medium-sized hardwood of Western Australia, growing between the Darling Ranges and the Kalgoorlie area. Most of the original stands were felled to make way for wheat farms. **2** Heartwood red-brown to chocolate brown. Sapwood pale brown. Texture relatively fine. Grain interlocked. **3** GD about 1120 kg/m³; ADD about 1050 kg/m³. **6** Lyctids NS; termites R; durability IG2, AG1; heartwood durable in regard to decay resistance but only moderately durable with respect to termites. **7** Provisionally S2 and SD3. **8** Mining timber, fencing, poles. **9** Confined to the eastern goldfields area of Western Australia.

Gum, scribbly *Eucalyptus haemastoma* Sm.
Eucalyptus micrantha DC.
Eucalyptus racemosa Cav.
Eucalyptus rossi
Eucalyptus signata

1 A medium-sized hardwood growing on poor coastal soils between Batemans Bay, New South Wales and Maryborough, Queensland. The name derives from the 'scribble' marks on the bark caused by a bark borer. **2** Heartwood pale pinkish brown. Sapwood distinctively paler and up to 50 mm wide. Texture moderately coarse. Grain often interlocked. Gum veins very common. Logs frequently of poor form.   **3** GD about 1150 kg/m³; ADD about 930 kg/m³.   **4** Because of the extremely high shrinkage, severe distortion can occur during drying. Shrinkage about 12 per cent radial, 18 per cent tangential; after reconditioning about 6 per cent radial, 8 per cent tangential. These figures are for *Eucalyptus micrantha*; those for *Eucalyptus haemastoma* are somewhat lower.   **6** Lyctids NS; termites R; durability IG3, AG2.   **7** S4, SD5. Some mechanical properties are listed on page 418.   **8** Because of its high shrinkage it is seldom milled. It makes a good fuel.

Gum, shining *Eucalyptus nitens* Maiden

1 A large hardwood of the high altitude country on both sides of the Victoria–New South Wales border and the mountain areas of eastern Victoria. Small quantities occur in the Barrington Tops and Ebor districts of northern New South Wales.   **2** Heartwood straw colour, with pink or yellow tints. Sapwood not always easy to distinguish. Texture medium. Grain straight. Pin-hole borer holes and associated black stains of 'pencil streak' are often present, giving the otherwise attractive timber a very speckled appearance. This staining has to be quite severe before it has an important effect on strength.   **3** GD about 1050 kg/m³; ADD about 700 kg/m³.   **4** Drying needs much care because of collapse and surface checking. Shrinkage about 5 per cent radial, 9 per cent tangential; after reconditioning about 3 per cent radial, 6 per cent tangential.   **6** Lyctids S; termites NR; durability IG4, AG3, M4.   **7** S4, SD4. Some mechanical properties are listed on page 418.   **8** General construction. Material free of discolouration could be considered for joinery, handles.   **9** A commercial species in southern New South Wales and north-eastern Victoria.

Gum, spotted *Corymbia maculata* Hook.
Corymbia citriodora
Eucalyptus henryi
Other common name: lemon-scented gum

1 A large hardwood of common occurrence on the poorer clay subsoils of the east coast from the Victoria–New South Wales border to the Maryborough district in Queensland. Its very attractive smooth bark and long leaves has led to it being planted as an ornamental tree in many parts of Australia.   **2** Heartwood pale to dark brown or chocolate. Sapwood, to 50 mm wide, is distinctively paler but there may be a zone of intermediate wood, which can be a complicating factor when preservative treatment is undertaken, since it is not easy to impregnate. Texture moderately coarse. Grain variable; the frequent presence of wavy grain produces an attractive fiddleback figure. Slightly greasy nature. Gum veins common. Northern material is usually slightly denser, stronger and more durable than southern.   **3** GD about 1150 kg/m³; ADD about 950 kg/m³.   **4** Needs care in drying to reduce the risk of checking on tangential surface. Collapse is slight. Shrinkage about 4.5 per cent radial, 6 per cent tangential.   **5** Not hard to work. Satisfactory for steam bending if straight-grained material is selected. The unseasoned wood is somewhat corrosive to aluminium nails and screws. For good bonding a pressure of about 1000 kPa and a temperature above 20°C are usually needed, for temperature and pressure become more critical with denser species; a low moisture content, preferably about 8–10 per cent, is also desirable. The high extractives content can be a problem with phenolic-type adhesives and spotted gum seems to be a little different to most other eucalypts in that the sapwood as well as the heartwood is affected.   6 Lyctids S; termites R; durability IG2, AG1, M4.   7 S2, SD2. Some mechanical properties are listed on page 418.   8 Heavy engineering construction, piles, poles, shipbuilding, agricultural machinery, flooring, plywood. It is the main Australian species for handles subject to high-impact forces (e.g. axe handles).   9 Relatively common in New South Wales and southern Queensland.

Gum, white, Dunn's *Eucalyptus dunnii* Maiden
Other common name: Killarney ash (in Queensland)

1 A large hardwood of the richer soils adjacent to the rainforests of the far north coast and coastal ranges of New South Wales and southern Queensland.   2 Heartwood pale brown. Sapwood not clearly differentiated from the heartwood. Texture medium and even. Grain straight. Gum veins common.   3 GD about 1100 kg/m^3; ADD about 800 kg/m^3.   4 Care needed to ensure slow drying in the early stages to avoid checks and splits. Shrinkage about 5 per cent radial, 10 per cent tangential.   5 Relatively easy to work. Glues well.   6 Lyctids S; durability IG4, M4.   7 S3 and provisionally SD4. Some mechanical properties are listed on page 418.   8 Building framework, joinery.   9 Generally only in districts of occurrence.

Gum, yellow *Eucalyptus leucoxylon* F. Muell.

1 A medium-sized hardwood of limited availability in western Victoria, extending into southern South Australia as far as the Eyre Peninsula.   2 Heartwood pale brown, with yellow or pink tints. Sapwood distinctively paler and to 25 mm wide. Texture medium. Grain usually interlocked.   3 GD about 1200 kg/m^3; ADD about 1010 kg/m^3.   4 Slow to dry but little degrade. Shrinkage about 3 per cent radial, 6 per cent tangential.   6 Lyctids S; termites R; durability IG2, AG2.   7 Provisionally S4 and SD5. Some mechanical properties are listed on page 418.   8 Poles, fencing, general construction.   9 Usually only in districts of occurrence.

Gum, York *Eucalyptus loxophleba* Benth.

1 A medium-sized hardwood of the wheat-growing districts of Western Australia.   2 Heartwood yellowish brown to dark brown. Texture fine and even. Grain interlocked, often giving an attractive figure.   3 GD about 1230 kg/m^3; ADD about 1070 kg/m^3.   7 S2 and provisionally SD2.   8 Mallets, mauls, poles, posts. Could be of interest for decorative woodware.   9 Only in districts of occurrence.

Hardwood, Johnstone River *Backhousia bancroftii* F. M. Bail, et F. Muell.

1 A medium-sized hardwood of the Cairns district of north Queensland. **2** Heartwood in various shades of brown, usually dark and often striped. Sapwood usually distinctively paler. Texture fine and even. Grain variable. Logs are usually relatively free of defects. **3** ADD about 990 kg/m³. **5** Rather difficult to work because of its extreme hardness. Difficult to glue. **6** Lyctids S; termites NR; durability IG3, AG2, M4. **7** S3, SD3. **8** A favoured flooring timber because of its extreme resistance to indentation as well as its attractive and richly coloured appearance. **9** Parquetry flooring in main metropolitan centres.

Hemlock, western *Tsuga heterophylla* (Raf.) Sarg.

1 A large softwood of the high rainfall areas of the west coast of Canada and extending south into the United States. It is one of the most important species of western Canada. **2** Heartwood straw to pale brown, sometimes with a pinkish tinge. Sapwood not easily distinguishable and to 25 mm wide. Texture relatively fine and even. Grain straight. The growth rings are prominent because of the darker bands of latewood, but less so than those of Douglas fir. Usually non-resinous. **3** ADD about 500 kg/m³. **4** The green wood has a much higher moisture content than that of Douglas fir and it is slower and more difficult to dry. Moisture content of green material can vary greatly. Care is needed to avoid surface checking. Shrinkage about 2.5 per cent radial, 5 per cent tangential. **5** Easy to work, except for the small hard knots. Glues satisfactorily. Holds nails well. The relative softness of the earlywood and its possible compression by the planer can lead to ridged material. **6** Lyctids NS; termites NR; durability IG4, AG4, M4; heartwood moderately difficult to impregnate with preservatives. **7** S6, SD6. Some mechanical properties are listed on page 418. **8** General construction purposes, internal joinery. **9** Amabilis fir (see p. 273) and grand fir (*Abies grandis* Lindl.) grow in association with western hemlock and a mixture, in which western hemlock predominates, is often sold in Australia as Canada pine or hem-fir. In the western United States, hem-fir may contain any of the following firs: amabilis fir (also called Pacific silver fir), Californian red fir (*Abies magnified*), grand fir, noble fir (*Abies procera*) and white fir (*Abies concolor*).

Hickory *Carya* spp.

1 A medium-sized hardwood of eastern North America. **2** Heartwood yellow-brown or pale reddish brown. Sapwood white and wide. Because the white colour is popular with buyers of handles and sporting goods (the main uses of hickory), sappy regrowth trees with very wide sapwood are a favoured source, yet, for material of similar density, there is no significant difference in strength or toughness between the heartwood and the sapwood. Texture medium but uneven because of the ring-porous nature of the wood, which produces a distinctive figure somewhat like that of ash (*Fraxinus* spp.). Grain often slightly interlocked. Woodpecker birds often drill holes in the bark and this can lead to streaks of discolouration in the wood. If the streaks are of only slight-to-moderate intensity, there is not much effect on the mechanical properties of the wood. Rapid-growth hickory with no more than 17 rings per 25 mm of diameter is generally the heaviest and strongest.   **3** ADD about 800 kg/m³.   **4** Dries quickly but careful stacking is necessary to avoid checking, cupping and twisting. Shrinkage about 4 per cent radial, 6.5 per cent tangential.   **5** Not easy to work but gives a smooth finish. Predrilling may be needed when nailing. Excellent for steam bending. Difficult to glue. Not a very suitable base for paint.   **6** Lyctids S; durability IG4; heartwood moderately resistant to impregnation with preservatives.   **7** Probably S4, SD4, but the strength properties can vary considerably because of the range of species involved. Some mechanical properties are listed on page 418.   **8** Its outstanding combination of high strength in bending, stiffness, shock resistance and hardness make it very suitable for the handles of striking tools, especially axe handles. Other uses include sporting goods (e.g. baseball bats), agricultural implements, ladder rungs, dowels, textile machinery, pump rods, furniture. The sawdust and chips are favoured for the smoking of meats.   **9** Commonly seen as axe handles.

Another group of *Carya* species have the common name pecan and are the source of the well-known edible nut. The wood is similar in appearance to hickory but lower in strength. It is occasionally imported in the form of veneer and used for limed finish furniture.

Horizontal   *Anodopetalum biglandulosum* A. Cunn. ex Hook. f.

1 A small and often severely misshapen tree growing in the very wet south-western part of Tasmania.   **2** Heartwood pinkish brown. Sapwood not easily distinguishable. Texture very fine and even. Grain variable. The general appearance is reminiscent of coachwood, which belongs to the same botanical family (Cunoniaceae).   **3** ADD about 700 kg/m³.   **4** Shrinkage about 3.5 per cent radial, 8 per cent tangential.   **5** Firm but not difficult to work.   **7** Provisionally S5, SD6.   **8** Handles, decorative turnery and woodware.   **9** Not a commercial timber.

Iroko   *Chlorophora excelsa* (Welw.) Benth. et Hook. f.

1 A large hardwood of tropical Africa.   **2** Heartwood pale yellow to brown, darkening on exposure to the air. Sapwood very pale yellow, distinctive from the heartwood, and varying in width from 50 to 100 mm, depending on the maturity of the tree. Texture rather coarse but even. Grain usually interlocked. Heartwood may contain hard deposits of calcium carbonate as a result of earlier wounding and this material is very destructive to saw teeth. The wood has some resemblance to teak.   **3** ADD about 660 kg/m³.   **4** Easy to dry but bluestain can be a problem. Shrinkage about 1.5 per cent radial, 2.5 per cent tangential.   **5** Difficult to work if mineral deposits present, otherwise satisfactory although the interlocked grain will require care in dressing. Glues satisfactorily. Predrilling for nails needed at board ends. Moderately satisfactory for steam bending. The sanding dust is likely to irritate the skin so efficient dust extraction equipment is needed. **6** Lyctids S; durability IG2; heartwood has good resistance to marine borers. **7** S5, SD6. Some mechanical properties are listed on page 418. **8** Furniture, decorative veneer, boat building, joinery, carving. **9** Occasionally seen in the form of decorative veneer.

Ironbark, grey *Eucalyptus paniculata* Sm.
Eucalyptus drepanophylla F. Muell. ex Benth.
Eucalyptus siderophloia Benth.

1 A large hardwood common along the coast of New South Wales and Queensland. **2** Heartwood colour varies considerably, from pale brown to dark chocolate brown and also dark red. If the wood was less difficult to work it would have considerable potential for heavy furniture because of its beautiful appearance. Perhaps techniques will be developed to make use of it as a decorative veneer now that favoured rainforest species are difficult to obtain. Texture moderately coarse and even. Grain usually interlocked. **3** GD about 1210 kg/m^3; ADD about 1120 kg/m^3. **4** Slow in drying and needs careful handling to avoid surface checking. Shrinkage about 4.5 per cent radial, 7.5 per cent tangential. **5** Because of its density it is hard to work. **6** Lyctids NS; termites R; durability IG1, AG1, M3. **7** S1, SD1. Some mechanical properties are listed on page 418. **8** Heavy engineering construction, poles, sleepers, flooring and decking, shipbuilding. **9** Relatively common in coastal New South Wales and southern Queensland.

Ironbark, red *Eucalyptus sideroxylon* A. Cunn. ex Woolls
Other common name: mugga

1 A medium-to-large tree occurring in north central Victoria, the inland slopes of New South Wales, and occasionally in the coastal districts of Victoria, New South Wales and Queensland. **2** Heartwood dark red. Sapwood pale yellow, to 25 mm wide. Texture medium and even. Grain interlocked. **3** GD about 1220 kg/m^3; ADD about 1130 kg/m^3. **4** Slow to dry. Care needed to minimise surface checking. Shrinkage about 3.5 per cent radial, 7 per cent tangential. **5** Hard to work because of high density and interlocked grain. **6** Lyctids S; termites R; durability IG1, AG1, M2. **7** S1, SD3. Some mechanical properties are listed on page 418. **8** Heavy engineering construction, poles, sleepers, etc. **9** Limited mainly to the districts of occurrence.

Ironbark, red, broad-leaved *Eucalyptus fibrosa* F. Muell. subsp.
Fibrosa, formerly *Eucalyptus siderophloia* auctt. austral.

1 A medium-to-large hardwood growing mainly in coastal districts of New South Wales and Queensland but extending inland as far as the western slopes in New South Wales. **2** Heartwood dark red. Sapwood yellow, to 25 mm wide. Texture moderately coarse and even. Grain often interlocked. **3** GD about 1210 kg/m^3; ADD about 1140 kg/m^3. **4** Slow to dry and needs care to avoid surface checking. Shrinkage about 4.5 per cent radial, 6.5 per cent tangential. **5** Because of its dense nature it is hard to work but has attractive appearance. **6** Lyctids NS; termites R; durability IG1, AG1. **7** S1, SD1. Some mechanical properties are listed on page 419. **8** Heavy engineering construction, poles, sleepers, flooring, bridge building. **9** Limited.

Ironbark, red, narrow-leaved *Eucalyptus crebra* F. Muell.

1 A large hardwood of the east coast from Sydney to Cairns, extending inland as far as the 500 mm rainfall areas of the western slopes and plains in New South Wales. **2** Heartwood dark red. Sapwood pale yellow, to 20 mm wide. Texture medium and even. Grain usually interlocked. **3** GD about 1160 kg/m^3; ADD about 1090 kg/m^3. **4** Slow to dry. Shrinkage about 3.5 per cent radial, 5 per cent tangential. This ironbark has greater resistance to surface checking than the other commercial ironbarks. **5** Hard to work because of its density and interlocked grain. **6** Lyctids NS; termites R; durability IG1, AG1. **7** S1, SD3. Some mechanical properties are listed on page 419. **8** Heavy engineering construction, poles, sleepers, wharfage. **9** Moderate quantities in New South Wales and Queensland.

Ironwood *Backhousia myrtifolia* Hook, et Harv.
Other common name: grey myrtle

1 A small hardwood of the coastal rainforests of northern New South Wales and southern Queensland. **2** Heartwood pinkish brown, darkening towards the centre of the tree. Sapwood narrow and hard to distinguish. Texture fine and even. Grain straight. **3** GD about 1100 kg/m^3; ADD about 1020 kg/m^3. **4** Slow to dry but little degrade. Shrinkage about 3.5 per cent radial, 7 per cent tangential. **5** Hard to work but turns cleanly to give a very smooth surface. **7** S1, SD2. Some mechanical properties are listed on page 419. **8** Chisel handles, mallets, turnery. Can be substituted for greenheart for fishing rods. **9** Not a commercial species.

Ironwood, Cooktown *Erythrophleum chlorostachys* (F. Muell.) Hennings ex Taub.

1 A small-to-medium hardwood, often of irregular shape, occurring in the far north of Queensland, the Northern Territory and Western Australia. **2** Heartwood bright red. Sapwood pale brown and may be 25 mm wide. Texture medium and even. Grain interlocked. **3** ADD about 1220 kg/m^3. **4** Inclined to check in drying. Shrinkage about 2 per cent radial, 3 per cent tangential. **5** Hard to work because of its density and interlocked grain but a very smooth finish can be produced. **6** Lyctids S; termites R, durability IG1, AG1. **7** S1 and provisionally SD1. Some mechanical properties are listed on page 419. **8** Fencing, sleepers, decorative turnery and woodware, knife handles; has potential for musical instruments. **9** Limited to districts of occurrence.

Ivorywood *Siphonodon australis* Benth.

1 A small-to-medium hardwood of the drier rainforests between the Clarence River in northern New South Wales and the Bundaberg district in Queensland. **2** Heartwood ivory white. Sapwood of similar colour and hard to distinguish. Texture very fine and even. Grain straight. **3** GD about 1110 kg/m³; ADD about 860 kg/m³. **4** Needs a lot of care in drying to minimise bluestain and checking. Slight collapse occurs. Shrinkage about 4 per cent radial, 9 per cent tangential. **5** Firm but easy to work and yields a very fine surface. **6** Lyctids S; durability IG4. **7** S4 and provisionally SD4. Some mechanical properties are listed on page 419. **8** Carving, turnery, inlay work, artificial limbs, manicure equipment. The sawdust is useful for polishing fine metal parts. **9** Not a commercial timber.

Jam, raspberry *Acacia acuminata* Benth.

1 A small hardwood of south-west Western Australia, between Albany and the Swan River. The unusual name comes from the odour of the wood when freshly cut. **2** Heartwood dark chocolate brown. Sapwood pale yellow. Texture fine and even. Grain interlocked, producing an attractive fiddleback figure. **3** ADD about 1100 kg/m³. **4** Shrinkage about 1 per cent radial, 2 per cent tangential. **6** Lyctids NS; termites R; durability IG1, AG1, M2. **7** Provisionally S2, SD2. **8** Turnery and decorative woodware, small items of furniture. **9** Not a commercial timber.

Jarrah *Eucalyptus marginata* Donn ex Sm.

1 A large hardwood of the south-west corner of Western Australia, in the 650–1250 mm rainfall area and on lateritic soils. **2** Heartwood dark red. Sapwood pale yellow. Texture relatively coarse but even. Grain slightly interlocked, sometimes producing a fiddleback figure. **3** GD about 1170 kg/m³; ADD about 820 kg/m³. **4** Little degrade in drying if handled carefully. Negligible collapse. Shrinkage about 5 per cent radial, 7.5 per cent tangential. **5** Considering its density it is relatively easy to work if tools are maintained in a sharp condition. The planer angle may need reducing to 15°. Glues satisfactorily. Satisfactory for steam bending. Care needed when nailing. **6** Lyctids S; termites R; durability IG2, AG2, M3. **7** S4, SD4. Some mechanical properties are listed on page 419. **8** General construction sleepers, poles, piles, flooring, panelling, joinery and heavy furniture. **9** One of the major species of Western Australia. Small quantities, mainly of flooring, are sold in the eastern states.

Jelutong *Dyera costulata* Hook. f.
Dyera lowii Hook. f.

1 A large hardwood of Malaysia and Indonesia. **2** Heartwood creamy colour, as is also the wide sapwood. Texture fine and even. Grain straight. Slight but distinctive odour. Appearance is affected by the slits of latex canals, which are about 10–20 mm long and often occur in clusters at 600–900 mm intervals. The latex is the principal ingredient of chewing gum. **3** ADD about 400 kg/m³. **4** Easy to dry but there is a risk of bluestain. Shrinkage about 1.5 per cent radial, 3 per cent tangential. **5** Easy to work. Gives a very smooth finish. Glues satisfactorily. Nails well. Good for carving. **6** Lyctids S; durability IG4, M4; heartwood relatively easy to impregnate with preservatives. **7** S7, SD8. Some mechanical properties are listed on page 419. **8** Pattern-making, carving, core stock, plywood, drawing boards, interior joinery. **9** Occasionally imported.

Kamarere *Eucalyptus deglupta* Bl.

1 A large hardwood, one of the few eucalypts growing naturally beyond Australia. It occurs in Papua New Guinea, Irian Jaya and Sulawesi. It is being planted extensively in the Philippines. **2** Heartwood pale to medium red-brown. Sapwood 20–40 mm wide, pale pink but not always distinctive from the heartwood. Texture rather coarse but even. Grain sometimes interlocked, with the production of a ribbon figure on the radial surface. Somewhat like karri in general appearance. **3** ADD of mature material about 700 kg/m³ but young plantation wood may be as low as 400 kg/m³. **4** Easy to dry if mature wood. Shrinkage about 3 per cent radial, 5 per cent tangential. **5** Relatively easy to work. Glues well. Splits readily so predrilling for nails may be necessary. **6** Lyctids S; termites NR; durability IG4, M4. **7** S4, SD4. Some mechanical properties are listed on page 419. **8** General construction purposes, plywood, handles, joinery, flooring. **9** Occasionally imported.

Kapur *Dryobalanops* spp., especially
Dryobalanops arjomatica Gaertn.

1 A large hardwood of the lowland forests of Malaysia and Indonesia. **2** Heartwood yellow, pink or reddish brown, darkening on exposure. Sapwood distinctively paler and 50–150 mm wide. Texture medium and even. Grain sometimes slightly interlocked, producing a small amount of figure on the radial surface. Freshly cut wood has a camphor-like odour. A camphor-like material is sometimes present in cavities in the wood but it is different from the true camphor, which is produced by the camphor laurel (*Cinnamomum camphora*), and it does not have the moth-repellent properties of the true camphor. **3** ADD about 750 kg/m³. **4** Slow to dry. Thick stock inclined to check. Shrinkage about 3 per cent radial, 6 per cent tangential. **5** The presence of silica makes it somewhat difficult to work when seasoned. Wet wood is blackened by contact with iron. Not very suitable for steam bending. Glues satisfactorily but extra care is needed with urea–formaldehyde and phenol–formaldehyde adhesives. Predrilling may be needed when nailing near extremities. **6** Lyctids NS; termites NR; durability IG3, AG2, M4. **7** S3, SD3. Some mechanical properties are listed on page 419. **8** Plywood, furniture, joinery. **9** Considerable quantities are imported, especially for windowsills.

Karri *Eucalyptus diversicolor* F. Muell.

1 One of Australia's tallest hardwoods, native to a very limited high rainfall area in the south-west corner of Western Australia, west of Albany. **2** Heartwood pale pink to reddish brown. Sapwood whitish and usually easy to distinguish. Texture somewhat coarse but even. Grain often interlocked. **3** GD about 1200 kg/m^3; ADD about 900 kg/m^3. **4** Careful handling is needed during drying to inhibit surface checking. Only slight collapse. Shrinkage about 4.5 per cent radial, 10 per cent tangential. **5** Not easy to work and planing angle may need to be reduced to 15°. Moderately suitable for steam bending. Some predrilling may be needed when nailing. Variable in gluability. Does not have a good reputation in regard to paint holding. **6** Lyctids NS; termites NR; durability IG3, AG2, M4. **7** S3, SD2. Some mechanical properties are listed on page 419. **8** General construction (for which it has the advantage, in Western Australia, of being available in long clear lengths and large sections), flooring, panelling, structural plywood, shipbuilding, sleepers. When preservative-treated it is favoured as a crossing timber, even when concrete is used as the main sleeper material. **9** One of the main timbers in Western Australia. Small quantities are marketed in the eastern states for flooring and roof truss material.

Kaudamu *Myristica* spp.
Other common name: nutmeg

1 A large hardwood of Fiji. Related species occur in Papua New Guinea and in northern Queensland. **2** Heartwood pale brown with orange or pink tinting. Sapwood distinctly paler, up to 50 mm wide. Texture medium and even. Grain usually straight. **3** ADD about 580 kg/m^3. **4** Shrinkage about 4 per cent radial, 8 per cent tangential. Relatively easy to dry. Needs care against bluestain and surface checking. **5** Easy to work. Peels readily. **6** Lyctids S; durability IG4; heartwood amenable to impregnation with preservatives. **7** Provisionally S7, SD7. **8** Joinery, furniture, plywood, turnery. **9** Seldom seen in Australia.

Kauri, East Indian *Agathis dammara* (A. B. Lamb.) L. C. Rich.
Synonym: *Agathis alba* (A. B. Lamb.) Foxw.
Other common names: bindang, damar minyak, Indonesian kauri, almaciga

1 A large softwood of South-East Asia and extending from Malaysia through to Papua New Guinea and the Philippines. The tree is often tapped to obtain a copal resin used in the manufacture of varnishes and lacquers. No odour or taste in the seasoned wood. **2** Heartwood pale yellowish brown, sometimes with a pinkish tinge. Sapwood often hard to distinguish from the heartwood. Texture very fine and even. Grain straight. No figure. Free of brittleheart. **3** GD about 800 kg/m^3; ADD about 550 kg/m^3. **4** Easy to dry but care needed to avoid bluestain. Shrinkage about 1.5 per cent radial, 3 per cent tangential. **5** Very easy to work. Excellent producer of veneer. Nails well.   **6** Lyctids NS; durability IG4; heartwood can be impregnated with preservatives.   **7** S7, SD7. Some mechanical properties are listed on page 419.   **8** Plywood, pattern-making, kitchen utensils, matches, joinery, vats, sounding boards for musical instruments, artificial limbs, instrument cases.   **9** Occasionally imported.

Kauri, Fijian *Agathis vitiensis* (Seem.) Drake
Other common name: dakua makadre

1 A medium-to-large softwood native to Fiji.   **2** Heartwood yellowish brown, sapwood slightly paler and of width ranging from 50 to 125 mm. Texture very fine and even. Grain usually straight. Some compression wood may be present.   **3** ADD about 550 kg/m³.   **4** Easy to dry but has some tendency to twist. Precautions needed against bluestain. Shrinkage about 3 per cent radial, 4.5 per cent tangential.   **5** Easy to work, although there may be some furriness.   **6** Lyctids NS; durability IG4; heartwood can be impregnated with preservatives.   **7** Provisionally S7, SD7.   **8** Plywood, joinery, furniture, flooring, turnery, boat building, kitchen equipment, vats, carving.   **9** Seldom seen in Australia.

Kauri, New Zealand *Agathis australis* (D. Don) Salisb.

1 A large softwood whose natural occurrence is limited to a small area of New Zealand, north of Auckland. Now scarce.   **2** Heartwood pale brown, sometimes pale reddish brown. Sapwood distinctively paler. Latewood slightly darker than earlywood but the growth rings are not prominent. Texture very fine and even. Grain straight. No odour.   **3** GD about 820 kg/m³; ADD about 560 kg/m³.   **4** Dries slowly, with little degrade. Shrinkage about 2.5 per cent radial, 4 per cent tangential.   **5** Easy to work. Good nailing and gluing properties. Very stable in service. Excellent base for coatings.   **6** Lyctids NS; durability IG2 (the best of the Kauris), M4; heartwood is resistant to impregnation with preservatives.   **7** S5, SD5. Some mechanical properties are listed on page 419.   **8** Vats, food preparation equipment, textile rollers, boat building.   **9** Because of its scarcity it is now rarely seen outside New Zealand.

Kauri, Queensland North Queensland kauri—*Agathis* microstachya J. F. Bail, et C. T. White
South Queensland kauri—*Agathis robusta* (C. Moore ex F. Muell.) F. M. Bail.
Other common name: Queensland kauri pine

1 A large softwood native to the Cairns and Maryborough districts, respectively.   **2** Heartwood pale cream to pale brown. Sapwood not visibly distinct. Texture fine and even. Grain straight. The wood is usually slightly darker than that of hoop pine and the presence of flecks in the rays as seen on the radial surface distinguishes it from both hoop and bunya pines.   **3** GD about 720 kg/m³; ADD about 480 kg/m³.   **4** Dries quickly with little degrade but needs protection against bluestain. Shrinkage about 2 per cent radial, 3.5 per cent tangential.   **5** Usually easy to work but sometimes compression wood is present. Glues well. Fair for steam bending.   6 Lyctids NS; termites NR; durability IG4, AG4, M4; heartwood relatively easy to impregnate with preservatives.   7 S7, SD8. Some mechanical properties are listed on page 419.   8 Plywood, furniture, joinery, pattern-making, vats, kitchen utensils, battery separators, turnery, violin bellies.   9 Mainly limited to north Queensland.

Vanikoro kauri, *Agathis macrophylla* (Lindl.) Mast., which grows on the Santa Cruz and Solomon Islands, is rather similar in appearance and properties and is occasionally imported.

Kempas *Koompassia malaccensis* Maing.
Koompassia excelsa Taub.
Koompassia grandiflora Kosterm.

1 A large hardwood native to Malaysia, Indonesia, the Philippines and Papua New Guinea, and usually growing in swampy ground.   2 Heartwood reddish brown, often with yellow streaks. Sapwood pale yellow or pinkish brown, to about 50 mm wide, and distinct from the heartwood. Texture coarse but even. Grain interlocked, giving some figure to the radial surface. Some brittleheart may be present in logs.   3 GD about 1000 kg/m^3; ADD about 850 kg/m^3.   4 Dries quickly but care needed to prevent splitting. The presence of 'included phloem' can reduce strength and promote the occurrence of splits during drying. Shrinkage about 2 per cent radial, 3 per cent tangential.   5 The interlocked grain can cause difficulty in working it. Unsuitable for turnery. Peels satisfactorily. May need predrilling for nails.   6 Lyctids S; termites NR; durability IG3, M4.   7 S2, SD2.   8 Plywood, flooring. When treated with preservative it is used for sleepers, bridges and wharfage.   9 Small quantities occasionally imported.

Keruing *Dipterocarpus* spp.
Other common names: apitong, eng, gurjun, yang, bagac

1 A large hardwood of South-East Asia, the Philippines and the Indian subcontinent.   2 Because of the large number of species that are included under this title, the heartwood colour varies considerably but is generally pale to dark reddish brown. The sapwood, 30–100 mm wide, is usually grey, yellowish or pale brown, and not always clearly distinguishable from the heartwood. Texture is moderately coarse but even. Grain is usually straight but may be slightly interlocked, resulting in some stripe figure on the radial surface. High resin content and strongly resinous odour.   3 GD about 950 kg/m^3; ADD about 750 kg/m^3. Because of the diversity of species involved, the density range can vary considerably from these figures.   4 Careful drying needed to avoid checks and end splits. Presteaming for several hours before drying helps to improve the rate of drying and lessens degrade. Kiln drying is helpful in expelling the volatile constituents of the resin, making it less mobile in the seasoned wood. Shrinkage is variable because of species range but averages about 3.5 per cent radial, 7 per cent tangential.   5 Can be difficult to work when dry because of the presence of both silica and resin. Sanding dust can irritate the skin. Nails satisfactorily but

glues variably. Its high resin content makes it a poor base for coatings. Unsuitable for steam bending. **6** Lyctids S; termites NR; durability IG3, AG3, M4; heartwood variable in its resistance to impregnation and there is the possibility of uneven distribution of preservative. **7** S3, SD3. Some mechanical properties are listed on page 419. **8** General construction. Preservative-treated material is used for poles, piles, sleepers, cross-arms. **9** Occasionally imported.

Koto *Pterygota bequaertii* De Wild.
Other common name: African ash

1 A large hardwood of the west African rainforests. **2** Heartwood pale straw, with white fleck of rays on the radial surface. Sapwood not readily distinguishable. Texture coarse. Grain slightly interlocked. Unpleasant odour when green but it disappears after drying. **3** ADD about 600 kg/m³. **4** Dries quickly with little degrade but precautions needed against bluestain. Shrinkage about 3.5 per cent radial, 7 per cent tangential. **5** Easy to work if tools kept sharp to overcome furring tendency. Nails and glues satisfactorily and is easily converted into veneer. **6** Lyctids S; durability IG4; heartwood amenable to impregnation with preservatives. **7** Possibly S6, SD7. **8** Decorative veneer, furniture, joinery. **9** Small quantities are imported in veneer form.

Kurrajong, flame *Brachychiton acerifolius* F. Muell.
Other common name: flame tree

1 A medium-sized hardwood of the coastal rainforests from the Illawarra district of New South Wales to north Queensland. **2** Heartwood white to cream. Sapwood wide and not distinctive from the heartwood. Texture coarse and even. Grain straight. Very soft. Rays prominent on radial surface. **3** GD about 800 kg/m³; ADD about 420 kg/m³. **4** Dries quickly without much degrade but precautions must be taken against bluestain. Shrinkage about 3 per cent radial, 8.5 per cent tangential; after reconditioning about 2.5 per cent radial, 7 per cent tangential. **5** Because of its 'woolly' nature it is important to keep tools sharp. **6** Lyctids S; durability IG4, AG4. **7** Provisionally less than S7 and SD8. Not for structural use. Some mechanical properties are listed on page 419. **8** Core stock, modelling, stage sets, hat blocks. **9** Seldom offered commercially.

Kwila *Intsia bijuga* (Colebr.) O. Ktze.
Intsia palembanica Miq.
Other common names: ipil, merbau, vesi

1 A large hardwood of wide distribution in South-East Asia and eastwards to Papua New Guinea, Philippines, Solomon Islands and Fiji. Occurs occasionally in north Queensland. **2** Heartwood may be bright yellow when first cut but becomes pale to dark reddish brown. Sapwood to 80 mm wide, pale yellow and usually distinct from the heartwood. Texture moderately coarse but even. Grain sometimes slightly interlocked, producing a ribbon figure on the radial surface. Characteristic oily odour when freshly cut. Rather greasy to the touch. The vessels contain a yellow substance that will stain textiles and concrete. Contact with iron under moist conditions will cause formation of a black stain. **3** GD about 1200 kg/m³; ADD about 850 kg/m³. **4** Dries slowly with little degrade. Shrinkage about 1.5 per cent radial, 2.5 per cent tangential. **5** It cuts cleanly but saw teeth tend to become clogged with a gummy material. The cutting angle of the planer needs to be reduced, especially on the radial surface. Predrilling may be needed when nailing. Glues reasonably satisfactorily except with casein. Sanding dust can be irritating to both skin and mucous membranes. Turns well. **6** Lyctids S; termites R; durability IG3, AG1, M3. **7** S2, SD3. Some mechanical properties are listed on page 420. **8** Furniture, flooring, decking, panelling, turnery, sills, boat building, cross-arms, carving, vats, window joinery, veneer. **9** Occasionally imported.

Lancewood, brown *Acacia doratoxylon* A. Cunn.

1 A small hardwood found in many parts of Australia and with typical *Acacia* wood. **3** ADD about 900 kg/m³. **7** Provisionally S3, SD4. **8** Not of commercial importance.

Laran *Anthocephalus chinensis* (Lam.) A. Rich, ex Walp.
Synonym: *Anthocephalus cadamba* (Roxb.) Miq.
Other common name: labula

1 A hardwood occurring mainly on the island of New Britain in Papua New Guinea. Also in the Philippines and other parts of South-East Asia. Said to be of very rapid growth and of interest as a possible plantation species. **2** Heartwood pale yellow. Sapwood whitish but not clearly distinct from the heartwood. Texture medium and even. Grain usually straight. No figure. **3** ADD about 430 kg/m³. **4** Easy to dry but precautions needed against bluestain. Shrinkage about 2 per cent radial, 4.5 per cent tangential. **5** Easy to work. Glues and nails well. **6** Lyctids S; durability IG3; heartwood relatively easy to impregnate with preservatives. **7** S6 and SD6 (for mature wood). **8** Interior joinery, core stock, containers. **9** Seldom seen in Australia.

Larch, European *Larix decidua* Mill.

1 A medium-sized softwood native to central and southern Europe but a common plantation species in cool temperature climates, including New Zealand. One of the few deciduous softwoods. **2** Heartwood pale reddish brown. Sapwood pale yellow-brown and narrow. Texture moderately fine but uneven. Grain straight. A prominent growth ring figure is defined by the denser and darker latewood. Knots are usually small, tight and numerous. **3** GD of plantation material about 750 kg/m³; ADD about 560 kg/m³. **4** Relatively easy to dry but care is needed to avoid splitting and twisting. Bluestain is seldom a problem and there is an absence of low density corewood. Shrinkage about 2 per cent radial, 5 per cent tangential. **5** Relatively easy to work, except at the knots. Tends to split when being nailed so predrilling near ends is needed. Does not hold nail plates well because of the considerable difference in density between earlywood and latewood. Has a slightly corrosive action on steel nails. Glues satisfactorily. The alternating bands of hard and soft tissue can lead to uneven wear in, say, flooring. Not a very good paint holder under exposed conditions. **6** Lyctids NS; durability IG4. Slowly grown European heartwood has good in-ground durability but the faster growth plantation material is considerably less durable. It is difficult to impregnate with preservatives. **7** S5, SD6. Some mechanical properties are listed on page 420. **8** Building framework, panelling, furniture. **9** Plantation grown timber is occasionally imported from New Zealand.

Larch, western *Larix occidentalis* Nutt.

1 A large softwood of the mountain areas of north-western United States, where it is found in association with Douglas fir. It extends across the border into Canada. **2** Heartwood yellowish brown. Sapwood yellowish white, usually only about 25 mm wide. Grain usually straight. Subject to ring shakes. Knots common but usually small. Growth rings prominent. **3** ADD about 600 kg/m³. **4** Shrinkage about 2.5 per cent radial, 5 per cent tangential. **6** Lyctids NS; durability IG2; heartwood probably difficult to impregnate with preservatives. **7** S5, SD5, although Canadian figures show dry material can be SD4. Some mechanical properties are listed on page 420. **8** Building framework, panelling, joinery. **9** Seldom imported under its own name but some may come in with shipments of Douglas fir.

Laurel, camphor *Cinnamomum camphora* Nees et Eberm.

1 A large hardwood widely distributed in South-East Asia, China and Japan. Early this century it was widely planted as an ornamental tree in eastern Australia but it is not now favoured because of the extreme viability of the seeds. It can be a problem tree on dairy farms because the grazed leaves give milk an unpleasant taste. On the north coast of New South Wales it is inhibiting the regrowth of rainforest species in some districts. The wood and leaves, when distilled, yield camphor. **2** Heartwood very variable in colour from pale to mid brown, often streaked with darker brown or red. Sapwood very wide and pale brown. Texture moderately fine and even. Grain usually interlocked. Characteristic camphor odour. Repellent to moths. **3** ADD about 550 kg/m³. **4** Easy to dry. Shrinkage about 2 per cent radial, 3.5 per cent tangential. **5** Easy to work. **6** Lyctids S. **7** SD6 and provisionally S6. **8** Clothes storage cabinets, decorative veneer (from highly figured roots, gnarled logs, etc.), carving. **9** Not in commercial quantities.

Leatherwood *Eucryphia lucida* (Labill.) Baill.
Synonym: *Eucryphia billardieri* Spach

1 A small hardwood of the high rainfall areas of western Tasmania. **2** Heartwood pinkish brown. Sapwood not clearly defined. Texture very fine and even. Grain usually straight. Growth rings visible but not conspicuous. **3** ADD about 740 kg/m³. **4** Easy to dry. Shrinkage about 5 per cent radial, 9.5 per cent tangential; after reconditioning about 4.5 per cent radial, 8 per cent tangential. **5** Moderately easy to work. Turns and glues well. Good for steam bending. **6** Lyctids NS; durability IG3. **7** Provisionally S5 and SD5. **8** Turnery, handles, small articles of furniture. **9** Not a commercial timber.

Lemonwood *Calycophyllum candidissimum* (Vahl) DC.

1 A small hardwood of the Caribbean region, mainly Cuba and Central America. **2** Heartwood brown. Sapwood distinctly paler. Most of the commercial timber is sapwood. Texture fine and even. Grain variable. **3** ADD about 800 kg/m³. **5** Relatively easy to work. Very good elasticity and resistance to splitting. **6** Durability IG3. **7** Provisionally S5 and SD5. **8** Fishing rods, archery bows, tool handles, turnery. **9** Not seen in Australia, except in made-up articles.

Lightwood *Acacia implexa* Benth.

1 A small-to-medium hardwood of scattered occurrence in coastal and tableland areas of eastern Australia. **2** Heartwood rich dark brown. Sapwood distinctively paler. Texture medium and even. Grain usually straight. **3** ADD variable, averaging about 800 kg/m³ (rather a contrast to its common name!). **4** Easy to dry. Shrinkage about 2 per cent radial, 4 per cent tangential. **5** Glues well. Has good resistance to shock. **7** Provisionally S4, SD5. **8** Handles, turnery. **9** Not a commercial timber.

Lignum-vitae *Guaiacum* spp., mainly
Guaiacum officinale L.

1 A small hardwood of the West Indies and tropical America. **2** Heartwood greenish brown. Sapwood narrow, yellow and distinct from the heartwood. It contains a resin that used to be an ingredient in medicines, hence the name 'wood of life'. It has the rare property of being self-lubricating when used as a bearing, thus having great value for underwater use. Texture fine and even. Grain interlocked, producing a ripple figure. Oily to the touch. **3** ADD about 1200 kg/m³. **4** Needs care in drying to prevent checks and splits. Dries very slowly. Shrinkage about 2 per cent radial, 4 per cent tangential. **5** Difficult to work because of its hardness and interlocked grain. Splits easily tangentially but much more resistant in the radial plane. Turns well. **6** Lyctids NS; durability IG2. **7** S1, SD1. Some mechanical properties are listed on page 420. **8** Bearings (especially for the propeller shafts of ships), mallet heads, rollers, turnery, pulleys and for lapping tungsten carbide steel cutters. **9** Very small quantities are imported.

Lumbayau *Heritiera* spp., principally
Heritiera javanica (Bl.) Kosterm.
Heritiera simplicifolia (Mast.) Kosterm.
Other common names: mengkulang, chumprag

1 A large hardwood of the Philippines, Indonesia, Malaysia and Thailand, belonging to the same genus as the Australian tulip oaks and having wood of rather similar appearance. **2** Heartwood reddish brown to brown, sometimes with dark streaks. Sapwood pale yellowish red or greyish yellow, not always readily distinguishable from the heartwood, and up to 120 mm wide. Texture moderately coarse and even. Grain straight or shallowly interlocked, giving some stripe figure to the radial surface. The rays are prominent and give a fine fleck figuring. Greasy to the touch. Brittleheart sometimes present. **3** ADD about 730 kg/m^3. **4** Dries quickly with little degrade if care is taken to minimise warping and surface checking. Shrinkage about 2 per cent radial, 4 per cent tangential. **5** Because of the presence of silica it soon dulls saws. Peels well. Nails and glues satisfactorily. Yields a smooth finish. **6** Lyctids S; termites NR; durability IG4, M4; heartwood moderately resistant to impregnation with preservatives. **7** S5, SD5. **8** Plywood, internal joinery, furniture, flooring, boat building. **9** Seldom seen in Australia.

Magnolia *Galbulimima belgraveana* (F. Muell.) T. A. Sprague
Synonym: *Galbulimima baccata* F. M. Bail.

1 A hardwood of the rainforests of north Queensland and Papua New Guinea. **2** Heartwood pale to dark brown. Sapwood greyish white. Texture medium and even. Grain straight. **3** ADD about 600 kg/m^3. **4** Easy to dry but precautions needed against bluestain. Shrinkage about 2 per cent radial, 4 per cent tangential. **5** Easy to work but extra care needed when gluing. **6** Lyctids S; durability IG4. **7** Provisionally S6 and SD6. **8** Plywood, mouldings. **9** Small quantities in northern Queensland.

Mahogany, African *Khaya* spp., especially
Khaya anthotheca (Welw.) C. DC.
Khaya grandifoliola C. DC.
Khaya ivorensis A. Chev.

1 A large hardwood mainly of west Africa but found eastward as far as Uganda and Tanzania. **2** Heartwood pinkish brown to dark reddish brown. Sapwood yellow-brown, not always distinct from the heartwood. Texture coarser than that of American mahogany because of the larger pores. Grain frequently interlocked, producing a stripe figure on the radial surface. Brittleheart often present in the logs. **3** ADD varies considerably with species, from about 530–700 kg/m^3, averaging about 570 kg/m^3. **4** Easy to dry, with little degrade. Shrinkage about 1.5 per cent radial, 3 per cent tangential. **5** Relatively easy to work unless a lot of interlocked grain is present. Brittleheart material will give a 'woolly' cut and needs very sharp tools. Nails and glues well. More resistant to indentation than American mahogany. Unsuitable for steam bending. Damp wood develops black stains in contact with iron. The sanding dust can irritate the skin so good dust extraction is needed. **6** Lyctids S; durability IG3. **7** S6, SD6. Some mechanical properties are listed on page 420. **8** Furniture, decorative veneer, panelling, joinery, boat building. **9** Seldom imported.

Mahogany, American *Swietenia mahagoni* Jack
Swietenia macrophylla King
Other common names: Cuban mahogany, Spanish mahogany,
Honduras mahogany

1 A large hardwood native to the West Indies, especially Cuba, and the adjacent mainland from Mexico to Brazil. **2** Heartwood yellow-brown to red-brown, darkening on exposure. Sapwood distinctively paler. The end of each growth ring is marked by paler wood, distinguishing it from other mahoganies. Texture moderately fine. Grain variable; interlocked material is sought for decorative veneer production. **3** ADD varies greatly, from about 400 to 850 kg/m^3. The average for the species is about 550 kg/m^3 but Cuban material averages about 700 kg/m^3. **4** Dries quickly with little degrade. Shrinkage about 1.5 per cent radial, 2.5 per cent tangential. **5** Easy to work but sharp tools are needed to avoid 'woolliness' in highly figured material. Nails and glues well. Moderately suitable for steam bending. **6** Lyctids S; durability IG3. **7** S5, SD6. Some mechanical properties are listed on page 420. **8** The original mahogany, whose importation to Europe at the beginning of the 18th century led to such progress in furniture design. Its working and finishing properties, stability and appearance make it one of the world's outstanding furniture timbers; it is now scarce. **9** Seldom seen in Australia.

Mahogany, brush *Geissois benthamii* F. Muell.
Other common name: red carabeen

1 A medium-to-large hardwood of the east coast rainforests from the Manning River, New South Wales to southern Queensland. **2** Heartwood pale to dark pinkish brown. Sapwood to 25 mm wide, yellowish white. Texture fine and even. Grain variable but little figure. The wood sometimes contains pockets of crystalline masses of calcium oxalate, which severely blunt saws and gap planer knives. This material often occurs in long streaks, somewhat like gum veins, presumably as a response to an earlier injury. **3** GD about 900 kg/m^3; ADD about 650 kg/m^3. **4** Relatively easy to dry but care is needed to avoid surface checking. Only slight collapse. Shrinkage about 3.5 per cent radial, 7.5 per cent tangential. **5** More difficult to work than its density would suggest. **6** Lyctids S; termites NR; durability IG4, M4. **7** Provisionally S5 and SD5. Some mechanical properties are listed on page 420. **8** Plywood, joinery, turnery, carving, handles. **9** Limited.

Mahogany, brush, northern *Geissois biagiana* (F. Muell.)
F. Muell. ex Engl.
Synonym: *Weinmannia biagiana* F. Muell.

1 A hardwood of the north Queensland rainforests. **2** Heartwood brown. Medium texture. Straight grain. **3** ADD about 640 kg/m^3. **6** Lyctids S; durability IG4. **7** Provisionally S5, SD5. **8** Joinery. **9** Limited to districts of occurrence.

Mahogany, miva *Dysoxylum muelleri* Benth.
Other common name: red bean

1 A medium-to-large hardwood of occasional occurrence in the coastal rainforests from the Illawarra district of New South Wales to the Gympie district of Queensland. **2** Heartwood dark reddish brown. Sapwood much paler and readily distinguishable. Texture moderately fine and even. Grain sometimes interlocked. The tangential surface has a fine tracery of soft tissue. **3** GD about 1100 kg/m³; ADD about 670 kg/m³. **4** Slow to dry but little degrade. Negligible collapse. Shrinkage about 3 per cent radial, 5 per cent tangential. **5** Easy to work but the sanding dust can be very irritating to mucous membranes. Glues well. **6** Lyctids S; durability IG2. **7** Provisionally S5 and SD6. Some mechanical properties are listed on page 420. **8** Furniture, veneer, panelling, window joinery, carving, turnery. **9** Scarce.

Mahogany, Philippine, red, dark *Shorea* spp., especially
Shorea agsaboensis Stern.
Shorea negrosensis Foxw.
Shorea polysperma Merr.
Other common names: dark red lauan, tanguile

1 A large hardwood of the Philippine rainforests. **2** Heartwood various shades of red. Sapwood to 50 mm wide, cream or pale grey, clearly defined from the heartwood. Texture coarse and even. Grain often interlocked, giving a ribbon figure on the radial surface. **3** ADD averages about 630 kg/m³. **4** Easy to dry, with little degrade. Shrinkage about 2 per cent radial, 4 per cent tangential. **5** Easy to work if tools kept sharp. Cutting angle may need reduction when dressing interlocked grain. Glues satisfactorily. Peels well. **6** Lyctids S; termites NR; durability IG4; AG3, M4. **7** Probably S5, SD6. Some mechanical properties are listed on page 420. **8** Plywood, furniture, joinery, boat building. **9** Considerable quantities are imported.

Mahogany, Philippine, red, light *Shorea, Pentacme* and
Parashorea spp., principally
Parashorea malaanonan (Blanco) Merr.
Parashorea plicata Brandis
Shorea almon Foxw.
Shorea squamata Dyer
Other common names: light red lauan, white lauan, almon, bagtikan, mayapis

1 The name embraces many large hardwoods of the Philippine rainforests, so its properties are quite variable. Just as the red merantis are divided into 'light red' and 'dark red', so are the Philippine mahoganies, whose wood is similar to that of the merantis. **2** Heartwood pale straw when first cut, turning to pale brown. Sapwood often not clearly differentiated in colour, to 50 mm wide. Texture coarse but even. Grain often interlocked, producing a stripe figure on the radial surface. Logs may contain brittleheart. Narrow concentric lines of resin ducts may be mistaken for growth rings. **3** ADD varies considerably, averaging about 530 kg/m³. **4** Dries quickly with little degrade in most species. Shrinkage variable, from about 2.5 per cent to 4.5 per cent radial, 5 per cent to 6.5 per cent tangential. **5** Relatively easy to work. Interlocked grain will need careful dressing. Unsuitable for steam bending. Nails and glues satisfactorily. **6** Lyctids S; termites NR; durability IG4; AG3, M4. **7** S6 and SD7. Some mechanical properties are listed on page 420. **8** Plywood, internal mouldings, joinery, furniture. **9** Large quantities are imported.

Mahogany, red *Eucalyptus resinifera* Sm.
Eucalyptus pellita F. Muell.

1 A large hardwood of the east coast from Sydney to Atherton in north Queensland. **2** Heartwood dark red. Sapwood distinctively paler. Texture medium and even. Grain slightly interlocked. The pin holes made by the ambrosia borer in the green timber are a common feature. **3** GD about 1150 kg/m³; ADD about 950 kg/m³. **4** Dries with little degrade if carefully stacked. Negligible collapse. Shrinkage about 4 per cent radial, 6 per cent tangential. **5** Relatively easy to work. Needs care in gluing. One of the best eucalypts for painting since the wood has good resistance to surface checking. May be 'ebonised' to a rich black colour by treatment with ferric chloride solution. **6** Lyctid S; termites R, durability IG2, AG1, M2. **7** S2, SD3. Some mechanical properties are listed on page 420. **8** Flooring, cladding, panelling, general construction, sleepers, poles. **9** Only limited quantities.

Mahogany, rose *Dysoxylum fraseranum* (A. Juss.) Benth.
Other common name: rosewood

1 A large hardwood of the east coast rainforests between the Hawkesbury River and north Queensland. **2** Heartwood reddish brown. Sapwood much paler. Relatively fine and uniform texture. Grain often interlocked. The soft tissue gives a slight figure to the tangential surface. Distinctive pleasant odour. **3** GD about 1120 kg/m³; ADD about 720 kg/m³. **4** Slow to dry, with some risk of surface checking. Only slight collapse. Shrinkage about 2.5 per cent radial, 4.5 per cent tangential. **5** Easy to work but it can be rather brittle and break away on sharp arrises. Predrilling of nail holes near ends may be necessary. The wood of many trees is liable to contain a sticky aromatic gum, which bleeds through the surface and interferes with the application of finishes. Kiln drying can help to drive off some of the gum before use. Provided the amount present is not abundant, sponging of the surface with methylated spirits half an hour before the application of the finish or adhesive should meet the problem. The sanding dust can be irritating to mucous membranes. Unsuitable for steam bending. **6** Lyctids S; termites R; durability IG2. **7** S5, SD5. Some mechanical properties are listed on page 420. **8** Furniture, panelling, joinery, turnery, carving, window frames and sills, decorative veneer. **9** Limited.

Mahogany, southern *Eucalyptus botryoides* Sm.
Other common name: bangalay

1 A large hardwood of the east coast from Bairnsdale in Victoria to Port Stephens in New South Wales. **2** Heartwood reddish brown (rather like Sydney blue gum). Sapwood distinctively paler. Texture medium and even. Grain interlocked. **3** GD about 1180 kg/m^3; ADD about 920 kg/m^3. **4** Slow in drying; susceptible to end splitting. Some collapse. Shrinkage about 5 per cent radial, 10 per cent tangential; after reconditioning about 4 per cent radial, 7 per cent tangential. **6** Lyctids NS; termites R; durability IG3, AG2. **7** S2, SD3. Some mechanical properties are listed on page 421. **8** General structural purposes, flooring. **9** Relatively common on south coast of New South Wales.

Mahogany, spur *Dysoxylum pettigrewianum* F. M. Bail.

1 A medium-to-large hardwood of the north Queensland rainforests. **2** Heartwood red-brown. Sapwood white. Texture moderately fine and even. Grain variable. Pleasant odour when freshly cut. **3** ADD about 870 kg/m^3. **5** Easy to work but may be difficult to glue. **6** Lyctids S; durability IG4. **7** Provisionally S3, SD4. **8** Flooring, panelling. **9** Limited to districts of occurrence.

Mahogany, swamp *Eucalyptus robusta* Sm.
Other common name: swamp messmate

1 A medium-sized hardwood of swampy coastal areas from Jervis Bay in New South Wales to central Queensland. **2** Heartwood red. Sapwood usually distinctively paler. Texture moderately coarse and even. Grain sometimes interlocked, producing an attractive striped figure on the quarter-cut surface. **3** ADD about 850 kg/m^3. **4** Very prone to collapse in drying. Shrinkage about 7 per cent radial, 9 per cent tangential. **6** Lyctids S; termites R; durability IG2. **7** Provisionally S3, SD4. **8** Because of drying degrade it is not favoured for general building purposes but could be satisfactory for fencing. **9** Not a commercial species.

Mahogany, white *Eucalyptus acmenoides* Schau.
Eucalyptus tenuipes
Eucalyptus umbra subsp. Cornea
Other common name: In Queensland it is sometimes called
'yellow stringybark' but this should not be encouraged because of the inevitable confusion with the true yellow stringybark, *Eucalyptus muellerana*.

1 A large hardwood of the east coast between Sydney and the Atherton district of north Queensland. **2** Heartwood yellow-brown, having a close resemblance to tallowwood. Sapwood narrow (less than 20 mm) and usually sufficiently paler to be distinguishable. Texture medium and even. Grain usually interlocked. Large holes caused by the larva of the *Zeuzera* wood moth are sometimes present and are a distinguishing feature. Mature logs occasionally contain 'water rings', tangential lines of detached wood, but gum veins are not common. The wood is very similar to that of tallowwood but it is distinguished by the occasional gum vein and the undulating pattern of grub markings. It is of a less greasy nature. **3** GD about 1200 kg/m³; ADD about 1000 kg/m³. **4** Slow to dry but little degrade or collapse. Shrinkage about 3.5 per cent radial, 6 per cent tangential. **6** Lyctids NS; termites R; durability IG1, AG1, M2. **7** S2, SD3. Some mechanical properties are listed on page 421. **8** Heavy engineering construction, poles, sleepers, shipbuilding. Not a good fuel. **9** An important commercial species in New South Wales and Queensland.

Makoré *Tieghemella heckelii* Pierre
Synonym: *Mimusops heckelii* Hutch, et Dalz.

1 A large hardwood of west Africa. **2** Heartwood pink to blood red or reddish brown, sometimes even with a slight purplish tinge. Sapwood usually distinctively paler. Texture fine to medium and even. Grain variable, sometimes giving a mottled figure to the radial surface. **3** ADD about 650 kg/m³. **4** Slow to dry but little degrade. Shrinkage about 2.5 per cent radial, 3 per cent tangential. **5** Because of the presence of silica, cutters and saws need frequent resharpening when working this timber. Predrilling may be needed when nailing near ends. Sanding dust likely to be irritating to the nose and throat. Glues satisfactorily. Not very suitable for steam bending. Wet timber in contact with iron will develop a blackish stain. **6** Lyctids S; termites R, durability IG2. **7** S5, SD6. Some mechanical properties are listed on page 421. **8** Decorative veneer, furniture, joinery, turnery. **9** Occasionally seen in the form of veneer.

Malakauayan *Podocarpus philippinensis* Foxw.

1 A medium-sized softwood of Luzon and Mindoro in the Philippines. **2** Heartwood pale yellow-brown overlaid with a grey-brown fleck. There may be bands of wood with a slightly orange tint. Said to be of finer texture than *Agathis alba* and also denser. **6** Lyctids NS. **8** Carving, household utensils, high-quality joinery. **9** Supplies have been offered to the local market.

Another Philippine podocarp is igem, *Podocarpus imbricatus* R. Br. or *Podocarpus javanicus* (Burm. f.) Merr. Its properties are, in general, similar to those of malakauayan. Small quantities are sometimes imported.

Malas *Homalium foetidum* (Roxb.) Benth.

1 A large hardwood native to Malaysia, Indonesia, the Philippines and Papua New Guinea. **2** Heartwood orange-brown to red-brown. Sapwood not readily distinguishable. Texture moderately fine and even. Grain variable. Characteristic iodine-like odour when freshly cut. **3** ADD about 800 kg/m³. **4** Some risk of checking during drying. Shrinkage about 2.5 per cent radial, 5 per cent tangential.   **5** Relatively easy to work. Glues satisfactorily. May need predrilling for nails.   **6** Lyctids NS; termites NR; durability IG3, M4; heartwood not difficult to impregnate with preservatives.   **7** S2, SD2. Some mechanical properties are listed on page 421.   **8** Heavy engineering construction, shipbuilding, flooring, poles, handles, joinery, turnery.   **9** Small quantities occasionally imported.

Mallee *Eucalyptus* spp.

1 The name 'mallee' is applied to those eucalypts that usually put forth a number of stems from the one bulbous root stock. They seldom grow to a large size, the height of the mature tree seldom exceeding 10 m. They are most frequently seen on poor sandy soils in inland areas where they perform a valuable role in checking soil erosion. Seventeen species of mallee are listed in Australian Standard AS/NZS 1148 *Timber—Nomenclature—Australian, New Zealand and Imported Species*.   **7** Seldom used in construction because of the small size of stem but the strength grouping would be about SD4, SD5.   **8** The main use for the wood is for fuel: mallee roots are especially favoured for the lounge room fireplace in those districts where it is available.

The blue mallee (*Eucalyptus fructicetorum* F. Muell. ex Miq.) of western New South Wales and Victoria has leaves that yield an oil with a high cineole content. Green mallee (*Eucalyptus viridis* R. T. Bak.) is also used as a source of eucalyptus oil.

Mallet, brown *Eucalyptus astringens* Maiden

1 There are a number of 'mallets' in Western Australia but brown mallet is the most important. It is a small-to-medium hardwood of the 300–400 mm rainfall belt of south-west Western Australia and its main value is in its bark, which is a valuable source of tannins for leather production and which can also be used for controlling the viscosity of the mud used when drilling for oil. The bark contains 40–57 per cent tannins and varies in thickness from 6 mm on young trees to 13 mm on mature stems.   **2** Heartwood pale red-brown to dark grey-brown with red streaks. Sapwood, to 30 mm wide, distinctly paler. Texture fine and even. Grain often interlocked.   **3** GD about 1120 kg/m³; ADD about 980 kg/m³.   **4** Easy to dry. Shrinkage about 4.5 per cent radial, 7 per cent tangential.   **5** Rather hard to work but dresses well. Satisfactory for steam bending.   **6** Lyctids NS; termites R; durability IG2, AG1.   **7** S1, SD2. Some mechanical properties are listed on page 421.   **8** General construction, handles, fuel.   **9** Limited to districts of occurrence.

Mangrove

Mangroves are a common feature of tidal shores in the warmer ocean waters and adjacent rivers. A brief description of the most common Australian species follows. All the mangroves are suitable for fuel. They are not available in normal commerce.

Black mangrove *Bruguiera gymnorhiza* (L.) Lam.

1 Grows in the saline water of tidal bays and rivers.   **2** Heartwood red. Texture fine.   **3** ADD about 960 kg/m³.   **4** Tends to check considerably in drying. Shrinkage about 2.5 per cent radial, 5.5 per cent tangential.   **5** Not difficult to work.   **6** Lyctids NS; durability IG3.   **7** Provisionally S3, SD3.   **8** Favoured for the smoking of fish. The bark is rich in tannins.

Grey mangrove *Avicennia marina* (Forssk.) Vierh. var. *australasica* (Walp.) Moldenke

1 It is common on estuarine mudflats.   **2** Heartwood grey-brown to very dark brown. Texture coarse. Grain interlocked.   **3** GD about 1150 kg/m³; ADD about 850 kg/m³.   **4** Slight collapse during drying. Shrinkage about 3.5 per cent radial, 4 per cent tangential.   **6** Lyctids NS; termites NR; durability IG4, M4.   **7** Provisionally S4, SD5. Some mechanical properties are listed on page 421.   **8** Often used for boat knees, posts, fuel.

Red mangrove *Rhizophora mucronata* (Lam.) Merr.

1 A seashore mangrove more common in tropical waters   **2** Heartwood bright pink to red.   **3** ADD about 980 kg/m³.   **4** Shrinkage about 2 per cent radial, 6 per cent tangential.   **6** Lyctids NS.   **7** Provisionally S3, SD4. Some mechanical properties are listed on page 421.   **8** Bark rich in tannins.

River mangrove *Aegiceras corniculatum* (L.) Blco.
  Synonym: *Aegiceras majus* Gaertn.

1 It is common on the tidal river flats from Sydney to Cape York and across to southern Asia.   **2** Heartwood white.   **3** ADD about 650 kg/m³.   **8** Used in oyster bed construction.

Maple, Queensland *Flindersia brayleyana* F. Muell.

1 A large rainforest hardwood of north Queensland. *Flindersia pimenteliana* F. Muell. (maple silkwood) is very similar. It also grows in Papua New Guinea.   **2** Heartwood pinkish brown to mid brown. Texture medium and even. Grain often interlocked, producing a wide variety of stripe and fiddleback figure.   **3** ADD about 580 kg/m³, although *F. pimenteliana* may be slightly denser (640 kg/m³).   **4** Easy to dry. Only very slight collapse. Shrinkage about 3 per cent radial, 7 per cent tangential.   **5** Easy to work but the presence of interlocked grain may require a reduction in planer angle. Nails and glues well. Buckles too readily to be suitable for steam bending. Fuming with ammonia produces a grey colour.   **6** Lyctids NS; termites NR; durability IG4, M4.   **7** SD6 and provisionally S6. Some mechanical properties are listed on page 421.   **8** An outstanding furniture wood, decorative veneer, rifle stocks, panelling, joinery.   **9** Limited supplies available in metropolitan centres.

Maple, rose *Cryptocarya erythroxylon* Maiden et Betche
Cryptocarya rigida Meissn.
Synonym: *Cryptocarya patentinervis* F. Muell. ex Benth.
Other common name: pigeonberry ash

1 A large hardwood of the coastal rainforests between the Hastings River in New South Wales and the Atherton district of north Queensland. **2** Heartwood pinkish brown. Sapwood usually distinctly paler. Texture medium and even. Grain sometimes slightly interlocked. The freshly cut surface has a distinctive odour somewhat akin to crushed celery. Occasionally subject to a gummy exudate. **3** GD about 980 kg/m³; ADD about 720 kg/m³. **4** Needs care in drying to prevent surface checking. Stack covers needed to prevent staining during drying. Negligible collapse. Shrinkage about 3.5 per cent radial, 7 per cent tangential. **5** Firm but easy to work. Satisfactory for steam bending. **6** Lyctids S; termites NR; durability IG4, M4. **7** S4, SD4. Some mechanical properties are listed on page 421. **8** Plywood, furniture, joinery, flooring. **9** Mainly as plywood.

Maple, scented *Flindersia laevicarpa* C. T. White et W. D. Francis

1 A medium-to-large hardwood of the north Queensland rainforests. **2** Heartwood pale pinkish brown. Has high sheen. Texture moderately fine and even. Grain straight. **3** ADD about 720 kg/m³. **4** Easy to dry. Negligible collapse. Shrinkage about 3 per cent radial, 6 per cent tangential. **5** Easy to work. Glues well. **6** Lyctids NS; termites NR; durability IG3, M4. **7** Provisionally S5, SD5. **8** Furniture, joinery, decorative veneer. **9** Scarce.

Maple, sugar *Acer saccharum* Marsh.
Other common name: rock maple (which is a more commonly accepted name for the wood)

1 A medium-to-large hardwood of eastern North America. Its sweet sap is the source of maple syrup. **2** Heartwood pale brown to pale red-brown. Sapwood creamy, but not always clearly differentiated from the heartwood, and up to 130 mm wide. Texture fine and even. Grain usually straight but wavy grain is sometimes present. Fine brown lines of tissue marking the extremities of the growth rings give a distinctive figure to the tangential surface. 'Bird's eye' figure is commonly associated with the rotary cut veneer and arises from localised sudden dips in the growth rings and the associated distortion of the fibres. **3** ADD about 730 kg/m³. **4** Slow to dry but little degrade. Shrinkage about 3 per cent radial, 6 per cent tangential. **5** Not easy to work so tool edges are soon blunted. Glues satisfactorily. Needs care in nailing. Takes finishes well. Good for turning and steam bending. Outstanding resistance to abrasion. **6** Lyctids S; durability IG4, M4. **7** S4, SD4. Some mechanical properties are listed on page 421. **8** Flooring (especially for bowling alleys, squash courts and ballrooms), shoe lasts, textile bobbins, musical instruments (e.g. piano actions), handles, laminated golf club heads, decorative veneer, furniture. **9** Seldom imported.

Mararie *Pseudoweinmannia lachnocarpa* (F. Muell.) Engl.
Synonym: *Geissois lachnocarpa* (F. Muell.) Maiden

1 A medium-sized hardwood of occasional occurrence in the coastal rainforests between Coffs Harbour in New South Wales and Atherton in north Queensland. **2** Heartwood rose-pink to mauve-brown. Sapwood distinctively paler. Texture fine and even. Grain straight. **3** GD about 1040 kg/m³; ADD about 840 kg/m³. **4** Care needed in drying to avoid end splits and surface checks. Collapse slight. Shrinkage about 3.5 per cent radial, 6 per cent tangential. **5** Easy to work. **6** Lyctids S; durability IG4. **7** S3 and provisionally SD3. Some mechanical properties are listed on page 421. **8** Bearings, mallets, chisel handles, carving, turnery, joinery. **9** Scarce.

Marfim, Pau *Balfourodendron riedelianum* Engl.

1 A medium-sized hardwood of Brazil, Paraguay and Argentina. **2** Heartwood white to pale yellow. Sapwood similar. Texture relatively fine and uniform. Grain generally straight. **3** ADD about 850 kg/m³. **4** Needs care in drying. Subject to bluestain. Shrinkage about 5 per cent radial, 10 per cent tangential. **5** Not hard to work. Finishes to a very smooth surface. Glues well but inclined to split in nailing. Sanding dust may irritate skin and mucous surfaces. **6** Durability IG4. **7** Provisionally S4, SD4. Some mechanical properties are listed on page 421. **8** Furniture, turnery, handles. **9** Small quantities occasionally imported.

Marri *Eucalyptus calophylla* R. Br. ex Lindl.

1 A large hardwood occurring in the jarrah and karri forests of south-west Western Australia. Valuable in honey production. **2** Heartwood pale brown. Sapwood to 40 mm wide, usually sufficiently paler to be distinguishable. Texture rather coarse but even. Grain slightly interlocked. Gum veins common. Logs usually sound right to the centre. **3** ADD about 850 kg/m³. **4** Shrinkage about 3.5 per cent radial, 6.5 per cent tangential. **5** Relatively easy to work. Nails satisfactorily. Good base for finishes. Satisfactory for steam bending. **6** Lyctids S; termites NR; durability IG3, AG3, M4. **7** S3, SD3. Some mechanical properties are listed on page 421. **8** General construction, handles, oars, sporting equipment. Preservative-treated material useful for piles, poles, posts. **9** Limited to Western Australia.

Matai *Podocarpus spicatus* R. Br.

1 A medium-sized softwood widely distributed throughout New Zealand, the main stands being in the central area of the north island. **2** Heartwood straw-yellow to orange-brown. Sapwood narrow and white. Texture very fine and even. Grain straight. Growth rings visible but not prominent. Some resin may be present. **3** GD about 1100 kg/m³; ADD about 610 kg/m³. **4** Easy to dry. Shrinkage about 2 per cent radial, 3.5 per cent tangential. **5** Easy to work. Peels well for veneer. May need predrilling for nails. Moderately suitable for steam bending. Glues satisfactorily. **6** Lyctids NS; termites R;

durability IG2; heartwood moderately resistant to impregnation with preservatives.   **7** S5, SD7. Some mechanical properties are listed on page 421.   **8** Furniture, internal and external joinery, sills, cladding, flooring, turnery.   **9** Seldom imported.

Medang tabak *Dactylocladus stenostachys* Oliv.
Other common name: jongkong

1 A large hardwood of Sabah, Sarawak and Indonesia.   **2** Heartwood yellow-brown, turning red-brown on exposure. Sapwood not clearly marked as its pale colour merges gradually into that of the heartwood. Texture moderately fine and even. Grain usually straight. Logs may contain brittleheart.   **3** ADD about 530 kg/m^3.   **4** Easy to dry but care needed to avoid bluestain. Shrinkage about 2 per cent radial, 4 per cent tangential.   **5** Easy to work, giving a very smooth finish. Unsuitable for steam bending.   **6** Lyctids NS; termites NR; durability IG4; heartwood easy to impregnate with preservatives.   **7** SD5 and provisionally S5.   **8** Joinery, utility furniture, plywood.   **9** Small quantities occasionally imported.

Meranti, red, dark *Shorea* spp.

1 The term 'meranti' is applied to a large number of species of *Shorea*, which is a dominant hardwood genus in Malaysia, Indonesia, the Philippines and Thailand. The term 'seraya' is common in Sabah, and 'lauan' in the Philippines, for very similar *Shorea* timber. A large number of South-East Asian species are likely to be included under dark red meranti or under alternative names, such as dark red seraya, dark red lauan or oba suluk.   **2** Heartwood reddish brown. Sapwood often wide, to 50 mm, and usually distinctively paler; it may have a grey tinge. Texture coarse but even. Grain usually interlocked, producing a stripe figure on the radial surface. Logs are less likely to contain brittleheart and pin-hole borer damage than those of light red meranti.   **3** ADD usually in the range 640–720 kg/m^3.   **4** Slower to dry than light red meranti. Shrinkage about 2 per cent radial, 4 per cent tangential.   **5** Relatively easy to work although some species may contain a little silica. Tools need to be kept sharp to avoid producing a 'woolly' surface. Nails and glues well. Unsuitable for steam bending.   **6** Lyctids S; termites NR; durability IG4, AG3, M4.   **7** S5, SD6. Some mechanical properties are listed on page 421.   **8** Plywood, joinery, furniture, panelling.   **9** Large quantities are imported.

Meranti, red, light *Shorea* spp.

1 Separation into light red meranti and dark red meranti is based more on wood density than on heartwood colour. Light red meranti trees grow to a large size.   **2** Heartwood is pale to mid red-brown. Sapwood yellow, pink or grey and usually easily distinguishable. Texture coarse but even. Grain interlocked, usually giving a ribbon or stripe figure to the radial surface. Brittleheart and pin-hole borer damage are common in the logs.   **3** ADD 400–640 kg/m^3.   **4** Easy to dry but precautions should be taken against bluestain. Shrinkage about 2 per cent radial, 4.5 per cent tangential.   **5** Relatively easy to work but may give a rather 'woolly' cut, so sharp tools are necessary. Glues satisfactorily. Unsuitable for steam bending.   **6** Lyctids S; termites NR; durability IG4, AG4, M4.   **7** S6, SD7. Some mechanical properties are listed on page 422.   **8** Plywood, internal mouldings and joinery, panelling.   **9** Large quantities are imported.

Meranti, white *Shorea* spp.

Numerous species of *Shorea* in South-East Asia are sold under this name.

1 In this instance the white seraya of Sabah is a quite different type of wood to white meranti and is virtually equivalent to light red Philippine mahogany.   **2** Heartwood white when freshly cut, darkening to a pale yellow-brown. Sapwood white, not distinct from the heartwood, and up to 60 mm wide. Texture moderately coarse, finer than the red meranti and white seraya. The grain is only shallowly interlocked, so there is no pronounced figure. The logs are generally very free of defects with only a slight amount of brittleheart and pin-hole borer damage. Because of the presence of a considerable amount of silica, the logs are difficult to saw and are usually peeled for veneer.   **3** ADD about 550 kg/m³.   **4** Shrinkage about 1.5 per cent radial, 2.5 per cent tangential.   **5** Very difficult to work because of the high silica content, so better reserved for plywood production where most of the cutting is carried out in the green condition.   **6** Lyctids S; termites NR; durability IG4, M4; heartwood can be impregnated with preservatives.   **7** S4, SD5. Some mechanical properties are listed on page 422.   **8** Plywood.   **9** Limited amounts are imported as plywood.

Meranti, yellow *Shorea* spp.

Other common name: yellow seraya

1 A large hardwood of Indonesia, Sarawak and the Philippines.   **2** Heartwood pale yellow to yellow-brown, sometimes with a greenish tinge. Sapwood usually distinctively paler. Texture moderately coarse but even. Grain slightly interlocked. The logs are likely to contain some brittleheart and pin-hole borer damage.   **3** ADD 550–650 kg/m³.   **4** Slower to dry than the other merantis but little degrade. Shrinkage about 1.5 per cent radial, 4 per cent tangential.   **5** Easy to work if tools are kept sharp to counteract the 'woolly' nature of the surface. Nails and glues satisfactorily. Dark stains may occur if wet wood is in contact with iron fixings.   **6** Lyctids S; termites R; durability IG4, M4.   **7** S5, SD6. Some mechanical properties are listed on page 422.   **8** Internal joinery, furniture.   **9** Small quantities are imported.

Merawan *Hopea* spp., including *Hopea papuana* Diels.

Other common name: light hopea

1 A medium-to-large hardwood of Papua New Guinea, Indonesia, Sarawak, Sabah and the Philippines.   **2** Heartwood yellowish brown to dark brown. Sapwood pale yellow but may not be distinctive from the heartwood. Texture moderately fine and even. Grain slightly interlocked. **3** ADD about 700 kg/m³. **4** Slow in drying. Needs precautions against checking and bluestain. Shrinkage about 2 per cent radial, 5.5 per cent tangential. **5** Relatively easy to work if tools are kept sharp. **6** Lyctids S; durability IG3. **7** S3, SD4. Some mechanical properties are listed on page 422. **8** General construction, boat building, sills, joinery, furniture. **9** Small quantities are imported.

Mersawa *Anisoptera* spp.
Other common name: palosapis

1 A large hardwood whose occurrence extends from South-East Asia across to the Philippines and Papua New Guinea. **2** Heartwood pale yellow or yellow-brown. Sapwood not clearly differentiated and up to 80 mm wide. Texture moderately coarse but even. Grain straight or only slightly interlocked. **3** GD about 1100 kg/m³; ADD about 680 kg/m³. **4** Slow in drying, with some risk of checking and formation of bluestain. Shrinkage about 2 per cent radial, 4 per cent tangential, although slightly higher figures have been quoted for Papua New Guinea material. **5** The presence of silica in the rays causes rapid blunting of cutting equipment but logs peel without difficulty. Not suitable for steam bending or turnery. Glues satisfactorily. Acidic finishes may give the wood a reddish hue. **6** Lyctids S; termites NR; durability IG4, AG3, M4. **7** Probably S6, SD6. **8** Plywood, flooring, general construction. **9** Small quantities are imported.

Messmate *Eucalyptus obliqua* L'Herit.
Other common name: messmate stringybark

1 A large hardwood of common occurrence in Tasmania and Victoria, and also in the tableland districts of New South Wales and southern Queensland. **2** Heartwood pale brown. Sapwood pale yellow, usually distinguishable from the heartwood. Texture moderately coarse but even. Grain sometimes interlocked. Growth rings visible but not prominent. Gum veins common. Heartwood may contain 2 per cent by weight of polyphenols, which are likely to stain alkaline surfaces brown. 'Pencil streak' stains sometimes present. **3** GD about 1080 kg/m³; ADD averages about 780 kg/m³. **4** Slow in drying and likely to check. Some collapse occurs. Shrinkage about 5 per cent radial, 11 per cent tangential; after reconditioning about 3.5 per cent radial, 6.5 per cent tangential. **5** Relatively easy to work. Glues well. Satisfactory for steam bending. Fuming with ammonia gives a grey colour to the surface. **6** Lyctids S; termites NR; durability IG3, AG3, M4. **7** S3, SD3. Some mechanical properties are listed on page 422. **8** General construction, furniture, flooring, panelling. **9** A common timber in districts of occurrence.

Messmate, Gympie *Eucalyptus cloeziana* F. Muell.

1 A large hardwood of scattered occurrence in coastal Queensland from Gympie to the Atherton district. **2** Heartwood yellow-brown.

Texture medium and even. Grain can be slightly interlocked. **3** ADD about 1000 kg/m³. **4** Easy to dry. Negligible collapse. Shrinkage about 3.5 per cent radial, 6 per cent tangential. **6** Lyctids NS; termites R; durability IG1, AG1. **7** S2, SD3. Some mechanical properties are listed on page 422. **8** General construction, sleepers, poles, bridges, etc. **9** Limited to districts of occurrence.

Morrell, red *Eucalyptus longicornis* F. Muell.

1 A medium-sized hardwood of the West Australian wheat-growing districts in the 250–300 mm rainfall zone. **2** Heartwood dark red to dark chocolate brown. Texture fine and even. Grain interlocked. **3** GD about 1170 kg/m³; ADD about 1020 kg/m³. **5** Rather difficult to work because of the interlocked grain. **6** Termites R; durability IG1. **7** S3 and provisionally SD3. **8** Fencing, timbering for mines, tool handles. Has a very attractive appearance. **9** Small quantities in districts of occurrence.

Mulga *Acacia aneura* F. Muell. ex Benth.

1 A small hardwood, often only of shrub size, which grows in the dry interior of Australia where annual rainfall is well below 250 mm per year. It acts as a soil binder and a source of subsistence fodder for stock when drought has destroyed normal pasture. Because of these important functions its use as a commercial timber should be discouraged. **2** There is a strong colour contrast between its golden yellow sapwood and the dark brown heartwood, so it has been a popular species for the production of wood articles for the tourist trade, often without proper drying of the timber, which leads to dissatisfaction for the purchaser. Texture fine and even. Grain usually straight. Heart shakes often present. **3** GD about 1200 kg/m³; ADD about 1100 kg/m³. **4** Needs slow drying to avoid splits and checks. If round logs are being dried for turnery the ends should be coated with varnish or paint to slow down moisture loss. Wood ornaments are often turned roughly to size in the green condition because it is much easier to work in that state and it will then dry more quickly. To avoid degrade it should receive a sealer coat before being set aside for some months to dry, after which it is finished to final shape. For larger sizes chemical seasoning methods may be worthwhile. **6** Lyctids NS; durability IG2. **7** Provisionally S1, SD1. **8** Turnery, fancy woodware. It was used by the Australian Aboriginals for boomerangs, spear shafts and ends, and for nulla-nullas. **9** Scarce.

Mutenye *Guibourtia arnoldiana* (De Wild, et Th. Dur.) J. Leonard

1 A medium-sized hardwood of the Congo region of west Africa. **2** Heartwood pale brown with frequent darker streaks, which sometimes have a reddish tinge. Sapwood dull grey with a yellow tinge and to 75 mm wide. Texture relatively fine and even. Grain straight. **3** ADD about 850 kg/m³. **4** Shrinkage about 2.5 per cent radial, 5 per cent tangential. **5** Not hard to work despite some silica present. Peels well if logs are preheated. May need predrilling for nails. Glues well as long as the occasional occurrences of gum are avoided.   **6** Lyctids S; durability IG3. Sapwood resistant to impregnation with preservatives. **7** Possibly S4, SD4.   **8** A substitute for walnut in furniture manufacture.   **9** Very small quantities sometimes imported.

Myall *Acacia pendula* A. Cunn. ex G. Don
Other common name: boree

1 A small hardwood of the rich alluvial soils on the inland plains of New South Wales and Queensland.   **2** Heartwood dark chocolate brown. Sapwood pale brown. Fine even texture. Grain interlocked. Pleasant violet-like odour when freshly cut.   **3** GD about 1280 kg/m³; ADD about 1100 kg/m³.   **4** Shrinkage low, about 3.5 per cent tangential.   **5** Very hard but it turns well.   **6** Lyctids NS; termites NR; IG2.   **7** Provisionally S1, SD2. Some mechanical properties are listed on page 422.   **8** It makes excellent fancy turnery but it is too valuable as a source of stock shelter and fodder to be cut for commercial timber.   **9** Not a commercial timber.

Myall, coast *Acacia glaucescens* Willd.

1 Of scattered occurrence on the coast and coastal ranges of New South Wales.   **3** ADD about 990 kg/m³.   **9** Not a commercial timber.

Nyatoh mainly *Palaquium* and *Payena* spp., but other genera of the Sapotaceae family are sometimes included

1 A large hardwood of South-East Asia and the Philippines.   **2** Heartwood pink to red-brown. Sapwood usually paler but not always readily distinguishable, up to 100 mm wide. Texture medium and even. Grain may be shallowly interlocked. The freshly cut surface may have a sour odour.   **3** Because of the range of possible species, ADD may vary considerably but it is generally within the range 600–700 kg/m³. **4** Care needed in drying to avoid end splits. Shrinkage about 2.5 per cent radial, 4 per cent tangential.   **5** Generally easy to work although gummy material can build up on the saw teeth. Susceptible to burn marks during sanding and turning. Some species contain silica. Nails well. Peels easily. Sanding dust can be irritating to mucous membranes. **6** Lyctids NS; durability IG4, M4.   **7** S4, SD4.   **8** Plywood, furniture, interior joinery.   **9** Limited quantities are imported.

Oak, bull *Casuarina luehmannii* R. T. Bak.

1 A small hardwood of the inland plains of New South Wales and Queensland, often growing in association with white cypress. Small quantities also occur in Victoria and South Australia.   **2** Heartwood dark red. Sapwood usually narrow and distinctively paler. Texture medium. Grain straight. Rays very prominent. Heart shakes likely.   **3** ADD about 1050 kg/m³.   **5** Very hard; Janka hardness exceeds 22 kN. **6** Lyctids NS; termites R; durability IG1; AG1.   **7** Provisionally S2, SD2.   **8** Because of its great resistance to indentation it makes excellent flooring. Suitable for roofing shingles and shakes, fancy turnery and wood ware, fencing, fuel.   **9** Seldom available commercially.

Oak, Caledonian *Carnarvonia araliifolia* F. Muell.

1 A medium-to-large hardwood of the north Queensland rain-forests. **2** Heartwood a rich brown colour. Sapwood much paler. Large ray figure. Texture moderately fine and even. Grain straight. **3** ADD about 690 kg/m³. **4** Easy to dry. **5** Easy to work. May need extra care in gluing. **6** Lyctids S; durability IG4, AG2. **7** Provisionally S4, SD5. **8** Decorative woodware, furniture, veneer. **9** Usually limited to districts of occurrence.

Oak, European *Quercus* spp. mainly
Quercus petraea Liebl.
Quercus robur L.

1 A medium-sized hardwood of wide occurrence in Great Britain and central and western Europe. **2** Heartwood pale yellow-brown, darkening with exposure. Sapwood, to 50 mm wide, creamy and usually distinctive. Texture coarse and rather uneven. Grain usually straight. The large ray figure of the radial surface is often referred to as 'silver grain'. The slower grown wood with narrow annual rings is comparatively soft and is the more suitable for furniture manufacture and veneer. **3** ADD about 700 kg/m³. **4** Drying is slow and uneven; forcing the rate can cause considerable degrade. Shrinkage varies considerably but averages about 3 per cent radial, 6 per cent tangential. **5** Relatively easy to work. Glues well. Very good for steam bending. Has corrosive effect on lead and iron. It is advisable to use only non-ferrous metal in contact with the wood to avoid the formation of black iron tannate stains if the wood becomes damp. Gives a dark grey colour when fumed with ammonia. **6** Lyctids S; durability IG2. **7** S5, SD5. Some mechanical properties are listed on page 422. **8** Furniture, decorative veneer, cooperage, flooring, carving, joinery, vats. **9** Seldom imported, except for special orders.

Oak, Japanese *Quercus* spp., principally
Quercus mongolica Fish. var. *grosseserrata* Rehd. et Wils.
Other common name: Pacific oak

1 A slow-growing deciduous hardwood of Japan. **2** Heartwood usually yellowish brown and paler than both the European oak and the American white oak, and softer. Texture moderately coarse. Grain usually straight. Characteristic oak rays. **3** ADD about 650 kg/m³. **4** Dries more rapidly, and with less risk of degrade, than the *Quercus* species described elsewhere. **5** Easy to work. Glues well. Logs peel easily. Corrodes lead and iron and it is advisable to use only non-ferrous metal in contact with the wood to avoid the formation of black iron tannate stains if the wood becomes damp. Good for steam bending. **6** Lyctids S; durability IG3. It has shown susceptibility to *Anobium* borer attack. **7** SD5 and provisionally S5. It is slightly weaker than European oak. **8** Furniture, decorative veneer, panelling, joinery. **9** Seldom imported.

Oak, New Guinea *Castanopsis acuminatissima* (Bl.) Rehd. and numerous *Lithocarpus* spp.

1 A hardwood mainly from the highland districts of Papua New Guinea. **2** Heartwood brown. Sapwood distinctly paler. Has the character of *Quercus* spp. but with a less aggressive ray figure. Texture relatively fine but uneven. Grain straight. **3** ADD variable because of the variety of species but in the 600–700 kg/m³ range. **4** Shrinkage about 3.5 per cent radial, 7 per cent tangential. **5** Reasonably easy to work. **6** Lyctids S; durability IG3. **7** S5 and provisionally SD5. Some mechanical properties are listed on page 422. **8** Plywood, decorative veneer, furniture, joinery, flooring, panelling, handles. **9** Small quantities occasionally imported.

Oak, silky, brown *Darlingia darlingiana* (F. Muell.) L. Johnson
Synonym: *Darlingia spectatissima* F. Muell.

1 A medium-to-large hardwood of the north Queensland rainforests. **2** Heartwood pale pinkish brown. Sapwood not always distinctively paler. Relatively fine texture. Straight grain. Typical silky oak ray figure. **3** ADD about 770 kg/m³. **4** Shrinkage about 2.5 per cent radial, 8 per cent tangential. **6** Lyctids S; durability IG4. **7** Provisionally S4, SD4. **8** Joinery, furniture, plywood. **9** Usually limited to districts of occurrence.

Oak, silky, crater *Musgravea stenostachya* F. Muell.

1 A medium-sized hardwood of the north Queensland rainforests. **2** Heartwood has rich reddish brown colour. Conspicuous ray figure. Texture medium. Grain straight. **3** ADD about 670 kg/m³. **4** Easy to season. **5** Easy to work. Peels well. Can be used for steam bending. **6** Lyctids S; durability IG4. **7** Provisionally S5, SD6. **8** Furniture, joinery, decorative veneer. **9** Usually limited to districts of occurrence.

Oak, silky, fishtail *Neorites kevediana* L. S. Sm.

1 A hardwood of the north Queensland rainforests. **2** Heartwood brown. Sapwood distinctively paler. Typical silky oak ray figure. Medium and even texture. Straight grain. **3** ADD about 970 kg/m³. **6** Durability IG4. **7** Provisionally S4, SD4. **8** Joinery, flooring. **9** Limited to districts of occurrence.

Oak, silky, mountain *Orites excelsa* R. Br.
Other common name: prickly ash

1 A medium-sized hardwood of the rainforests of the coastal ranges from the Hunter River in New South Wales to southern Queensland. **2** Heartwood pinkish brown. Sapwood whitish. Texture rather coarse but even. Grain straight. Rays not large but numerous and prominent. **3** GD about 990 kg/m³; ADD about 600 kg/m³. **4** Needs care in drying to prevent checking of the tangential surface. Collapse is negligible. Shrinkage about 2 per cent radial, 6.5 per cent tangential. 5 Easy to work. Good for steam bending. Nails and glues well. 6 Lyctids NS; durability IG4. 7 S5, SD5. 8 Plywood, furniture, joinery, cooperage. Unsuitable for handles because very fine splinters are inclined to break away from the rays. 9 Limited.

Oak, silky, northern *Cardwellia sublimis* F. Muell.

1 A large hardwood of the north Queensland rainforests. 2 Heartwood pinkish brown, darkening on exposure. Texture rather coarse. Grain straight. Rays prominent. 3 ADD about 550 kg/m^3. 4 Back-cut boards dry much faster than those quarter cut so sorting of material before drying is advisable. Shrinkage about 1.5 per cent radial, 4.5 per cent tangential. Negligible collapse. 5 Relatively easy to work. If bleaching is carried out the ammonia and hydrogen peroxide method is satisfactory on silky oaks but reddish streaks may persist. These can be substantially removed by a final application of 10 per cent oxalic acid solution. The extractives include gummy carbohydrates, which can affect the strength of adhesive bonds. 6 Lyctids S; termites NR; durability IG4, M4. 7 S6, SD7. 8 Furniture, plywood, joinery. 9 The most readily available of the silky oaks.

Oak, silky, red *Stenocarpus salignus* R. Br.
Other common name: beef wood

1 A medium-sized hardwood of occasional occurrence in the coastal rainforests between the Illawarra area of New South Wales and southern Queensland. 2 Heartwood dark red. Sapwood much paler. Texture moderately coarse. Grain straight. Prominent rays. 3 GD about 1110 kg/m^3; ADD about 830 kg/m^3. 4 Care needed against surface checking during drying. Some collapse occurs. Shrinkage about 3 per cent radial, 7.5 per cent tangential; after reconditioning about 2 per cent radial, 4.5 per cent tangential. 5 Not difficult to work. The sanding dust can be irritating to mucous membranes so good ventilation of the workplace is important. 6 Lyctids S, durability IG4. 7 S3, SD3. Some mechanical properties are listed on page 422. 8 Decorative turnery and woodware, plywood, joinery. 9 Limited.

Oak, silky, southern *Grevillea robusta* A. Cunn. ex R. Br.

1 A medium-sized hardwood of the coastal rainforests between the Clarence River in New South Wales and the Maryborough district of Queensland. Has been planted extensively as a garden and street tree in many parts of Australia, even in relatively dry inland towns. It is not a suitable species for plantation silviculture because it is especially productive of phytotoxins, which inhibit growth of its own kind (the phenomenon known as 'allelopathy'). 2 Heartwood pinkish brown with prominent rays of darker colour. Sapwood paler but not always clearly distinguishable. Texture medium. Grain straight. 3 GD about 1100 kg/m^3; ADD about 620 kg/m^3. 4 Shrinkage about 2 per cent radial, 5 per cent tangential. 6 Lyctids S; durability IG4. 7 Provisionally S6, SD5. Some mechanical properties are listed on page 422. 8 Plywood, furniture, joinery. 9 Scarce.

Oak, silky, spotted *Buckinghamia celsissima* F. Muell.

1 A medium-sized hardwood of the north Queensland rainforests. **2** Heartwood pale brown. Sapwood white. Texture relatively fine and even. Grain straight. Prominent ray figure. **3** ADD about 930 kg/m³. **4** Needs care in drying. **5** Firm to work. **6** Durability IG4. **7** SD3 and provisionally S3. **8** Decorative woodware, feature flooring. **9** Only in districts of occurrence.

Oak, tulip, blush *Argyrodendron actinophyllum* (F. M. Bail.) H. L. Edlin subsp. *Actinophyllum*
Synonyms: *Heritiera actinophylla* (F. M. Bail.) Kosterm.
Tarrietia actinophylla F. M. Bail.
Other common name: booyong

1 A large hardwood of the rainforests between Gloucester in New South Wales and Gympie in Queensland. **2** Heartwood pale brown. Sapwood not readily distinguishable and can be very wide. The rays are a prominent feature, Texture coarse but even. Grain usually straight. **3** GD about 1050 kg/m³; ADD about 810 kg/m³. **4** Careful drying needed to minimise staining, end splitting and checking of the tangential surface; it should be carried out with full protection from the weather. The use of eucalypt stickers in stacks exposed to rain can cause staining of the tulip oak at each bearing, so it is important either to cover the stacks against rain penetration or use stickers of tulip oak. Large logs may contain a central core of dark brown wood (often referred to as 'black heart'), which is of very attractive appearance but very difficult to dry free of checking. Collapse is slight and reconditioning might only accentuate the surface checking. Shrinkage about 4.5 per cent radial, 8.5 per cent tangential. **6** Lyctids S, termites NR; durability IG4, M4. The impregnation of sapwood with aqueous preservatives needs careful control to ensure even penetration. **7** Provisionally S3, SD3. Some mechanical properties are listed on page 422. **8** Plywood, flooring, panelling, furniture, handles, bent work, drop-hammer boards. **9** Mainly in districts of occurrence.

Oak, tulip, brown *Argyrodendron trifoliolatum* F. Muell.
Synonyms: *Heritiera trifoliolata* (F. Muell.) Kosterm.
Tarrietia argyrodendron Benth.
Other common name: white booyong

1 A large hardwood of the rainforests between the Manning River in New South Wales and the Cairns district of north Queensland. **2** Heartwood brown. Sapwood not readily distinguishable and often very wide. The core of the log may contain 'black heart' similar to that referred to in the description of blush tulip oak. Texture coarse and even. Grain sometimes slightly interlocked. In general appearance it is virtually identical to blush tulip oak. **3** GD about 1050 kg/m³; ADD about 850 kg/m³. **4** Careful drying under cover is needed to minimise staining, checking and splitting. Collapse negligible. Shrinkage about 3 per cent radial, 6.5 per cent tangential. **5** Not easy to work. Some predrilling desirable when nailing near extremities. Suitable for steam bending. **6** Lyctids S; termites NR; durability IG4, M4. Sapwood needs careful control to achieve even penetration of aqueous preservatives. **7** S2, SD2. Some mechanical properties are listed on page 422. **8** Plywood, flooring, panelling, furniture, handles, general construction. **9** Mainly in districts of occurrence.

Oak, tulip, red *Argyrodendron peralatum* (F. M. Bail.) H. L. Edlin ex I. H. Boas
Synonyms: *Heritiera peralata* (F. M. Bail.) Kosterm.
Tarrietia argyrodendron Benth. var. *peralata* F. M. Bail.

1 A large hardwood of the north Queensland rainforests. **2** Heartwood pink to red-brown. Sapwood whitish but there is often a band of intermediate wood, perhaps 200 mm wide, which may be considered almost equivalent to sapwood in borer susceptibility. Texture coarse but even. Grain usually straight. Attractive 'water wave' figure on tangential face and ray fleck on radial face, as with the other tulip oaks. **3** ADD about 800 kg/m³. **4** Needs careful drying under cover to avoid staining and surface checking. Shrinkage about 4.5 per cent radial, 9 per cent tangential. **5** Not easy to work. Peels well. Glues satisfactorily. Good for steam bending. **6** Lyctids S; termites NR; durability IG4, M4. **7** S3, SD4. Some mechanical properties are listed on page 422. **8** Plywood, furniture, panelling, flooring, internal joinery, handles. **9** Mainly in districts of occurrence.

Oak, white, American *Quercus* spp.

1 A common medium-sized hardwood of central North America. **2** Heartwood pale yellow-brown to mid-brown, sometimes with a pink tinge. Sapwood almost white, but not always clearly differentiated. Texture coarse. Grain usually straight. Large rays. **3** ADD about 750 kg/m³. **4** Slow to dry and tends to check and split along the rays. Shrinkage about 3 per cent radial, 5 per cent tangential. **5** Relatively easy to work to a smooth finish. Glues satisfactorily. Very good for steam bending. Tends to corrode iron and lead; it is advisable to use only non-ferrous metal in contact with the wood to avoid the formation of black iron tannate stains if the wood becomes damp. **6** Lyctids S; termites NR; durability IG4, M4. **7** Provisionally S6, SD6. Some mechanical properties are listed on page 422. **8** Furniture, flooring, carving. Because of the impermeability of the heartwood it is highly esteemed for vats and casks for the maturing of wine and spirits. **9** Only imported for special orders.

Obeche *Triplochiton scleroxylon* K. Schum.

1 A large west African hardwood. **2** Heartwood white to pale yellow. Sapwood similar and up to 150 mm wide. Texture medium and even. Grain slightly interlocked, producing some stripe figure on the radial surface. **3** ADD about 370 kg/m³. **4** Dries quickly but bluestain can be troublesome. Shrinkage about 2 per cent radial, 3 per cent tangential. **5** Easy to work. Glues satisfactorily. Too soft to be a good nail holder. Just fair for steam bending. The sanding dust can irritate mucous membranes. **6** Lyctids S; durability IG4. **7** Weak, not a structural timber. Some mechanical properties are listed on page 422. **8** Plywood, internal joinery, furniture. **9** Seldom imported.

Osage-Orange *Madura pomifera* Schneid.

1 A small North American hardwood said to have been used by the Indians for bows and clubs. Small quantities have been grown in Australia by archery enthusiasts. **2** Heartwood orange-brown. Sapwood pale yellow. Texture relatively fine and even. Grain variable. The pronounced growth rings produce an attractive figure. **3** ADD about 950 kg/m³. **5** Difficult to glue. Dresses to a very smooth surface. Very pliable. **6** Lyctids S; durability IG2. **7** Provisionally SD3. Some mechanical properties are listed on page 423. **8** Archery bows, walking sticks, decorative woodware. **9** Not commercially available.

Padauk, African *Pterocarpus soyauxii* Taub.

1 A medium-sized hardwood of west Africa. **2** Heartwood dark red. Sapwood pale brown or grey and varying considerably in width from narrow to 200 mm. Texture rather coarse because of the large pores. Grain straight or slightly interlocked. Slight odour when freshly cut. **3** ADD variable, 650–800 kg/m³. **4** Slow in drying but shows little degrade. Shrinkage about 3 per cent radial, 4 per cent tangential. **5** Relatively easy to work. The sanding dust can be irritating to mucous surfaces. Nails satisfactorily. **6** Lyctids S; durability IG2; heartwood moderately resistant to impregnation with preservatives. Sapwood has moderate resistance to impregnation. **7** Possibly S4, SD3. **8** Furniture, turnery, tool handles, knife handles, flooring, carving. **9** Rarely imported.

Padauk, Burma *Pterocarpus macrocarpus* Kurz.
Other common name: pradoo (in Thailand)

1 A medium-sized hardwood of Burma and Thailand. **2** Heartwood pinkish brown to rich orange-brown. Sapwood greyish. Texture medium and even. Grain often interlocked, producing a ribbon figure on the radial surface. **3** ADD about 850 kg/m³. **4** Slow in drying, with a tendency to form face checks. Shrinkage about 2 per cent radial, 4 per cent tangential. **5** Hard to work when dried but it machines well if care is taken when dressing the radial surface. Turns well. Glues satisfactorily. **6** Lyctids S; durability IG2. **7** Possibly S2, SD3. **8** Tool handles, flooring, furniture. **9** Rarely imported.

Palaquium *Palaquium* spp.
Other common name: sacau (in Fiji)

1 There is another group of *Palaquium* species in Fiji with the common name 'bauvudi'. Rainforest hardwoods of wide distribution from Thailand, Indonesia, the Philippines, Papua New Guinea, the Solomon Islands and Fiji. Not to be confused with the nyatoh of South-East

Asia, which also embraces *Palaquium* species. **2** Heartwood pinkish brown to reddish brown. Sapwood pale pink, to 50 mm wide. Texture moderately fine and even. Grain sometimes interlocked, producing a ribbon figure on the radial surface. **3** ADD variable because of the range of species involved, from about 450–900 kg/m³, averaging about 550 kg/m³. Sacau is at the top end of the range, bauvudi about the average. **4** Dries quickly with little degrade. Shrinkage about 1.5 per cent radial, 4 per cent tangential for lower density species, to about 5 per cent radial, 6.5 per cent tangential for higher density material. **5** Silica may be present to make some species hard on tool edges but the wood is usually easy to work. Glues well. May need extra care in nailing. **6** Lyctids S; durability IG4. **7** Strength varies very considerably, ranging from S3, SD2 for heavy material (e.g. sacau) to S6, SD7 for low-density wood (e.g. bauvudi). **8** Plywood, interior joinery, turnery, carving. The higher density species are more suitable for general structural purposes. **9** Seldom imported.

Pear *Pyrus communis* L.

1 A small hardwood, the wild pear of Europe and northern Asia. **2** Heartwood pale pinkish brown. Sapwood very similar. Texture very fine and even. Grain variable. **3** ADD about 700 kg/m³. **4** Needs to be dried slowly and carefully to avoid twisting. Shrinkage about 4 per cent radial, 7 per cent tangential. **5** Easy to work. Gives a very smooth finish. Turns well and is much favoured for carving. **6** Lyctids NS; durability IG4. **7** Possibly S5, SD5. **8** Drawing instruments, carving, wood engraving, printing blocks, tool handles, turnery, picture frames, musical instruments (e.g. recorders), shafts of billiard cues, furniture and decorative veneer. Favoured in the manufacture of glassware for lights, being used to provide special shapes; the wood blocks are used in the wet condition and the requirement is fine grain and ability to hold a lot of water. **9** Not available commercially in Australia.

Penda, brown *Xanthostemon chrysanthus* (F. Muell.) F. Muell. ex Benth.

1 A large hardwood of the north Queensland rainforests. Red penda (*Xanthostemon whitei* Gugerli) has similar properties but is of redder colour. **2** Heartwood pale to dark brown. Texture relatively fine and even. Grain interlocked. **3** ADD about 1030 kg/m³. **4** Careful drying needed to prevent twisting and checking. Shrinkage about 4 per cent radial, 6 per cent tangential. **5** Hard to work. **6** Lyctids NS; termites NR; durability IG2, AG1, M2. **7** Provisionally S2, SD2. **8** Building framework, flooring. **9** Mainly in districts of occurrence.

Peppermint, broad-leaved *Eucalyptus dives* Schau.

1 A medium-sized hardwood of eastern and southern Victoria, and southern New South Wales. The leaves are rich in piperitone-type eucalyptus oil but most of the world's supply now comes from plantations in South Africa. The oil has important industrial uses. **2** Heartwood pale pinkish brown. Sapwood paler but not sharply differentiated. Texture medium and even. Grain often interlocked. Gum veins common. **3** GD about 1100 kg/m³; ADD about 820 kg/m³. **4** Difficult to dry without internal checks. Considerable collapse. Shrinkage about 6 per cent radial, 11 per cent tangential; after reconditioning about 3 per cent radial, 5 per cent tangential. **5** Not hard to work. **6** Lyctids S; termites NR; durability IG3, AG2, M4. **7** S3, SD4. Some mechanical properties are listed on page 423. **8** Because of shrinkage problems it is generally used only for lower quality building framework. **9** Not a commercial species.

River peppermint (*Eucalyptus elata* Dehnh.; synonym: *Eucalyptus andreana* Naud.) is a relatively common species on the south coast of New South Wales with somewhat similar properties but it is less troublesome in drying. Its strength grouping is provisionally S4, SD4.

Peppermint, narrow-leaved *Eucalyptus australiana* R. T. Bak. et H. G. Sm.
Eucalyptus radiata Sieb. ex DC.
Eucalyptus phellandra R. T. Bak. et H. G. Sm.

1 This is probably the best group of the peppermints, which are not held in high regard as timber producers because of heavy gum veining, high shrinkage and often severe collapse. The leaves, especially of *Eucalyptus radiata*, are rich in eucalyptus oil of phellandrene type, used in soap-making, perfumery and disinfectants. Medium-to-large hardwoods of the mountain country of eastern Victoria and southern New South Wales. **2** Heartwood pale pinkish brown. Sapwood slightly paler but not sharply differentiated. Texture medium and even. Grain sometimes interlocked. Gum veins common. **3** GD about 1100 kg/m³; ADD about 800 kg/m³. **4** Difficult to dry without incurring degrade. Considerable collapse. Shrinkage about 6 per cent radial, 12 per cent tangential; after reconditioning about 4 per cent radial, 7 per cent tangential. **5** Not hard to work. **6** Lyctids S; termites NR; durability IG3, AG3, M4. **7** S4, SD4. Some mechanical properties are listed on page 423. **8** General construction purposes. **9** Seldom offered commercially.

Pepperwood *Cinnamomum laubatii* F. Muell.

1 A medium-sized hardwood of the Queensland rainforests between Mackay and Atherton. **2** Heartwood straw to golden brown, sometimes with darker stripes. Sapwood may not be sharply differentiated. Texture relatively fine and even. Grain usually straight. **3** ADD about 480 kg/m³. **4** Easy to dry. Negligible collapse. Shrinkage about 2 per cent radial, 5 per cent tangential. **5** Soft and easy to work. Glues well. **6** Lyctids S; durability IG4. **7** Provisionally S7, SD8. **8** Plywood, joinery. **9** Mainly in districts of occurrence.

Pernambuco wood *Guilandina echinata* (Lam) Spreng.
Synonym: *Caesalpinia echinata* Lam

1 A large hardwood of coastal Brazil. **2** Heartwood orange-red, darkening on exposure. The sapwood is narrow and of much paler colour. Texture fine and even. Grain usually straight. **3** ADD variable, averaging about 1100 kg/m^3. **4** Liable to check in drying. Shrinkage probably large, at least 4 per cent radial, 8 per cent tangential. **5** Very hard but not difficult to work and gives a very smooth finish. Suitable for turnery and carving. The sanding dust is reputed to be irritating, so good ventilation of the workshop is required. **6** Lyctids S; termites R; durability IG1. **7** Probably S1. **8** This is the species usually demanded for violin and cello bows but it is now scarce and expensive. **9** Only seen in Australia in musical instruments. Species such as grey ironbark and turpentine would be worthy of a trial as a substitute.

Persimmon *Diospyros virginiana* L.

1 A small-to-medium hardwood of south-eastern United States. **2** Heartwood pale to dark brown. Sapwood cream to yellowish brown but not always clearly differentiated. Texture moderately fine and uniform. Grain straight. **3** ADD about 830 kg/m^3. **4** Needs much care in drying to prevent checking. Shrinkage about 4.5 per cent radial, 6.5 per cent tangential. **5** Rather difficult to work and needs special techniques for gluing. **6** Lyctids S. **7** S5, SD4. **8** Has high shock resistance and is the traditional species for golf club heads. Also used for shoe lasts, textile machinery, woodworking plane stocks, handles. **9** Small amounts sometimes imported by sporting equipment manufacturers.

The Japanese timber kaki (*Diospyros kaki* L. f.) is very similar to the American persimmon but the heartwood is almost black, with streaks of orange, yellow or pink. Air-dry density about 770 kg/m^3. Used for the same purposes.

Pine, black *Prumnopitys amara* (El.) de Laub.
Synonym: *Podocarpus amarus* Bl.

6 Lyctids NS; durability IG4.

Pine, brown *Podocarpus elatus* R. Br. ex Endl.

1 Black and brown pine have very similar timber and are medium-sized softwoods, now rare in the forests but often planted as ornamental trees in eastern Australia. Black pine is native to the rainforests of north Queensland, Papua New Guinea and Indonesia, while brown pine used to be seen in the rainforests between the Illawarra region of New South Wales and the Cairns district of north Queensland. Very little brown pine now remains in NSW forests. **2** Heartwood golden brown. Sapwood narrow and distinctively paler. Texture very fine and even. Grain straight. Growth rings inconspicuous. **3** ADD about 600 kg/m^3 for brown pine and 500 kg/m^3 for black pine. **4** Easy to dry.

Shrinkage about 1.5 per cent radial, 3.5 per cent tangential.   **5** Easy to work. Turns and glues well.   **6** Lyctids NS; durability M3; heartwood is relatively easily impregnated with preservatives.   **7** S6, SD7. Some mechanical properties of black pine from Papua New Guinea are listed on page 423.   **8** Furniture, plywood, turnery, carving, kitchen utensils, musical instruments (e.g. piano keys, violin bellies).   **9** Scarce.

Pine, bunya *Araucaria bidwillii* Hook.

1 A large softwood whose natural occurrence is limited to the Gympie and Yarraman districts of southern Queensland.   **2** Heartwood pale brown. Sapwood not clearly distinguishable. The wood is almost identical to that of hoop pine but is slightly pinker and of lower density. Texture very fine and even. Grain straight.   **3** GD about 720 kg/m³; ADD about 460 kg/m³.   **4** Dries rapidly but precautions against bluestain are necessary. Shrinkage about 2 per cent radial, 4 per cent tangential.   **5** Easy to work. Glues well.   **6** Lyctids NS; termites NR; durability IG4, AG4, M4; heartwood is relatively easy to impregnate with preservatives.   **7** S6, SD5. Some mechanical properties are listed on page 423.   **8** Plywood, joinery, furniture.   **9** Only in southern Queensland.

Pine, Caribbean *Pinus caribaea* Mor. var. *bahamensis* (Griseb.) B. et G.
Pinus caribaea Mor. var. *caribaea*
Pinus caribaea Mor. var. *hondurensis* (Seneclauze) B. et G.

1 A medium-sized softwood native to Central America, Cuba and the Bahamas but the timber seen in Australia is from local plantations in Queensland and northern New South Wales. Trial plantings have done well on Melville Island in the Northern Territory near Darwin.   **2** Heartwood yellow to golden brown. Sapwood usually distinctively paler. Texture rather coarse and uneven. Grain usually straight. Growth rings prominent. High resin content.   **3** GD about 990 kg/m³; ADD about 500 kg/m³.   **4** Easy to dry but precautions against bluestain are necessary. Shrinkage about 2 per cent radial, 4 per cent tangential.   **5** The presence of resin can be a nuisance during the sawing of the log because it builds up on saws and other equipment. Nails and glues satisfactorily. Barely suitable for steam bending. Poor resistance to heavy impact loads.   **6** Lyctids NS; termites R; durability IG4, AG4, M4.   **7** Provisionally S6, SD6. Some mechanical properties are listed on page 423.   **8** General construction, flooring.   **9** Mainly in Queensland and northern New South Wales.

Another Caribbean pine, or Caribbean pitch pine, closely related to *Pinus caribaea*, is *Pinus oocarpa* Schiede, which is native to Central America. It is hard, heavy and strong for a pine, the density of mature wood even reaching 700 kg/m³, but that of fast-growth plantation wood would be considerably less. The resin content is high, which improves its durability, but does make it more suitable for structural rather than decorative uses. Little information is available on its mechanical and physical properties but it is being tried out in many tropical countries as a possible plantation species.

Pine, celery-top *Phyllocladus asplenifolius* (Labill.) Hook. f.
Synonym: *Phyllocladus rhomboidalis* L.C. et A. Rich.

1 A medium-size softwood of high rainfall areas in Tasmania.
2 Heartwood pale yellow to pale brown. Sapwood narrow and not
clearly distinguishable. Texture fine and even. Grain usually straight.
Growth rings conspicuous and very close together. No taste or
odour. **3** GD about 1050 kg/m³; ADD about 650 kg/m³. **4** Dries
without much degrade. Shrinkage about 1.5 per cent radial, 3.5 per cent
tangential. **5** Because of the frequent presence of compression wood
it may not be easy to work. Excellent for steam bending. **6** Lyctids
NS; termites R; durability IG3, AG2. **7** S4, SD5. Some mechanical
properties are listed on page 423. **8** Vats (especially for acid storage),
boat building, garden furniture, joinery, kitchen utensils, turnery,
carving. **9** Scarce.

Pine, Corsican *Pinus nigra* Arnold var. *maritima* (Ait.) Poir.
Synonym: *Pinus laricio* Poir.

1 Native to southern Europe; because of its hardiness under severe
weather conditions it has been used as a plantation species for
problem sites in Australia and New Zealand, but only on a small
scale. **2** Heartwood pinkish brown. Sapwood distinctively paler.
Texture medium and even. Grain usually straight. Growth rings
prominent. The wood is similar in general behaviour to radiata pine
but usually has smaller and more closely spaced knots and is free of
cone holes. **3** GD about 990 kg/m³; ADD about 550 kg/m³. **4** Dries
rather slowly. Very prone to bluestain. Shrinkage about 3 per cent radial,
5.5 per cent tangential. **5** Easy to work. **6** Lyctids NS; durability
IG4, AG4, M4; heartwood only moderately resistant to impregnation
with preservatives. **7** Provisionally S7, SD6. Some mechanical
properties are listed on page 423. **8** General construction, flooring
panelling, poles. **9** Seldom offered commercially.

Pine, hoop *Araucaria cunninghamii* Ait. ex D. Don

1 A large softwood native to the rainforests of northern New South
Wales and Queensland, and also occurring in the mountain regions
of Papua New Guinea. **2** Heartwood pale yellow-brown. Sapwood,
to 150 mm wide, almost white. Texture very fine and even. Grain
straight. Compression wood often occurs, generally indicated by bands
of darker coloured wood. Growth rings inconspicuous. **3** GD about
680 kg/m³; ADD about 530 kg/m³. **4** Easy to dry but care needed
to avoid bluestain. Shrinkage about 2.5 per cent radial, 3.5 per cent
tangential. Plantation thinnings are inclined to twist due to spiral
grain; for best results it may be desirable to use a high temperature
drying technique under restraint after plasticisation by a presteaming
treatment. **5** Easy to work. Knots do not machine as easily as those of
Pinus species. Unsuitable for steam bending. Glues well. **6** Lyctids NS;
termites NR; durability IG4, AG4, M4; heartwood variable in resistance
to impregnation with preservatives. In tropical and semitropical areas
the hoop pine borer (*Calymmaderus* spp.) may attack it; complete

enclosure by other materials or coating with paint or varnish will give protection. **7** S6, SD5. Some mechanical properties are listed on page 423. **8** Plywood, particleboard, furniture, match splints and boxes (makes the best box), battery separators, joinery, flooring, panelling. **9** Mainly in Queensland.

The Norfolk Island pine, *Araucaria heterophylla* (Salisb.) Franco, produces wood of similar appearance although it may not be quite as strong. It is used as a general purpose timber in Norfolk Island. Its strength grouping is provisionally S6, SD6.

Pine, Huon *Dacrydium franklinii* Hook. f.

1 A medium-sized softwood of the high rainfall areas of south-western Tasmania. **2** Heartwood pale straw, becoming yellow after long exposure. Sapwood very narrow and hard to distinguish. Texture very fine and even. Grain straight. Growth rings closely spaced. A characteristic odour, due to the essential oil methyl eugenol, present when wood freshly cut; distillation gives a yield of about 3 per cent of oil. Rather greasy to the touch. Material with a 'birds-eye' figure sometimes obtainable. **3** GD about 960 kg/m^3; ADD about 520 kg/m^3. **4** Easy to dry without degrade. Shrinkage about 2.5 per cent radial, 3 per cent tangential. **5** Easy to work. Turns, nails and finishes well. Gluing with resorcinol and epoxies sometimes presents difficulties. Good for steam bending. **6** Lyctids NS; termites R; durability IG3, AG3, M4. **7** S6, SD6. **8** Boat building, turnery, carving, pattern-making, kitchen utensils, outdoor furniture. The oil extracted from the wood has been used as a lens-grinding fluid; it has a repellent effect against mosquitoes but unfortunately the odour is nauseating to some people. **9** Scarce.

Pine, King William *Athrotaxis selaginoides* D. Don

1 A medium-to-large softwood of the high rainfall areas of western Tasmania. **2** Heartwood pink to pale reddish brown, which fades on exposure. Sapwood narrow and not readily distinguishable. Texture fine but uneven due to the harder latewood. Grain straight. Growth rings prominent due to the considerably darker latewood. Compression wood common. **3** GD about 620 kg/m^3; ADD about 400 kg/m^3. **4** Shrinkage about 1.5 per cent radial, 4 per cent tangential. **5** When free of compression wood it is easy to work and steam bend. Resin exudation sometimes occurs and it may interfere with its acceptance for musical instruments. Glues satisfactorily. **6** Lyctids NS; termites R; durability IG2, AG2, M4. **7** S7, SD8. Some mechanical properties are listed on page 423. **8** Boat building, vats, external joinery and furniture, sounding boards for pianos and violins. **9** Scarce.

Pine, klinki *Araucaria hunsteinii* K. Schum.
Synonym: *Araucaria klinkii* Lauterb.

1 A large softwood of the highlands of Papua New Guinea. **2** Heartwood straw to pale brown. Sapwood not readily distinguishable. Texture very fine and even. Grain straight. The wood is virtually identical to that of hoop pine but the density is slightly lower. One way of identifying it from hoop pine is to apply a few drops of concentrated hydrochloric acid: it gives an intense green colour.   **3** ADD about 450 kg/m³.   **4** Easy to dry but precautions against bluestain are essential. Shrinkage 2.5 per cent radial, 4 per cent tangential.   **5** Easy to work.   **6** Lyctids NS; termites NR; durability IG4, M4; heartwood relatively easy to impregnate with preservatives.   **7** S6, SD6. Some mechanical properties are listed on page 423.   **8** Plywood, battery separators, ice-cream spoons, furniture, joinery.   **9** Usually seen only as plywood in Australia.

Pine, loblolly *Pinus taeda* L.

1 A fast-growing, medium-sized softwood native to the south-eastern states of the United States. It is being grown in plantations in Queensland and northern New South Wales and also in the north of the north island of New Zealand.   **2** Heartwood pale reddish brown. Sapwood yellowish white and wide. High resin content. Texture fine but uneven. Grain straight.   **3** GD about 970 kg/m³; ADD about 550 kg/m³ for the usual plantation logs but can be as high as 630 kg/m³ for mature trees.   **4** Easy to dry but needs protection against bluestain. Shrinkage about 3 per cent radial, 5 per cent tangential.   **5** Relatively easy to work but compression of the earlywood by the planer may lead to a slightly ridged surface. Nails tend to follow the growth rings.   **6** Lyctids NS; termites NR; durability IG4, AG4, M4; heartwood of plantation material difficult to impregnate with preservatives. Sapwood less permeable than that of radiata pine but it accepts a satisfactory loading of preservative for most purposes.   **7** S6, SD6. Some mechanical properties are listed on pages 423 and 424.   **8** General framing purposes, plywood, joinery.   **9** Mainly in Queensland and northern New South Wales.

Pine, longleaf *Pinus palustris* Mill.
Other common name: pitch pine

1 A common softwood of the south-eastern states of the United States but it is seldom planted in Australia.   **2** Heartwood pinkish brown to orange-brown. Sapwood pale yellow, about 50 mm wide in mature trees but much wider in young growth. Growth rings prominent. Texture medium but uneven. Grain straight. Denser and harder than most pines. High resin content.   **3** ADD about 660 kg/m³.   **4** Dries relatively slowly and needs careful handling to avoid splits and surface checks. Shrinkage about 2.5 per cent radial, 4 per cent tangential.   **5** Its working properties are similar to those of Douglas fir. Nails satisfactorily. Glues satisfactorily as long as resin content is not excessive. Not really suitable for steam bending.   **6** Lyctids NS; termites NR; durability IG4, AG4, M4; heartwood resistant to impregnation with preservatives.   **7** S5, SD5. Some mechanical properties are listed on page 424.   **8** Essentially a structural timber and one of the strongest softwoods.   **9** Rarely seen in Australia.

Pine, maritime *Pinus pinaster* Ait.
Synonym: *Pinus maritima* Poir.

1 A medium-sized softwood native to south-western Europe and north-western Africa but its major forestry development is on the Atlantic coast of southern France, Spain and Portugal. It is able to reach commercial size on poor sandy coastal soils and for this reason considerable areas have been planted in Western Australia on land too low in nutrients to support radiata pine. It is not a favoured species for plantation development when reasonable soils are available. **2** Heartwood pale reddish brown. Sapwood pale yellow. Texture rather coarse and uneven. Grain straight. Resinous. **3** ADD about 600 kg/m³. **4** Shrinkage about 3 per cent radial, 5 per cent tangential. **5** Relatively easy to work but knots and resin pockets are common. **6** Lyctids NS; termites R; durability IG4, AG4, M4. **7** Provisionally S6 and SD6. Some mechanical properties are listed on page 424. **8** General construction. If preservative-treated it can be used for posts, poles and mining timber. **9** Only in Western Australia.

Pine, Parana *Araucaria angustifolia* (Bert.) O. Ktze.

1 A large softwood of south-eastern Brazil and adjacent areas of Paraguay and Argentina. **2** Heartwood yellow to brown with some orange streaks. Sapwood pale yellow. Texture fine and uniform. Grain straight. It is one of the very few woods that is not acidic; at times it can give an alkaline reaction. Pin knots are sometimes common. **3** ADD about 550 kg/m³. **4** Careful drying is needed because of the considerable amount of growth stresses often present. Precautions are needed against bluestain. Darker coloured wood dries slowly and is more prone to splitting. Shrinkage about 4 per cent radial, 7 per cent tangential. **5** It is usually easy to work but some material is full of stresses and will distort severely while being sawn or machined. Glues and finishes well. Care needed in nailing. **6** Lyctids NS; durability IG4; heartwood moderately resistant to impregnation with preservatives. **7** S5, SD6. Some material is rather brittle so its use as a beam should probably be avoided. Some mechanical properties are listed on page 424. **8** Internal joinery, turnery, plywood. **9** Only occasionally imported.

Pine, patula *Pinus patula* Schlecht. et Cham.

1 A medium-sized softwood, native to Mexico; it has been tried as a plantation species in many countries in the south temperate zone. Only small areas have been planted in Australia. **2** Heartwood pale brown. Sapwood pale yellow-brown and wide. Texture medium and uneven. Grain straight. Growth rings prominent. Liable to contain many small, lens-shaped resin pockets. **3** GD about 830 kg/m³; ADD about 470 kg/m³. **4** Easy to dry but prone to bluestain. Shrinkage about 2 per cent radial, 4.5 per cent tangential. **5** Easy to work except for the frequent resin pockets. **6** Lyctids NS; durability IG4, AG4, M4. **7** Provisionally S7, SD7. **8** General construction. **9** Scarce.

Pine, radiata *Pinus radiata* D. Don
Other common name: Monterey pine

1 A large softwood native to a very limited area of the west coast of
North America but planted widely in the world's south temperate zone,
especially in South Africa, Chile, New Zealand and Australia, mainly
because of its ease of propagation, speed of growth, adaptability to a
relatively wide range of soils and relative freedom from disease. Its
vigorous early growth enables it to overcome competing weed growth.
It is a species for the cooler climates, being unsuitable for the subtropics
and the more humid coastal areas. Its rate of growth is four to ten
times that of the eucalypt hardwoods native to the cool tableland areas
where it is being grown in eastern Australia and it produces a wood
that is more acceptable to the construction industry. The bark is rich
in tannins that are suitable for use in the manufacture of adhesives;
it also contains some wax, which may have a possible use in water
repellents. 2 Heartwood pale yellow-brown. Sapwood wide and not
always clearly distinguishable visually. Texture fine but uneven. Grain
usually straight except for a central core of about 100 mm diameter,
which has a pronounced spirality; this spirality can cause considerable
twisting during drying if the stack is not adequately weighed down.
This potentially troublesome core is generally confined to the first
ten growth rings, where the wood has shorter fibres and abnormally
low density. The spirality increases in the first few years and then
gradually decreases until the grain is nearly parallel to the tree's axis
by the 15th ring. Growth rings prominent due to the darker colour of
the latewood. 3 GD about 800 kg/m³; ADD varies considerably with
the maturity of the tree, ranging from about 450 kg/m³ to 580 kg/m³
but averaging about 500 kg/m³. The first few rings of growth may have
a density as low as 350 kg/m³. Density increases by about 30 per cent
during the first 20 years, and reaches a relatively constant value in the
wood laid down after 25 years. 4 Easy to dry, except for the twist-
prone core. Very prone to bluestain during the warmer months. The
staining fungi can enter the log almost as soon as it is felled, so rapid
logging and processing are needed for a large part of the year. Because
of its rapid drying rate it is usually kiln dried directly from the green
condition. Presteaming for several hours before drying improves the
stability of the seasoned product. Material dried at a relatively high
temperature (e.g. 135°C) is more stable than that dried at 100°C but
long periods at an elevated temperature should be avoided because
of an adverse effect on strength. Wood of very high initial moisture
content is inclined to have a greater amount of reaction wood.
Shrinkage about 3 per cent radial, 4.5 per cent tangential. 5 Easy
to work except for the knots. Nails satisfactorily. Material high in
resin content (Plate 43) is difficult to glue. Clear material can be
painted satisfactorily but knots, resin streaks and the bands of dense
latewood are inclined to bleed sufficient resin to mar exterior coatings
if material high in resin content is so used (Plate 44); such material
should be reserved for structural purposes. Unsuitable for steam
bending because of the difficulty of obtaining an even curve. Prone
to surface checking when exposed uncoated to the weather or when

coated only with stain-type finishes, which are less protective against moisture penetration; on quarter-cut material the surface checking occurs mainly at rays and resin canals, while on back-cut boards the fissures are mainly in the vicinity of the junction between latewood and earlywood. Unlike the eucalypts, radiata pine does not cause appreciable staining of alkaline surfaces, such as concrete paths and fibre-cement cladding.   **6** Lyctids NS; termites NR; durability IG4, AG4, M4; heartwood resistant to impregnation with preservatives. The wide, readily impregnated sapwood enables a substantial cylinder of preservative-treated wood to be provided in round timber.   **7** S6, SD6. Some mechanical properties are listed on page 424. Following the publication of Ditchburne, Kloot and Rumball's paper (see below) in 1975, the strength grouping of radiata pine was raised. However, it should be kept in mind that the sampling on which this report was based was from trees more than 20 years old and not less than 250 mm breast height in diameter; material containing pith was largely ignored. If the trend of utilisation continues towards a much earlier use of plantation material for structural members, involving a greater proportion of low-density material, it would seem prudent to make further surveys or, alternatively, base the grading of the structural material on mechanical rather than visual methods, to ensure that it meets the assigned stress ratings.   **8** General construction, flooring, panelling, furniture, joinery, plywood, particleboard, fibreboard, paper. When preservative-treated it is used for cladding, decking, external trim, poles, piles, fencing and sleepers.   **9** Because of the large areas being planted in Australia and New Zealand, this species is destined to be the major general purpose timber in Australia.

Further reading

Australian National University (1970). *Pinus radiata*. Proceedings of symposium. August 1970. 2 vols. Canberra: ANU.

Beesley, J. and Rumball, B. L. (1977). Observations on the decay resistance of the impermeable heartwood of CCA-treated radiata pine. Technology paper 12. Melbourne: CSIRO Division of Building Research.

Boyd, J. D. (1964). The strength of Australian pole timbers; item 4, radiata pine poles. Technology paper 32. Melbourne: CSIRO Division of Forest Production.

Ditchburne, N., Kloot, N. H., Rumball, B. (1975). The mechanical properties of Australian-grown *Pinus radiata* D. Don. Technology paper 9. Melbourne: CSIRO Division of Building Research.

Pine, slash *Pinus elliottii* Engelm. var. *elliottii*
Pinus elliottii Engelm. var. *densa* Little et Dorman

1 A medium-sized softwood native to south-eastern United States, where it is one of the 'southern pine' group. It is an important plantation species in Queensland and, to a lesser extent, in New South Wales and New Zealand. The tree can vary widely in form and is not very suitable for windy sites. The wood often has a considerable density gradient.   **2** Heartwood pale reddish brown. Sapwood pale yellow and not clearly marked from the heartwood. Texture relatively coarse.

Grain straight. Growth rings prominent. Resin flow is very abundant.
3 GD about 1000 kg/m³; ADD varies considerably with maturity of
the tree, from about 450 to 630 kg/m³, averaging about 530 kg/m³.
4 Easy to dry but prone to bluestain. Shrinkage about 3 per cent radial,
5 per cent tangential. **5** Relatively easy to work but the high resin
content can cause a build up of rubbish on the processing equipment
when handling unseasoned timber. Nails tend to follow the growth
rings. As with radiata pine, material high in resin should be directed
to structural purposes because of its effect on finishes and adhesives.
6 Lyctids NS; termites R; durability IG4, AG4, M4; heartwood difficult
to impregnate with preservatives. The sapwood is slightly less permeable than that of radiata pine. **7** Provisionally S5, SD5. Some
mechanical properties are listed on page 424. Figures for mature US
material are given for comparison with young plantation material of
local origin. **8** General construction, flooring, panelling, plywood.
9 Mainly in Queensland and northern New South Wales.

Pine, sugar *Pinus lambertiana* Dougl.

1 A large softwood native to California and southern Oregon, on the
west coast of the United States. **2** Heartwood pale brown. Sapwood
creamy. Texture moderately coarse. Grain straight. A prominent
characteristic is the resin canals, which are prominent as dark brown
lines on the tangential surface. **3** ADD about 400 kg/m³. **4** Easy to
dry. Shrinkage about 2 per cent radial, 3.5 per cent tangential. **5** Easy
to work. Holds its shape well. Good base for paint. Nails and glues
well. **6** Lyctids NS; durability IG4. **7** Provisionally SD8 and below
S7. Not a structural timber. Some mechanical properties are listed
on page 424. **8** Pattern-making, joinery. **9** Very small quantities
are imported.

Pine, white, New Zealand *Dacrycarpus dacrydioides* A. Rich.
Other common name: kahikatea

1 A medium-sized softwood native to both islands of New Zealand
but now found mainly on the west coast of the south island. Timber
from lowland areas is mainly white sapwood but that from hilly
country may contain some yellow heartwood. **2** Texture very fine
and even. Grain straight. No taste or odour. **3** GD about 820 kg/m³;
ADD about 450 kg/m³. **4** Easy to dry but precautions against
bluestain are necessary. Shrinkage about 2.3 per cent radial, 4.5 per
cent tangential. **5** Easy to work, nail, turn. **6** Lyctids NS; durability
IG4, M4. Sapwood particularly susceptible to *Anobium* borer attack
and needs to be preservative-treated when used for structural and
decorative uses. **7** S7, SD7. Some mechanical properties are listed on
page 424. **8** Cladding, joinery, plywood, kitchen utensils. **9** Seldom
seen in Australia.

Pine, white, western *Pinus monticola* Dougl. ex D. Don

1 A medium-to-large softwood of western North America from
British Columbia to California. **2** Heartwood pale brown. Sapwood

creamy. Texture fine but uneven. Grain straight. Only slightly resinous. **3** ADD about 430 kg/m³. **4** Easy to dry but precautions are needed against bluestain. Shrinkage about 2.5 per cent radial, 4 per cent tangential. **5** Easy to work. Glues and nails well. Good base for paint. **6** Lyctids NS; durability IG4, M4. **7** Probably SD7. Weak in bending and shock resistance. Some mechanical properties of North American material are listed on page 424. **8** Joinery, pattern-making. **9** Seldom seen in Australia.

Pine, yellow, Siberian *Pinus cembra* L. var. *sibirica* (Du Tour) Loud.
Pinus koraiensis Sieb. et Zucc.
Other common name: Keddar

1 A softwood of the colder parts of northern Asia. **2** Heartwood yellowish brown to reddish brown. Sapwood much paler. Grain straight. Texture variable, dependent on rate of growth. Pleasant odour. **3** ADD about 420 kg/m³. **6** Lyctids NS. **8** General internal joinery use. **9** Occasional shipments are received from northern Europe.

Pine, yellow, western *Pinus ponderosa* Dougl.
The Australian standard name is now 'ponderosa pine'.

1 A large softwood of western North America, in British Columbia, Oregon, Washington and California. Small areas have been planted in Australia but it has not been very successful under local conditions. It tolerates a severe climate but it has slow initial growth and tends to have a very pronounced taper. **2** Heartwood yellow to reddish brown. Sapwood wide and pale yellow. Texture medium. Grain generally straight. The latewood is sharply defined. Resinous. **3** GD of young plantation wood about 960 kg/m³; ADD about 400 kg/m³. **4** Easy to dry but precautions against bluestain are necessary. Shrinkage about 2.5 per cent radial, 4.5 per cent tangential. **5** Easy to work. Nails and glues well. **6** Lyctids NS; durability IG4, AG4, M4. **7** Provisionally SD8. Some mechanical properties are listed on pages 424 and 425. **8** Pattern-making, joinery. **9** Limited.

Jeffrey pine (*Pinus jeffreyi* A. Murr.) grows in association with western yellow pine in its native habitat and has rather similar properties.

Pinkwood *Eucryphia moorei* F. Muell.

1 A medium-sized hardwood of occasional occurrence in the damp coastal gullies of the south coast of New South Wales. **2** Heartwood pale pinkish brown. Sapwood narrow and not readily distinguishable. Texture fine and even. Grain generally straight. The wood has a resemblance to coachwood. **3** ADD about 600 kg/m³. **6** Lyctids NS. **7** Provisionally S7, SD8. **8** Turnery, joinery. **9** Not a commercial timber.

Pittosporum *Pittosporum* spp., especially *Pittosporum undulatum* Vent.

1 A small hardwood common as understorey trees in the wetter areas of coastal New South Wales and Queensland but usually too small to be of commercial interest. **2** Heartwood cream to pale yellow. Sapwood similar. Texture very fine and even. Grain usually straight. **3** ADD about 850 kg/m³. **6** Lyctids probably NS. **7** Provisionally S4, SD4. **8** Artificial limbs, kitchen utensils, carving, turnery, marquetry. **9** Not a commercial timber.

Planchonella, red *Planchonella* spp., especially *Planchonella torricellensis* (K. Schum.) H. J. Lam

1 A rainforest hardwood of Papua New Guinea, the Solomon Islands and Fiji. **2** Heartwood pink to pinkish brown with some dark markings. Sapwood paler but not always clearly distinguishable. Texture moderately fine and even. Grain usually straight. **3** ADD about 590 kg/m³. **4** Dries quickly with little degrade. Shrinkage about 2 per cent radial, 5 per cent tangential. **5** Easy to work to a smooth finish. Glues and nails well. **6** Lyctids S; termites NR; durability IG4, M4; heartwood difficult to impregnate with preservatives. **7** S5, SD5. Some mechanical properties are listed on page 425. **8** Building framework, flooring, panelling, joinery, turnery. **9** Seldom seen in Australia.

Poplar *Populus* spp., especially varieties of *Populus euramericana* (Dode) Guinier
See also eastern cottonwood, page 268.

1 Poplars are hardwoods of wide distribution in the Northern Hemisphere. The development of very fast-growing hybrids largely based on *Populus euramericana* attracted the attention of tree growers and considerable areas were planted in Australia in the 1960s, but the unfortunate entry of *Melampsora* rust fungi in 1972, despite quarantine precautions, dampened the initial enthusiasm for poplar growing. The rust damages the leaves, which then fall off, causing a much slower rate of growth and often leading to the death of the leading shoot. Rust-resistant clones have been developed. **2** Heartwood pale brown. Sapwood white to cream and up to 80 mm wide in fast-growing stems (about three growth rings). Texture fine but sometimes slightly uneven because of the harder latewood. Grain straight. **3** GD about 740 kg/m³; ADD about 440 kg/m³ for young fast-grown wood to 540 kg/m³ for mature trees. **4** Dries quickly but prone to bluestain. Shrinkage about 2.5 per cent radial, 5.5 per cent tangential. **5** Its woolly nature makes it rather difficult to work unless tools are kept sharp. Glues and nails well. **6** Lyctids S; termites NR; durability IG4. **7** Provisionally S7, SD8. Some mechanical properties are listed on page 425. Further investigation of mechanical properties is needed. **8** Match splints, plywood, artificial limbs, brake blocks, wood wool. **9** Limited to districts of growth.

Poplar, pink *Euroschinus falcata* Hook. f. var. *falcata*

1 A medium-sized hardwood of occasional occurrence in the coastal rainforests between the Hastings River in New South Wales and north Queensland. **2** Heartwood pinkish grey with yellow streaks.

Sapwood white. Texture fine and even. Grain slightly interlocked. Distinctive silken sheen. **3** GD about 800 kg/m³; ADD about 450 kg/m³. **4** Dries quickly but is very susceptible to bluestain. Shrinkage about 2 per cent radial, 4 per cent tangential. **5** Difficult to dress smoothly because of its woolly nature. Glues well. **6** Lyctids S; termites NR; durability IG4, M4. **7** Provisionally S7, SD7. Not a structural timber. Some mechanical properties are listed on page 425. **8** Brake blocks, internal joinery, core stock. **9** Rare.

Possumwood *Quintinia sieberi* A. DC.

1 A small hardwood of the coastal ranges of New South Wales and southern Queensland. **2** Heartwood pale brown. No distinct sapwood. Very fine texture. Grain slightly interlocked. Some ray figure. **3** ADD about 530 kg/m³. **5** Easy to work. **7** Provisionally S6, SD6. **8** Turnery, carving. **9** Not a commercial timber.

Purpleheart *Peltogyne* spp.

1 A medium-sized hardwood of the northern part of South America. **2** Heartwood brown when freshly cut but rapidly changing to a purple colour. Sapwood grey. Texture medium and even. Grain variable. **3** ADD varies considerably with species but averages about 880 kg/m³. **4** Dries well with little degrade. Shrinkage about 2 per cent radial, 4 per cent tangential. **5** Not easy to work. Needs predrilling for nails. Fair for steam bending. **6** Lyctids S; durability IG2. **7** S2, SD3. Some mechanical properties are listed on page 425. **8** Decorative veneer, turnery, marquetry, flooring, storage of chemicals, billiard cue butts. **9** Not seen in Australia.

Pyinkado *Xylia xylocarpa* (Roxb.) Taub.
Synonym: *Xylia dojabriformis* Benth.

1 A large hardwood of South-East Asia. **2** Heartwood dull reddish brown. Sapwood pale brown and narrow. Texture moderately fine and even. Grain variable. Gummy exudations often present. **3** ADD about 950 kg/m³. **4** Dries slowly, with little degrade. Shrinkage about 3.5 per cent radial, 6 per cent tangential. **5** Usually worked green because of the difficulty of handling it when dry, when it rapidly blunts cutting edges. **6** Lyctids S; durability IG2. **7** Possibly S2, SD3. **8** Bridges, wharfage, marine piling, railway sleepers, flooring. **9** Not seen in Australia.

Quandong, brown *Elaeocarpus coorangooloo* J. F. Bail, et C. T. White
Elaeocarpus ruminatus F. Muell.
Other common name: caloon

1 A medium-sized hardwood of the Queensland rainforests between Mackay and Atherton. **2** Heartwood pale brown or yellow-brown sometimes with stripes of darker colour, more noticeable on the radial surface. Texture moderately fine and even. Grain often interlocked, producing a ribbon figure on the radial surface. **3** ADD about 610 kg/m³. **5** Easy to work. Glues well. **6** Durability

IG2. **7** Provisionally S6, SD7. **8** Decorative veneer, plywood, joinery, furniture. **9** Mainly in districts of occurrence.

Quandong, silver *Elaeocarpus grandis* F. Muell.
Other common names: blueberry ash, blue fig

1 A medium-sized hardwood of occasional occurrence in the coastal rainforests between the Nambucca River in New South Wales and north Queensland. **2** Heartwood white to cream. Sapwood similar and up to 100 mm wide. Texture moderately fine and even. Grain straight. **3** GD about 750 kg/m^3; ADD about 500 kg/m^3. **4** Rather slow to dry and prone to bluestain but little other degrade. Shrinkage about 1.5 per cent radial, 4.5 per cent tangential. **5** Very easy to work. Nails and glues well. Good for steam bending. **6** Lyctids S; termites NR; durability IG4, M4; heartwood relatively easy to impregnate with preservatives. **7** S5, SD6. Some mechanical properties are listed on page 425. **8** Decorative veneer, plywood, joinery, furniture, oars, boat building. **9** Mainly in districts of occurrence.

Raintree *Samanea saman* (Jacq.) Merr.
Synonyms: *Pithecellobium saman* (Jacq.) Benth.
Enterolobium saman Prain
Other common name: monkey pod wood

1 A medium-sized hardwood native to central America and the north of South America but planted widely in many tropical countries, especially as a fast-growing shelter tree in coffee and cocoa plantations. **2** The wood from young trees is pale brown, mainly sapwood, and easy to work but that from mature trees may be dark chocolate brown heartwood, which can be difficult to work. Texture very coarse. Grain interlocked. **3** ADD about 560 kg/m^3. **6** Lyctids S. **7** S7, SD8. Not a structural timber. **8** Very commonly used for fancy woodware for the tourist souvenir trade in tropical countries. **9** Seen only in finished articles.

Ramin *Gonystylus* spp., especially *Gonystylus bancanus* (Miq.) Baill.
Other common names: melawis, mavota

1 A medium-sized hardwood of the coastal swamp forests from South-East Asia across to Fiji. **2** Heartwood straw colour. Sapwood of similar colour and up to 60 mm wide. Texture medium and even. Grain straight or shallowly interlocked. Very little figure. The green timber has an unpleasant odour but this disappears when it is dry. **3** ADD about 650 kg/m^3. **4** Dries quickly. Prone to bluestain, end splits and surface checking. Shrinkage about 2.5 per cent radial, 5.5 per cent tangential. **5** Easy to work to a smooth finish. Predrilling may be needed when nailing near ends. Peels well although the veneer is inclined to be brittle. Unsuitable for steam bending because of excessive buckling. If any inner bark is present on material being processed, the fine splinters from it can cause skin irritation. **6** Lyctids S; termites NR; durability IG4, AG4, M4; heartwood relatively easy to impregnate with preservatives. **7** Possibly S4, SD4. Some mechanical properties are listed on page 425.   **8** Flooring, mouldings (very popular for picture frames), dowels, handles, turnery, carving, plywood.   **9** Considerable quantities are imported.

Rauli *Nothofagus* spp., especially *Nothofagus procera* (Poepp. et Endl.) Oerst.

1 A medium-sized hardwood of central Chile.   **2** Heartwood reddish brown. Sapwood paler but not always distinctly different. Texture fine and even. Grain straight.   **3** ADD about 580 kg/m^3.   **4** Not difficult to season. Shrinkage about 3 per cent radial, 6 per cent tangential.   **5** Easy to work, giving a smooth finish. Glues satisfactorily. Moderately good for steam bending.   **6** Lyctids S; durability IG3; heartwood moderately resistant to impregnation with preservatives.   **7** S5, SD6. Some mechanical properties are listed on page 425.   **8** Furniture, flooring, joinery, plywood.   **9** Seldom imported.

Redwood *Sequoia sempervirens* (D. Don) Endl.
Other common name: Californian redwood

1 A slow-growing softwood and one of the largest trees in the world; native to the damper regions of the Californian coast. Very selective of site. A small amount has been planted in New Zealand and occasional small shipments of the timber come from there.   **2** Heartwood pale to dark reddish brown. Sapwood narrow and creamy. Texture fine and usually even because there is little difference between the earlywood and latewood. Grain straight. Not resinous.   **3** ADD about 450 kg/m^3.   **4** Slow in drying but little degrade. Dark stains sometimes develop during drying due to migration of extractives. Shrinkage about 1.5 per cent radial, 2.5 per cent tangential. At times the longitudinal shrinkage is greater than normally expected. Plantation material from New Zealand is prone to some distortion and collapse during seasoning.   **5** Easy to work. Sanding dust can be irritating to the nose. Use non-ferrous fixings. Glues satisfactorily. Good base for coatings.   **6** Lyctids NS; termites R; durability IG2, AG1, M4; heartwood resistant to impregnation with preservatives. Good resistance to acids.   **7** S6, SD7 for mature material. Wood from small stems would be weaker. Some mechanical properties are listed on page 425.   **8** Cladding, panelling, external joinery, outdoor furniture, windows, greenhouses, plywood, vats, tanks, fill for cooling towers, pattern-making.   **9** Significant quantities are imported.

Rimu *Dacrydium cupressinum* Soland.

1 A large softwood native to both islands of New Zealand.   **2** Heartwood yellowish brown or reddish brown, with irregular darker streaks. Sapwood pale brown. There is often an intermediate zone of brown wood. Texture fine and even. Grain straight. Growth rings narrow and not sharply defined.   **3** GD about 960 kg/m^3; ADD about 600 kg/m^3.   **4** Heartwood should be separated from sapwood when being dried because it dries much more slowly. Little degrade. Shrinkage about 3 per cent radial, 5 per cent tangential.   **5** Moderately easy to work. Needs care in nailing. Good base for paint. Glues and steam bends satisfactorily. **6** Lyctids NS; durability IG4, M4; heartwood resistant to impregnation with preservatives. Sapwood and intermediate wood are attractive to the *Anobium* borer. **7** S6, SD7. Some mechanical properties are listed on page 425. **8** Flooring, cladding, furniture, joinery, plywood. **9** Very small quantities are imported.

Rosarosa *Heritiera ornithocephala* Kosterm.

1 A large hardwood of Fiji. **2** Heartwood reddish brown. Sapwood much paler. Texture medium and even. Grain usually interlocked. **3** ADD about 850 kg/m³. **4** Shrinkage about 4 per cent radial, 8 per cent tangential. Relatively easy to dry. Inclined to check on tangential face. Some collapse. **5** Relatively easy to work. Inclined to split in nailing. **6** Lyctids S; durability IG3. **7** Not known but it is quite a strong timber. **8** General building construction, flooring, panelling. **9** Seldom seen in Australia.

Rosewood, Brazilian *Dalbergia* spp., principally
Dalbergia nigra Fr. All.
Other common names: palisander, Rio rosewood. The name
palisander is often given to genera other than *Dalbergia* with
wood resembling that of the real Brazilian rosewood. Brazilian
rosewood should not be confused with Indian rosewood
(also *Dalbergia* spp.) or the rosewood of South-East Asia
(*Pterocarpus indicus* Willd.), both described below.

1 A hardwood of south-eastern Brazil. **2** Heartwood colour varies considerably; that of young trees is brown, while the dark purplish brown wood with black streaks sought by furniture manufacturers is confined to old trees. Sapwood wide and white. Texture medium. Grain generally straight. Freshly cut wood has a slight odour of roses. Rather waxy to the touch. Sanding dust may be a skin irritant. **3** ADD about 860 kg/m³. **4** Needs careful drying to avoid splits and checks. **5** Not easy to work. Planer cutting angle needs to be low. Turns excellently. Care needed when gluing. Gives a very smooth finish. **6** Lyctids S; durability IG2. **7** S4, SD3. **8** High-quality furniture, decorative veneer, knife handles, turnery, musical instruments, brush backs, billiard cue butts. **9** Usually seen only in decorative veneer and imported furniture.

Rosewood, Indian *Dalbergia latifolia* Roxb.
Dalbergia sissoo Roxb.

1 A medium-to-large hardwood of limited occurrence in India and South-East Asia. **2** Heartwood dark purplish brown with darker streaks, rather similar to Brazilian rosewood but usually with a more interlocked grain. Sapwood distinctively paler. Texture relatively fine. **3** ADD about 850 kg/m³. **4** Needs careful drying to avoid checks and splits. **5** Because of its very considerable hardness it is difficult to work and rapidly dulls cutting edges. Sanding dust may be a skin irritant. **6** Lyctids S; termites R; durability IG1. **7** Possibly S5,

SD5. Some mechanical properties are listed on page 425. **8** Furniture, decorative veneer, musical instruments, turnery. **9** Seldom seen in Australia.

Rosewood, New Guinea *Pterocarpus indicus* Willd.
Other common names: Amboyna wood, narra and 'rosewood' prefixed by the name of the producing country

1 A medium-sized hardwood of scattered occurrence in South-East Asia and the Philippines and eastward as far as the Solomon Islands. **2** Heartwood can be either golden brown or a dark blood-red. Sapwood to 60 mm wide and pale yellow. Texture medium. Grain variable. The freshly cut wood has a fragrant odour. Often highly figured. **3** ADD varies considerably but averages about 650 kg/m^3. **4** Easy to dry but slow. Shrinkage about 1 per cent radial, 2 per cent tangential. **5** Relatively easy to work but low cutter angle needed for the planer. Turns well. Nails and glues satisfactorily. **6** Lyctids S; termites R; durability IG3, AG2. **7** S4, SD5. Some mechanical properties are listed on page 425. **8** Furniture, veneer, turnery, panelling, knife handles. Some trees produce very highly figured burrs, which are used in the European furniture trade under the name 'Amboyna wood'. **9** Small quantities are sometimes imported.

Rosewood, scentless *Synoum glandulosum* (Sm.) A. Juss.

1 A small-to-medium hardwood of the coastal rainforests between Milton in New South Wales and Bundaberg in Queensland. A closely related species, *Synoum muelleri* C. DC., grows in the Cairns district. **2** Heartwood reddish brown, similar to rose mahogany but without its characteristic odour. Sapwood pale brown and not always sharply differentiated. Texture moderately fine and even. Grain straight. **3** GD about 1020 kg/m^3; ADD about 700 kg/m^3. **4** Easy to dry. Slight collapse. Shrinkage about 4 per cent radial, 7 per cent tangential. **5** Easy to work. Rather difficult to glue. **6** Lyctids S. **7** Provisionally S6, SD6. Some mechanical properties are listed on page 425. **8** Joinery, turnery, carving. **9** Seldom milled.

Saffronheart *Halfordia kendack* (Montr.) Guill.
Halfordia scleroxyla F. Muell.

1 A medium-sized hardwood of the coastal rainforests of Queensland and northern New South Wales. Related species with similar properties grow in Papua New Guinea. **2** Heartwood pale yellow. Sapwood not readily distinguishable. Texture fine and even. Grain variable. Rather greasy to touch. **3** GD about 1130 kg/m^3; ADD about 950 kg/m^3. **4** Needs careful initial drying to avoid checks and splits. Very slow in drying. No collapse. Quarter sawing is advisable. Shrinkage about 4 per cent radial, 7 per cent tangential. **6** Lyctids NS; termites R; durability IG1, AG1. **7** S1 and provisionally SD2. Some mechanical properties are listed on page 425. **8** Bearings, textile rollers, turnery, carving, fishing rods. **9** Seldom milled.

Sal *Shorea robusta* Gaertn. f.

1 A large hardwood of major commercial importance in India.
2 Heartwood yellowish brown. Sapwood pale brown. Texture medium and even. Grain interlocked, giving a stripe figure to the radial surface. **3** ADD 800–880 kg/m³. **4** Slow to dry, with risk of surface checks and end splits. Shrinkage about 4 per cent radial, 7 per cent tangential. **5** Difficult to work when dried but cuts cleanly. Cutting angle needs to be reduced to prevent tearing out on the radial surface. **6** Lyctids S; termites R; durability IG1, AG1. **7** Possibly S3, SD3. **8** Heavy construction, railway sleepers, piling, vats. **9** Not seen in Australia.

Salwood, brown *Acacia aulacocarpa* A. Cunn. ex Benth.
Other common name: brown wattle (in Papua New Guinea)

1 A small-to-medium hardwood of the rainforests of the central and north Queensland coast and in western Papua. Occasional trees are found in northern New South Wales. **2** Heartwood brown, often streaked with darker markings. Sapwood pale yellow to pale brown. Texture rather coarse but even. Grain straight. **3** ADD about 800 kg/m³. **4** Easy to dry. Shrinkage about 1.5 per cent radial, 4 per cent tangential. **5** Firm but relatively easy to work. Bends and glues well. **6** Lyctids S; durability IG3. **7** S5, SD5. Some mechanical properties are listed on page 425. **8** Furniture, veneer, joinery, turnery. **9** Only in north Queensland.

Sandalwood *Santalum spicatum* (R. Br.) A. DC.
Santalum lanceolatum R. Br.

1 A small hardwood of south-west Western Australia. Most sandalwood was destroyed in clearing the land for wheat growing. Occasionally found in other parts of inland Australia. **2** Heartwood pale yellow to pale brown. Sapwood creamy. Texture very fine and even. Grain variable. Freshly cut wood has a distinctive odour. **3** ADD about 950 kg/m³. **4** Shrinkage about 2.5 per cent radial, 3.5 per cent tangential. **7** Provisionally S3, SD3. **8** The wood was exported to China for many years to be burnt as joss sticks on ceremonial occasions. Also used for carving and the making of trinket boxes. The sandalwood oil obtained by distillation of the wood is used in soap, perfumes and medicines. **9** Scarce.

Sapele *Entandrophragma cylindricum* (Sprague) Sprague

1 A large hardwood of the wetter regions of west and central Africa, and growing as far east as Uganda. **2** Heartwood reddish brown or purplish brown. Sapwood pale yellow and up to 100 mm wide. Texture fine and even. Grain usually interlocked, producing a narrow and uniformly distributed stripe on the radial surface. The wood has a slight cedar-like odour when freshly cut. Logs are liable to contain ring shakes. **3** ADD about 650 kg/m³. **4** Slow to dry. Careful handling needed to minimise twisting and warping; quarter cutting is desirable for better performance. Shrinkage about 2 per cent radial, 4 per cent tangential. **5** Because of the interlocked grain extra care in dressing is required, otherwise it is relatively easy to work. Glues very well. Nails satisfactorily. Unsuitable for steam bending. **6** Lyctids S; durability IG3. **7** S4, SD5. Some mechanical properties are listed on page 425. **8** Decorative veneer, furniture, panelling. **9** Small quantities occasionally imported.

Sassafras *Doryphora sassafras* Endl.
Daphnandra micrantha (Tul.) Benth.—also known as socket sassafras

1 A medium-to-large hardwood of the coastal rainforests from the Hunter River in New South Wales to southern Queensland. **2** Heartwood greenish yellow to grey brown. Sapwood paler but not readily distinguishable. Texture fine and even. Grain straight. No figure. The freshly cut wood has a distinctive odour. **3** GD about 950 kg/m³ (*Doryphora*); 1020 kg/m³ (*Daphnandra*). ADD about 600 kg/m³ (*Doryphora*); 650 kg/m³ (*Daphnandra*). **4** Easy to dry but prone to bluestain. Shrinkage about 2.5 per cent radial, 6 per cent tangential. The dark heart material sometimes present is difficult to season without considerable checking and splitting. **5** Firm but easy to work. Glues well. Its uniform surface provides a good base for paints. **6** Lyctids NS; termites NR; durability IG4, M4; heartwood relatively easy to impregnate with preservatives. **7** S5, SD5. Some mechanical properties are listed on pages 425 and 426. **8** Plywood, joinery, turnery. **9** Limited.

Sassafras, northern *Doryphora aromatica* (F. M. Bail.) L. S. Sm.
Daphnandra dielsii Perk.
Daphnandra repandula F. Muell.

1 A medium-to-large hardwood of the north Queensland rainforests. **2** Heartwood yellow to greyish yellow. Sapwood not clearly defined. Texture very fine and even. Grain variable. Strong odour when freshly cut. **3** ADD range about 600 kg/m³. **4, 5** General behaviour similar to sassafras. **6** Lyctids NS; termites NR; durability IG4, M4. **7** S6, SD6. **8** Joinery, plywood. **9** Mainly in north Queensland.

Sassafras, southern *Atherosperma moschatum* Labill.

1 A medium-sized hardwood of the high rainfall areas of Tasmania. **2** Heartwood various shades of brown. Sapwood white or greyish. Texture fine and even. Grain straight. Usually no pronounced figure. **3** GD about 700 kg/m³; ADD about 630 kg/m³. **4** Easy to dry. Shrinkage about 2.5 per cent radial, 6.5 per cent tangential. **5** Easy to work. Good for turnery and steam bending. **6** Lyctids NS; termites NR; durability IG4. **7** Provisionally S6, SD5. Some mechanical properties are listed on page 426. **8** Turnery, brush stocks, handles, textile bobbins, shoe heels, bungs for casks, carving. Because of its very low tannin content it is the best Australian species for clothes pegs. **9** Scarce.

Satinash, cherry *Eugenia luehmannii* F. Muell.
Synonym: *Syzygium luehmannii* (F. Muell.) L. Johnson.

1 A medium-to-large hardwood of the rainforests from northern New South Wales to north Queensland. 2 Heartwood pale brown or grey-brown. Sapwood not clearly differentiated. Texture fine and even. Grain often interlocked. 3 ADD about 700 kg/m³. 4 Easy to dry. 5 Relatively easy to work. Glues well. 6 Lyctids S; durability IG4. 7 Provisionally S5, SD6. 8 Flooring, structural framing. 9 Limited to Queensland districts of occurrence.

Satinash, Eungella, red *Eugenia* spp.

1 A hardwood of the central and northern Queensland rainforests. 2 Heartwood pink to red. 3 ADD about 770 kg/m³. 4 Needs careful drying to avoid checking. 5 Hard to work. 6 Lyctids S; durability IG4. 7 Provisionally S4, SD5. 8 Flooring, structural framework. 9 Limited to districts of occurrence.

Satinash, Eungella, white *Eugenia* spp.

1 A hardwood of the central and northern Queensland rainforests. 2 Heartwood pale grey. 3 ADD about 720 kg/m³. 4 Slow to dry and needs careful handling to prevent checking. 5 Hard to work. Glues well. 6 Lyctids S; durability IG4. 7 Provisionally S4, SD4. 8 Flooring, structural framework. 9 Limited to districts of occurrence.

Satinash, grey *Syzygium gustavioides* F. M. Bail.
Other common name: watergum

1 A large hardwood of the rainforests in the Atherton district of north Queensland. 2 Heartwood greyish yellow. Sapwood not clearly defined. Texture relatively fine and even. Grain often interlocked. The extractives include appreciable amounts of triterpenes, which give a slightly greasy feel to the wood and can reduce the strength of the bond obtained with adhesives. 3 ADD about 700 kg/m³. 4 Slow in drying but little degrade. Shrinkage about 2.5 per cent radial, 5.5 per cent tangential. 5 Not easy to work. Unsuitable for steam bending. Glues satisfactorily. 6 Lyctids S; termites NR; durability IG3, M4. 7 S5, SD6. Some mechanical properties are listed on page 426. 8 Building framework, flooring, plywood. 9 Probably the most commonly available of the satinashes but usually confined to north Queensland.

Satinash, Kuranda *Eugenia kuranda* F. M. Bail.

1 A large hardwood of the north Queensland rainforests. 2 Heartwood brown, sometimes with almost a purplish tint in the inner heartwood. White lines indicative of the vessels. Distinct sheen. Sapwood not clearly differentiated. Texture relatively fine and even. Grain straight. 3 ADD between 800 and 900 kg/m³. 4 Dries without significant degrade. Shrinkage about 3.5 per cent radial, 7 per cent tangential. 6 Lyctids S; durability IG4. 7 S3, SD3. 8 Flooring, building framework. 9 Usually only in districts of occurrence.

Satinash, lillipilli *Acmena smithii* (Poir.) Merr. et Perry
Synonym: *Eugenia smithii* Poir.
Other common name: lillipilli

1 A small-to-medium hardwood of common occurrence in the damper areas of the coastal forests of Victoria, New South Wales, Queensland and even in the Northern Territory. Seldom milled. **2** Heartwood pinkish grey to pale brown. Sapwood not distinctive. Texture moderately fine to even. Grain often interlocked. **3** ADD about 700 kg/m³. **4** Slow to dry. **5** Presence of interlocked grain makes it rather difficult to dress. **6** Lyctids S; durability IG3. **7** Provisionally S5, SD6. **8** Building framework, flooring, joinery. **9** Usually only in districts of occurrence.

Satinash, New Guinea *Syzygium* spp., especially *Syzygium buettnerianum* (K. Schum.) Niedenzu
Other common name: New Guinea watergum

1 A large hardwood of Papua New Guinea. **2** Heartwood brown to reddish brown. Sapwood distinctively paler. Texture moderately fine and even. Grain often interlocked. **3** ADD about 750 kg/m³. **4** Dries slowly. Care needed to prevent surface checking on the tangential surface. Shrinkage about 2.5 per cent radial, 6 per cent tangential. **5** Relatively easy to work. Glues well. Predrilling may be needed when nailing near ends. **6** Lyctids S; durability IG3. **7** S3, SD3. Some mechanical properties are listed on page 426. **8** Building framework, joinery, flooring. **9** Not seen in Australia.

Satinash, rose *Eugenia francisii* F. M. Bail.
Synonym: *Syzygium francisii* (F. M. Bail.) L. Johnson

1 A large hardwood occurring in wet areas of southern Queensland. **2** Heartwood pinkish brown. Sapwood not clearly distinguishable. Texture moderately fine and even. Grain usually straight. **3** GD about 900 kg/m³; ADD about 700 kg/m³. **4** Needs careful drying to avoid warping. Quarter cutting is advisable. Some collapse occurs. Shrinkage about 4 per cent radial, 8 per cent tangential; after reconditioning about 2.5 per cent radial, 5.5 per cent tangential. **5** Not hard to work. **6** Lyctids S; durability IG3. **7** Provisionally S5, SD5. Some mechanical properties are listed on page 426. **8** Building framework, handles. **9** Only in districts of occurrence.

Satinay *Syncarpia hillii* F. M. Bail.
Other common name: Fraser Island turpentine

1 A large hardwood occurring mainly on Fraser Island off the south Queensland coast. **2** Heartwood reddish brown. Sapwood usually distinctively paler. Texture relatively fine and even. Grain rather interlocked, giving some ribbon figure to the radial surface, which also has a subdued ray fleck. The wood resembles turpentine but is easier to work. Logs generally have very few defects. **3** ADD about

840 kg/m³.   **4** The tangential surface is susceptible to surface checking during drying, so quarter cutting is desirable for ease of seasoning as well as good appearance. Collapse occurs. Shrinkage about 4.5 per cent radial, 10 per cent tangential; after reconditioning about 3 per cent radial, 6 per cent tangential.   **5** Care needed when dressing because of the interlocked grain. Fuming with ammonia produces a greyish plum colour. Rather difficult to glue. Good for firm carving.   **6** Lyctids NS; termites R; durability IG2, AG1, M2.   **7** S3, SD3. Some mechanical properties are listed on page 426.   **8** Flooring, panelling, decorative veneer, chisel handles, mallet heads, heavy furniture.   **9** Limited and only in Queensland.

Satinheart, green *Geijera salicifolia* Schott
Other common names: axegapper, scrub wilga

1 A large hardwood of occasional occurrence in the rainforests of northern New South Wales, Queensland and Papua New Guinea.   **2** Heartwood yellowish brown with stripes of lighter colour. Sapwood narrow and not clearly defined. Texture very fine and even. Grain usually straight.   **3** ADD about 1000 kg/m³.   **4** Shrinkage about 4.5 per cent radial, 6.5 per cent tangential.   **5** Very hard, therefore difficult to dress.   **6** Lyctids S; durability IG2.   **7** Provisionally S2 and SD3.   **8** Heavy construction, fishing rods.   **9** Seldom offered commercially.

Sen *Acanthopanax ricinifolius* Seem.

1 A medium-sized hardwood of Japan.   **2** Heartwood pale grey-brown. Sapwood white. Texture medium but somewhat uneven. Grain straight. Has a prominent growth ring figure on tangential surface.   **3** ADD about 560 kg/m³.   **4** Dries readily but shrinks considerably.   **5** Easy to work but rather brittle. Peels and slices readily.   **6** Durability IG4.   **7** Not a strong timber, possibly SD6.   **8** Decorative veneer, furniture.   **9** Not seen in Australia.

Sepetir *Copaifera* spp.
Pseudosindora spp.
Sindora spp.

1 A medium-to-large hardwood of South-East Asia.   **2** Heartwood pale pinkish brown to dark reddish brown, sometimes with a golden tint. Streaks of darker colour may occur, producing an attractive figure, especially on the tangential surface. Sapwood pale grey-brown, sometimes with a pinkish tinge; it can be very wide, even to 300 mm. Texture moderately fine and even. Grain usually straight. The wood may be slightly oily to the touch. Freshly cut surfaces have a spicy odour.   **3** ADD ranges from 640 to 720 kg/m³ because of the differing species involved and averages about 680 kg/m³.   **4** Slow in drying but usually there is little degrade. Shrinkage about 2 per cent radial, 3 per cent tangential.   **5** Can be rather difficult to work. Even though no silica is present, the wood soon dulls tool edges and a gummy substance builds up on saw teeth. Turns satisfactorily and gives a very smooth finish. Only moderately suitable for steam bending. **6** Lyctids S; termites NR; durability IG4, M4. **7** S4 and SD5. Some mechanical properties are listed on page 426. **8** Joinery, furniture, flooring, veneer. **9** Small quantities occasionally imported.

Sheoak, river *Casuarina cunninghamiana* Miq.

1 A medium-to-large hardwood, the largest of the Australian casuarinas, of common occurrence on the banks of the coastal rivers in New South Wales, Queensland and the Northern Territory but seldom milled because of its value in bank erosion control. **2** Heartwood pinkish grey to pale chocolate. Sapwood distinctively paler. Texture moderately fine. Grain usually straight. Rays very prominent. **3** GD about 970 kg/m³; ADD about 770 kg/m³. **4** Care needed in drying to avoid splitting. Some collapse. Shrinkage about 3 per cent radial, 8 per cent tangential; after reconditioning about 2 per cent radial, 5 per cent tangential. **6** Lyctids NS; durability IG2. **7** Provisionally S3, SD4. Some mechanical properties are listed on page 426. **8** Ornamental turnery, decorative woodware, fencing, roof shingles, excellent fuel. **9** Not a commercial timber.

Sheoak, rose *Allocasuarina torulosa* Ait.
Other common name: forest oak

1 A small-to-medium hardwood that is a common understorey tree in the coastal eucalypt forests of New South Wales and Queensland. **2** Heartwood dark red. Sapwood cream and to 25 mm wide. Texture moderately fine. Grain usually straight. Rays very prominent. **3** GD about 1160 kg/m³; ADD about 920 kg/m³. **4** Careful drying needed to avoid splits. Shrinkage about 1.5 per cent radial, 6 per cent tangential. **6** Lyctids NS; durability IG2. **7** Provisionally S2, SD2. Some mechanical properties are listed on page 426. **8** Decorative woodware and turnery, flooring, panelling, roofing shingles and shakes, fuel. **9** Small quantities are converted into roofing shakes in New South Wales, and have been used for the re-roofing of numerous historic buildings.

Sheoak, Western Australian *Casuarina fraserana* Miq.

1 A medium-sized hardwood occurring in the jarrah forests of south-west Western Australia. **2** Heartwood red-brown. Texture moderately fine and even. Grain straight. Rays not as prominent as those of river sheoak and rose sheoak. **3** ADD about 720 kg/m³. **4** Shrinkage about 1.5 per cent radial, 4.5 per cent tangential; after reconditioning about 1 per cent radial, 2 per cent tangential. **5** Relatively easy to work. Good for steam bending. **6** Lyctids NS; durability IG2. **7** Provisionally S6 and SD6. **8** Furniture, decorative woodware and turnery, roofing shingles, flooring, panelling. Until the advent of the aluminium cask it was a favoured species for beer barrels. **9** Small quantities, confined to Western Australia.

Silkwood, bolly *Cryptocarya oblata* F. M. Bail.
Other common name: tarzali silk wood

1 A large hardwood of the north Queensland rainforests. **2** Heartwood pinkish brown, very similar to Queensland maple. Sapwood, to 100 mm wide, distinctively paler. Texture medium and even. Grain straight. Slightly greasy to the touch. **3** ADD about 560 kg/m³. **4** Dries easily without degrade if carefully stacked. Shrinkage about 3 per cent radial, 7 per cent tangential. **5** Easy to work. Glues well. Unsuitable for steam bending. **6** Lyctids S; durability IG4. **7** Provisionally S7, SD7. **8** Furniture, panelling, turnery, decorative veneer, joinery, carving. **9** Small quantities in north Queensland.

Silkwood, red *Palaquium galactoxylum* (F. Muell.) H. J. Lam
Synonym: *Lucuma galactoxylon* F. Muell.
Other common name: Cairns pencil cedar

1 A medium-to-large hardwood of the north Queensland rainforests. **2** Heartwood mid-brown, sometimes with darker streaks. Texture slightly coarse but even. Grain often slightly interlocked. Little figure. **3** ADD about 560 kg/m³. **4** Shrinkage about 1 per cent radial, 3.5 per cent tangential. **5** Easy to work. Glues well. **6** Lyctids S; durability IG4. **7** Provisionally S6, SD7. **8** Furniture, joinery. **9** Small quantities in north Queensland.

Silkwood, silver *Flindersia acuminata* C. T. White
Other common name: Putt's pine

1 A medium-sized hardwood of the north Queensland rainforests. **2** Heartwood pale yellow, sometimes with brown markings. Sapwood not distinctive. Texture medium and even. Grain often interlocked, giving a ripple figure to the radial surface. **3** ADD about 530 kg/m³. **4** Easy to dry. Shrinkage about 2 per cent radial, 4 per cent tangential. **5** Easy to work. Glues well. Peels and slices readily. Fuming with ammonia produces an attractive grey colour. **6** Lyctids S; durability IG3. **7** Provisionally S7, SD7. **8** Furniture, decorative veneer, panelling, joinery, boat building. **9** Small quantities in north Queensland.

Siris, red *Albizia toona* F. M. Bail.

1 A medium-sized hardwood of the Queensland rainforests between Mackay and the Endeavour River. **2** Heartwood dark red with some yellow streaks. Sapwood white and up to 50 mm wide. Texture moderately coarse but even. Grain often interlocked. **3** ADD about 720 kg/m³. **4** Needs careful drying to avoid surface checking. Shrinkage about 2 per cent radial, 4.5 per cent tangential. **5** Easy to work. Glues well. **6** Lyctids S; durability IG3. **7** Provisionally S5, SD6. **8** Furniture, flooring, panelling, decorative turnery, joinery. **9** Mainly in districts of occurrence.

Siris, yellow *Albizia xanthoxylon* C. I. White et W. D. Francis

1 A medium-sized hardwood of the rainforests of north Queensland. **2** Heartwood golden brown. Texture moderately coarse but even. Grain sometimes slightly interlocked, giving some ripple figure to the radial surface. Slightly greasy nature. **3** ADD about 610 kg/m³. **4** Dries quickly but care needed to avoid surface checking. **5** Easy to work but the sanding dust is an irritant. Because of its somewhat greasy nature some extra care in surface preparation is desirable when gluing. **6** Lyctids S; durability IG3. **7** Provisionally S6, SD7. **8** Sills, joinery, panelling, boat building. **9** Mainly in districts of occurrence.

Spruce–pine–fir

1 While the Douglas fir, western hemlock and western red cedar of western Canada and north-western United States have been imported for many years, a species mixture is sometimes sold as spruce–pine–fir (SPF). This group of species constitutes the largest area of softwood forest in Canada, in cold climate areas where growth rates are slow and the mature tree seldom exceeds 30 m in height and 350 mm in diameter. Occurrence extends across the border into the United States. The name may incorporate any of the following species:

- alpine fir *Abies lasiocarpa* (Hook.) Nutt.
- balsam fir *Abies balsamea* (L.) Mill.
- jack pine *Pinus banksiana* Lamb
- lodgepole pine *Pinus contorta* Dougl.
- black spruce *Picea mariana* (Mill.) Britt., Stern et Pogg.
- Engelmann spruce *Picea engelmannii* (Parry) Engelm.
- red spruce *Picea rubens* Sarg.
- white spruce *Picea glauca* (Moench.) Voss

These species vary in availability from area to area, so the number likely to be present in a particular parcel could vary considerably. **2** Heartwood can be almost white but it may have a pale reddish brown colour. The whitish sapwood is often wide and hard to distinguish visually from the heartwood. Texture medium. Grain usually straight. Knots usually small. Little odour and said to be non-tainting. **3** ADD about 360 kg/m³ for alpine fir, 400 kg/m³ for balsam fir, 430 kg/m³ for white spruce, 460 kg/m³ for red spruce, Engelmann spruce, black spruce and lodgepole pine, and 500 kg/m³ for jack pine. **4** Easy to dry. Shrinkage about 2–3 per cent radial, about 3.5–4.5 per cent tangential. May need protection against bluestain. **5** Easy to work, glue and coat with finishes. **6** Lyctids NS; durability IG4; heartwood resistant to impregnation with preservatives. **7** There appears to be some difference in strength between Canadian and US material, at least in some species. Ratings would probably be:

1. alpine fir SD7 (Canada), SD8 (USA)
2. balsam fir SD7 (Canada), SD8 (USA)
3. jack pine SD7 (both sources)
4. lodgepole pine SD6 (Canada), SD7 (USA)

5. black spruce SD6 (both sources)
6. Engelmann spruce SD6 (Canada), SD7 (USA)
7. red spruce SD6 (both sources)
8. white spruce SD7 (both sources)

Since the timber will be required to be used in Australia in the seasoned condition for structural purposes, only the SD rating is relevant. Because of the different ratings involved it is important to know what is in the species mix provided, unless the material is already branded with the ordered stress grade. The ratings when sold as 'spruce–pine–fir' would be SD7 for Canadian material, SD8 for other sources. **8** Building framework, panelling, internal joinery. **9** Quantities have been imported from western Canada.

Spruce, Sitka *Picea sitchensis* (Bong.) Carr.

1 A large softwood of the west coast of North America, from northern California to Alaska. **2** Heartwood pale pinkish brown. Sapwood creamy but not always very distinct from the heartwood, and up to 150 mm wide in young trees. Texture relatively fine. Grain usually straight but fast-growth logs can have quite a lot of spiral grain around the pith. **3** ADD about 430 kg/m³. **4** Easy to dry. Kiln drying temperatures above 60°C should be avoided for structural timber because of a significant effect on strength properties. Shrinkage about 2 per cent radial, 4 per cent tangential. **5** Easy to work. Glues and nails satisfactorily. **6** Lyctids NS; durability IG4, M4; heartwood difficult to impregnate evenly with preservatives. **7** S7, SD6. Some mechanical properties are listed on pages 426 and 427. **8** Joinery, oars, sounding boards for musical instruments, masts, spars, boat building. Because of its relatively high strength-to-density ratio it has been a favoured species for light aircraft construction. **9** Small quantities are imported.

Spruce, Taiwan *Picea morrisonicola* Hayata

1 A medium-sized softwood native to Taiwan. **2** Heartwood pale yellow, darkening to brown on exposure. Sapwood not clearly differentiated. Texture fine but uneven. Grain straight. Growth rings conspicuous. **3** GD about 880 kg/m³; ADD about 500 kg/m³. **4** Easy to dry. Shrinkage about 2.5 per cent radial, 4 per cent tangential. **5** Easy to work. **6** Lyctids NS. **8** Building framework, furniture, joinery. **9** Small quantities sometimes imported.

Stringybark, blackdown *Eucalyptus sphaerocarpa* L. Johnson et D. Blaxell

1 A medium-sized hardwood limited to the Blackdown Tableland about 150 km west-south-west of Rockhampton in Queensland. **2** Heartwood brown. Sapwood paler. Texture medium and even. Grain slightly interlocked. **3** ADD about 1000 kg/m³. **4, 5** Relatively easy to dry and work. **6** Lyctids NS; termites R; durability IG2; AG1. **7** S3 and provisionally SD3. **8** General construction purposes, cross-arms, flooring, cladding. **9** Mainly in the area of occurrence.

Stringybark, blue-leaved *Eucalyptus agglomerata* Maiden

1 A medium-sized hardwood of the central and south coast and tablelands of New South Wales but not plentiful. It is being tried on a small scale as a plantation species. **2** Heartwood pale brown. Sapwood slightly paler. Texture medium and even. Grain usually straight. Growth rings indistinct. **3** GD about 1070 kg/m³; ADD about 880 kg/m³. **4** Some collapse occurs during drying. Shrinkage about 4.5 per cent radial, 7 per cent tangential; after reconditioning about 2 per cent radial, 3.5 per cent tangential. **5** Not difficult to work. Glues satisfactorily. **6** Lyctids NS; termites NR; durability IG3, AG3, M4. **7** S2, SD3. Some mechanical properties are listed on page 427. **8** Building framework, poles, flooring. Could have potential for structural plywood. **9** Limited.

Stringybark, brown *Eucalyptus baxteri* (Benth.) Maiden et Blakely
Eucalyptus blaxlandii Maiden et Cambage
Eucalyptus capitellata Sm.

1 A medium-sized hardwood of the mountain ranges around Adelaide in South Australia, the Grampian mountains in western Victoria, and the Great Dividing Range in Victoria and New South Wales. Of more importance in Victoria than elsewhere. **2** Heartwood pale brown. Sapwood may not be clearly defined. Texture medium and even. Grain variable. Gum veins common. **3** GD about 1080 kg/m³ for *E. blaxlandii* and 1140 kg/m³ for *E. capitellata*; ADD varies with species and climate, from about 800 kg/m³ in the south to 950 kg/m³ in the north. **4** Care needed in drying to minimise degrade. Considerable collapse occurs. Shrinkage about 5 per cent radial, 10 per cent tangential; after reconditioning about 4 per cent radial, 6 per cent tangential. Less in northern material. **5** Not difficult to work. **6** Lyctids NS; termites NR; durability IG3, AG2, M4. **7** S3, SD3. Some mechanical properties are listed on page 427. **8** Building framework, fuel. **9** Mainly in Victoria.

Stringybark, Darwin *Eucalyptus tetrodonta* F. Muell.

1 A small-to-medium hardwood widely distributed in coastal areas of the Northern Territory, in the Kimberley region of Western Australia, and on Cape York Peninsula in north Queensland. It is one of the few hardwoods of the Northern Territory to grow to a useful millable size and is probably its main potential commercial hardwood species. **2** Heartwood pale reddish brown. Sapwood yellow and distinctive. Texture moderately fine and even. Grain slightly interlocked. **3** ADD about 1050 kg/m³, but Queensland material has been reported as 1170 kg/m³. **4** Shrinkage about 4.5 per cent radial, 6 per cent tangential. **6** Lyctids S; termites R; durability IG1, AG1. **7** S1, provisionally SD2. Some mechanical properties are listed on page 427. **8** Building framework, poles (if the sapwood is preservative-treated). **9** Limited areas of occurrence.

Stringybark, diehard *Eucalyptus cameronii* Blakely et McKie

1 A large hardwood of occasional occurrence on the eastern edge of the northern tablelands of New South Wales. **2** Heartwood yellowish brown. Sapwood paler but not clearly distinguishable. Texture moderately fine and even. Grain usually straight. **3** GD about 1000 kg/m³; ADD about 770 kg/m³. **4** Needs care in drying to minimise checks and splits. Collapse occurs. Shrinkage about 6 per cent radial, 9 per cent tangential; after reconditioning about 4 per cent radial, 6 per cent tangential. **6** Durability IG3. **7** Provisionally S5, SD5. Some mechanical properties are listed on page 427. **8** Building framework. **9** Very limited.

Stringybark, red *Eucalyptus macrorhyncha* F. Muell. ex Benth.

1 A medium-sized hardwood of scattered occurrence on the tablelands and inland slopes in New South Wales and Victoria. A closely related species is Youman's stringybark. **2** Heartwood pale reddish brown. Sapwood distinctively paler and to 50 mm wide. Texture medium and even. Grain often interlocked. **3** GD about 1060 kg/m³; ADD about 900 kg/m³. **4** Some collapse occurs on drying. Shrinkage about 5.5 per cent radial, 10 per cent tangential; after reconditioning about 3 per cent radial, 5 per cent tangential. **6** Lyctids S; termites R; durability IG3, AG2, M3. **7** S3, SD4. Some mechanical properties are listed on page 427. **8** Building framework, fencing. **9** Mainly in districts of occurrence.

Stringybark, silvertop *Eucalyptus laevopinea* R. T. Bak.

1 A medium-sized hardwood of the coastal fall of the tablelands, mainly in northern New South Wales. **2** Heartwood pale brown, sometimes with a pinkish tint. Sapwood not clearly marked and to 50 mm wide. Texture medium and even. Grain usually straight. Growth rings indistinct. Relatively free of gum veins. **3** GD about 1030 kg/m³; ADD about 860 kg/m³. **4** Dries readily but some collapse and checking occurs. Shrinkage about 5 per cent radial, 8 per cent tangential; after reconditioning about 3.5 per cent radial, 6 per cent tangential. **5** Not hard to work. Glues well with phenolics so has potential for structural plywood and glued-laminated members. Very similar to blackbutt in general behaviour. **6** Lyctids NS; termites NR; durability IG3, AG3, M4. **7** S2 and provisionally SD2. Some mechanical properties are listed on page 427. **8** Building framework, preservative-treated posts and poles. Has potential for structural plywood. **9** Relatively common in northern New South Wales.

Stringybark, white *Eucalyptus eugenioides* Sieb. ex Spreng.
Eucalyptus globoidea Blakely, *Eucalyptus phaeotricha*

1 A medium-sized hardwood of common occurrence on the coast and adjacent tableland areas from eastern Victoria northward to south Queensland. **2** Heartwood pale brown with a pinkish tinge. Sapwood

347

paler but not sharply differentiated; usually narrow. Texture medium and even. Grain often interlocked. **3** GD about 1100 kg/m³; ADD increases with northward occurrence, from about 820 to 900 kg/m³. **4** Needs careful drying. Some collapse occurs. Shrinkage about 5 per cent radial, 9 per cent tangential; after reconditioning about 3 per cent radial, 5.5 per cent tangential. **5** Unsuitable for steam bending. **6** Lyctids NS; durability IG3, AG2, M3. **7** S3, SD3. Some mechanical properties are listed on page 427. **8** Building framework, preservative-treated posts and poles. **9** A common east coast species.

Stringybark, yellow *Eucalyptus muellerana* Howitt

1 A medium-to-large hardwood of the tableland areas of southern New South Wales. Some also in eastern Victoria. Probably the best of the stringybarks for wood quality. **2** Heartwood yellowish brown with a pink tinge. Sapwood usually sufficiently paler to be clearly distinguishable. Texture medium and even. Grain often interlocked. **3** GD about 1100 kg/m³; ADD about 870 kg/m³. **4** Dries readily but care needed to minimise checking and splitting. Some collapse occurs. Shrinkage about 4.5 per cent radial, 7.5 per cent tangential; after reconditioning about 3 per cent radial, 5 per cent tangential. **5** Unsuitable for steam bending. **6** Lyctids NS; termites R; durability IG3, AG2, M3. **7** S3, SD3. Some mechanical properties are listed on page 427. **8** Building framework, sleepers, poles, piles, cross-arms, flooring. **9** Common on the south coast of New South Wales.

Stringybark, Youman's *Eucalyptus youmanii* Blakely et McKie

1 A small-to-medium tree of the New England area of the northern tablelands of New South Wales. Its main feature is the high rutin content of the leaves. Rutin, a yellow crystalline powder, is a glycoside used for the treatment of blood vessel problems, such as varicose veins and haemorrhoids. The leaves may contain 15–25 per cent of rutin, while those of *Eucalyptus macrorhyncha* may contain 10–12 per cent. Alpine ash also contains some, about 4 per cent, but this is too small an amount to be of commercial interest. The young growing tips contain about twice that in the mature leaves. Trees at high altitude give the best yield.

Sucupira *Bowdichia* spp.
Diplotropis spp.
Ferreirea spectabilis Fr. All.
Other common name: tatabu

1 A large hardwood of Brazil and Guyana. **2** Heartwood dark brown with paler vessel lines, very similar to that of black bean. Sapwood pale and readily distinguishable. Texture moderately coarse. Grain variable. No odour or taste. **3** ADD 900–1000 kg/m³. **4** Care needed in drying to avoid degrade. Shrinkage about 3.5 per cent radial, 6 per cent tangential. **5** Not easy to work because of its density and grain variability. **7** Probably S2. **8** Turnery, decorative veneer. **9** Small quantities occasionally imported.

Sugi *Cryptomeria japonica* D. Don

1 A medium-sized softwood of Japan and Taiwan. The tree is of very ornamental appearance and there are many garden specimens in Australia. 2 Heartwood brown, with streaks of light and dark shades. Sapwood not clearly marked. A dark-coloured resin sometimes present. Texture very fine and even. Grain straight. 3 ADD about 400 kg/m³. 4 Care needed in drying to avoid checks and splits. Shrinkage about 2 per cent radial, 4 per cent tangential. 5 Presence of resin may have a blunting effect on tools. Knots usually frequent, making it difficult to dress to a smooth surface. Needs care in nailing. 6 Lyctids NS; durability IG2. 7 Possibly SD8. Not a structural timber. 8 Decorative woodware, panelling. 9 Not seen in Australia.

Sycamore *Acer pseudoplatanus* L.

1 A medium-to-large European hardwood. 2 Heartwood creamy, darkening on exposure. Sapwood not clearly separated. Texture fine and even. Grain sometimes wavy, producing a fiddleback figure. 3 ADD about 600 kg/m³. 4 Needs protection against bluestain during drying. Shrinkage probably in the vicinity of 2 per cent radial, 4 per cent tangential. 5 Relatively easy to work, except where grain is very wavy. Glues satisfactorily. Good for carving and turnery, and for steam bending if carefully selected for straightness of grain. 6 Lyctids NS; durability IG4; heartwood not difficult to impregnate with preservatives. Sapwood may suffer *Anobium* borer attack. 7 S5, SD6. Some mechanical properties are listed on page 427. 8 Decorative veneer, furniture, textile rollers, kitchen utensils, violin backs. 9 Usually only seen in Australia in made-up articles or veneer.

Sycamore, pink *Ceratopetalum virchowii* F. Muell.

1 A medium-sized hardwood of the rainforests of north Queensland. 2 Heartwood pinkish brown. Sapwood is similar and not visually distinguishable. Texture fine and even. Grain straight. Some figure on tangential surface owing to bands of soft tissue. 3 ADD about 700 kg/m³. 4 Dries with little degrade or collapse. Shrinkage about 3 per cent radial, 4.5 per cent tangential. 5 Easy to work. 6 Durability IG4. 7 Provisionally S5, SD5. Some mechanical properties are listed on page 427. 8 Furniture, joinery, plywood. 9 Limited to Queensland.

Sycamore, satin *Ceratopetalum succirubrum* C. T. White

1 A medium-sized hardwood of the rainforests of north Queensland. 2 Heartwood pinkish brown. Sapwood may not be clearly distinguishable. Texture fine and even. Grain straight. 3 ADD about 620 kg/m³. 4 Needs careful stacking for drying to avoid twisting. Negligible collapse. Shrinkage about 3 per cent radial, 4.5 per cent tangential. 5 Easy to work. Glues well. 6 Lyctids S; durability IG4. 7 Provisionally S6, SD6. Some mechanical properties are listed on page 427. 8 Furniture, joinery, decorative veneer. 9 Limited to Queensland.

349

Sycamore, silver *Cryptocarya glaucescens* R. Br.
Other common name: jackwood

1 A medium-sized hardwood of the coastal rainforests of New South Wales and Queensland. **2** Heartwood pale brown. Sapwood not clearly distinguishable. Texture fine and even. Grain sometimes interlocked. **3** GD about 920 kg/m^3; ADD about 630 kg/m^3. **4** Easy to dry. Negligible collapse. Shrinkage about 3 per cent radial, 7 per cent tangential. **5** The dry wood rapidly dulls cutting edges. Glues well. **6** Lyctids NS; termites NR; durability IG4, M4. **7** S5 and provisionally SD4. Some mechanical properties are listed on page 427. **8** Plywood, joinery, turnery, carving, flooring. **9** Scarce.

Tallowwood *Eucalyptus microcorys* F. Muell.

1 A large hardwood of the coast and coastal ranges between the Hunter River in New South Wales and the Maryborough district of Queensland. **2** Heartwood yellowish brown with a tinge of olive green. Sapwood usually distinctively paler. Texture moderately coarse but even. Grain often interlocked. Among its extractives are appreciable amounts of triterpenes, which give a greasy feel to the wood and can affect the strength of the bond obtainable with adhesives. A distinguishing characteristic, very unusual for a eucalypt, is the complete absence of gum veins. Pin-hole borer marks are often present, as are the fibre separations known as 'water rings'. **3** GD about 1230 kg/m^3; ADD about 990 kg/m^3. **4** Slow in drying. Collapse is negligible. Shrinkage about 4 per cent radial, 6 per cent tangential. **5** Reasonably easy to work, considering its density. Gluing can present some problems because of the wood's greasy nature; it may be worthwhile to wash the surface with 10 per cent sodium hydroxide before the application of adhesive. Moderately suitable for steam bending. Usually has good resistance to surface checking when exposed to the weather. **6** Lyctids S; termites R; durability IG1, AG1, M3. **7** S2, SD2. Some mechanical properties are listed on page 427. **8** Heavy engineering structures, sleepers, bridges, wharfage, flooring, cladding, sills, cross-arms, poles, piles, cooling towers. **9** A common species in New South Wales and southern Queensland.

Tamarind, pink *Jagera pseudorhus* (A. Rich.) Radlk.
Synonym: *Cupania pseudorhus* A. Rich.
Other common names: foambark, fern-leaved tamarind

1 A small hardwood of the eastern Australian rainforests from the Manning River in New South Wales to north Queensland. **2** Heartwood pale pinkish brown. Texture medium and even. Grain straight. The wood and bark contain saponins, which result in a considerable amount of froth when shaken with water. **3** ADD about 850 kg/m^3. **5** Easy to work and carve. Inclined to split in nailing. **7** Provisionally S5 and SD5. **8** Joinery, turnery, carving. **9** Seldom milled.

Taun *Pometia* spp., principally *Pometia pinnata* Forst.
Pometia tomentosa (Bl.) Teysm. et Binn.
Other common name: malugay

1 A large hardwood of wide distribution, from Sri Lanka eastwards through South-East Asia, the Philippines and Papua New Guinea to Samoa. **2** Heartwood reddish brown. Sapwood pale pink to pale reddish brown, not always clearly differentiated from the heartwood, and to 50 mm wide. An identifying feature is that the shavings produce froth when shaken with water. Texture moderately coarse and even. Grain straight or shallowly interlocked, producing some ribbon figure. No taste or odour in the seasoned wood. **3** ADD varies from about 680 kg/m³ for Papua New Guinea material to 850 kg/m³ for Malaysian wood. **4** Careful drying needed to avoid bluestain, warping and surface checking. Shrinkage about 3.5 per cent radial, 5.5 per cent tangential. **5** Relatively easy to work but the sanding dust may be irritating to mucous membranes. Glues and nails well. Good for steam bending. **6** Lyctids S; termites NR; durability IG3, AG2, M4. **7** S4, SD4. Some mechanical properties are listed on page 428. **8** Furniture, flooring, cladding, carving, boat building, joinery, handles, plywood. **9** Small quantities are imported.

Tawa *Beilschmiedia tawa* (A. Cunn.) Benth. et Hook. f.

1 A medium-sized hardwood of wide distribution on the north island of New Zealand. **2** Heartwood pale brown but the inner parts of mature stems can be very dark brown, referred to as 'black heart', which has considerably enhanced durability and is difficult to impregnate with preservatives. Sapwood is white. Texture fine and even. Grain straight. **3** GD about 1070 kg/m³; ADD about 720 kg/m³. **4** Easy to dry but precautions needed against bluestain. Slight collapse. Shrinkage about 3.5 per cent radial, 7 per cent tangential. **5** Relatively easy to work but planer knives tend to blunt quickly. Predrilling may be needed when nailing. **6** Lyctids S; durability IG4; heartwood readily impregnated with preservatives, except the 'black heart' material. **7** S4, SD4. Some mechanical properties are listed on page 428. **8** Furniture, turnery, handles, joinery, flooring, clothes pegs. **9** Not seen in Australia.

Teak *Tectona grandis* L. f.

1 A large hardwood of wide occurrence, from the Indian subcontinent to Burma, Thailand and Vietnam. Plantations are being established in a number of tropical countries, including Papua New Guinea. **2** Heartwood golden brown, often with dark markings. Sapwood pale yellow, to 25 mm wide, and easily distinguished. The wood contains an oleo-resin, which gives it a greasy feel and a distinctive odour to freshly cut material. Texture uneven, being alternately smooth and coarse because of the wood's ring-porous nature. Grain usually straight. The freshly cut wood can be very variable in colour, with blotches and streaks, but prolonged exposure to light modifies the more extreme variations. **3** ADD about 670 kg/m³ for mature wood but plantation material may be as low as 550 kg/m³. **4** Dries slowly and with little degrade. There can be wide variations in drying rate between individual boards. Some collapse may occur if high kiln temperatures are used. Shrinkage about 1.5 per cent radial, 2.5 per cent tangential. **5** Usually relatively easy to work but silica can be present and this will necessitate frequent sharpening of tools. Peels easily. Nails satisfactorily but gluing sometimes presents difficulties because of the oily nature of the wood, and it is important to have freshly dressed surfaces. Good resistance to acids. Not corrosive to metal fixings. Unsuitable for steam bending because of excessive buckling. Sanding dust is irritating to the skin for some people. White inclusions of calcium oxalate sometimes appear as flecks in the vessels, lowering the value of veneers thus affected. **6** Lyctids S; termites R; durability IG2, AG1. **7** S4, SD5. Some mechanical properties are listed on page 428. **8** Furniture, decorative veneer, garden furniture, ship's decking. **9** Becoming scarce.

Tea-tree, broad-leaved *Melaleuca leucadendron* (L.) L.
Melaleuca quinquenervia (Cav.) S. T. Blake
Melaleuca viridiflora Sol. ex Gaertn.

1 A medium-sized hardwood common on low-lying coastal areas subject to occasional flooding in New South Wales, Queensland and the Northern Territory, extending to Papua New Guinea and across to Malaysia. The tree is often heavily branched, so this feature plus its location, often in swampy ground, makes it of limited interest for sawmill logs. The bark has a lot of cork-like tissue interspersed with layers of fibrous material. When steam distilled, the leaves and twigs yield cajeput oil (largely cineole), which has a pleasant odour and taste and is used in pharmaceuticals, soaps and perfumes. Other smaller species of tea-tree (e.g. *Melaleuca linariifolia* Sm. and *Melaleuca alternifolia* Cheel) yield a more valuable oil. **2** Heartwood pinkish brown. Sapwood, to 35 mm wide, usually distinctively paler. Texture fine and even. Grain often interlocked. **3** GD about 1070 kg/m³; ADD about 750 kg/m³. **4** Needs care in drying to minimise checking and warping. Collapse slight. Shrinkage about 3.5 per cent radial, 7 per cent tangential. **5** Tends to dull tools. Glues satisfactorily. **6** Lyctids S; durability IG3, M3. **7** S4 and provisionally SD4. Some mechanical properties are listed on page 428. **8** General construction, flooring, boat knees (cut from the natural shapes of tree branches), oyster rack structural members (with bark left on). The bark is used for lining fernery baskets and for making bark paintings consisting of a collage of pieces of differing colour and shape. The cork from the bark can be used for infants' pillows and mattresses, having the advantage of easy washing and sterilisation while at the same time being open enough to allow ready access of air, virtually avoiding the risk of accidental suffocation. Small stems of tea-tree with bark intact make an attractive fencing material.

Terminalia, brown *Terminalia brassii* Exell

1 A large hardwood of the coastal swamps of Papua New Guinea.
2 Heartwood pale brown or yellowish brown. Sapwood pale
yellow. Texture coarse and even. Grain straight. 3 ADD about
450 kg/m³. 4 Easy to dry but precautions necessary against bluestain.
Shrinkage about 2 per cent radial, 4.5 per cent tangential. 5 Easy to
work. 6 Lyctids S; durability IG4. 7 S6, SD7. Some mechanical
properties are listed on page 428. 8 Plywood, internal joinery. 9 Small
quantities occasionally imported.

There are many other terminalias in Papua New Guinea varying
in air-dry density from about 450 to 750 kg/m³, and suitable for
general construction, plywood and joinery. They vary in colour
and are usually so described (e.g. red-brown terminalia, pale yellow
terminalia, yellow-brown terminalia). They are somewhat similar
to the merantis in appearance. The sapwood is susceptible to lyctid
borer attack. Their strength grouping varies from S4, SD5 to S6, SD6,
depending on the density.

Tingle, red *Eucalyptus jacksonii* Maiden

1 A large hardwood of limited occurrence in the south-west
corner of Western Australia, where it grows west of Albany in
association with karri, marri and yellow tingle. 2 Heartwood pale
red to reddish brown. Texture moderately coarse but even. Grain
straight. 3 GD about 1070 kg/m³; ADD about 770 kg/m³. 4 Some
collapse can occur in drying. Shrinkage about 6 per cent radial,
10 per cent tangential; after reconditioning about 3 per cent radial,
5 per cent tangential. 6 Lyctids NS; durability IG3, AG3. 7 S4,
SD4. 8 Furniture, panelling. 9 Rare.

Tingle, yellow *Eucalyptus guilfoylei* Maiden

1 A large hardwood of the south-west corner of Western Australia,
west of Albany. More plentiful than red tingle. 2 Heartwood yellow-
brown. 4 Does not collapse during drying. 6 Lyctids NS; durability
IG2, AG1. 7 S2, SD2. 8 General structural purposes. 9 Limited
to districts of occurrence.

Totara *Podocarpus totara* D. Don ex Lamb.

1 A large softwood occurring on both islands of New Zealand but
most common in central areas of the north island. 2 Heartwood
pinkish brown. Sapwood distinctively paler. Texture very fine and
even. Grain straight. Heart rot is common and because of the risk of
brittleness the timber is more suitable for use in compression than
tension. 3 GD about 950 kg/m³; ADD about 480 kg/m³. 4 Dries
slowly. There is some evidence that the heat of kiln drying drives
off some of the heartwood extractives responsible for its good
durability, so for external applications air drying may be desirable.
Shrinkage about 2 per cent radial, 5 per cent tangential. 5 Easy
to work. Tends to split very readily, so careful nailing is required.

Heartwood extractives may slow down the rate of drying of paint coatings. **6** Lyctids NS; durability IG2. Sapwood not susceptible to *Anobium* borer attack. **7** S7, SD8. Some mechanical properties are listed on page 428. **8** Joinery, garden furniture, vats, boat building, turnery. **9** Not seen in Australia.

Touriga, red *Calophyllum costatum* F. M. Bail.

1 A large hardwood of the rainforests between Innisfail and Cooktown in north Queensland. **2** Heartwood red with a purple tinge; it tends to fade considerably with long exposure. Sapwood to 30 mm wide, pale brown and distinctive. Texture moderately coarse but even. Grain sometimes interlocked. **3** ADD about 730 kg/m³. **4** Needs careful drying to inhibit twisting and end-splitting. Negligible collapse. Shrinkage about 3.5 per cent radial, 6 per cent tangential. **5** Easy to work unless there is a lot of interlocked grain present. Glues well. **6** Lyctids NS; termites NR; durability IG4, M4. **7** Provisionally S5, SD5. Some mechanical properties are listed on page 428. **8** Joinery, plywood. **9** Limited to areas of occurrence.

Tuart *Eucalyptus gomphocephala* DC.

1 A large hardwood occurring in a narrow strip of limestone country between the coast and the Darling Range in the south-west corner of Western Australia. **2** Heartwood pale yellow-brown. Texture fine and even. Grain very interlocked. **3** GD about 1250 kg/m³; ADD about 1030 kg/m³. **4** Slow to dry and prone to checking. Only slight collapse. Shrinkage about 3 per cent radial, 7 per cent tangential. **5** The very interlocked grain makes it difficult to dress smoothly. Although rich in tannins it is said to have little corrosive effect on metals. **6** Lyctids S; termites R; durability IG2, AG1, M4. **7** S3, SD3. Some mechanical properties are listed on page 428. **8** General building purposes, flooring. **9** Very limited.

Turpentine *Syncarpia glomulifera* (Sm.) Niedenzu
Synonym: *Syncarpia laurifolia* Ten.
Other name: luster (in Queensland)

1 A large hardwood of the richer soils with high rainfall on the east coast between Sydney and Cairns. Its name is derived from the small amount of oleo-resin in the inner bark but it belies the character of the wood, which is probably the most difficult Australian timber to burn. **2** Heartwood reddish brown. Sapwood distinctly paler. Texture fine and even. Grain often interlocked. No gum veins. Its general appearance is rather similar to that of the redder types of brush box. Sometimes it has a discoloured dark brown heartwood, which has a lower resistance to impact forces but otherwise seems satisfactory. **3** GD about 1130 kg/m³; ADD about 930 kg/m³. **4** Slow in drying. Tangential surfaces may check. Some collapse is common. Shrinkage about 6 per cent radial, 12 per cent tangential; after reconditioning about 4 per cent radial, 7 per cent tangential. **5** Because of the presence of silica the dry wood very quickly blunts cutting edges. Satisfactory for steam bending. Not easy to glue. The extractives produce dark brown stains on alkaline surfaces, such as concrete and fibre cement. **6** Lyctids NS; termites R; durability IG2, AG1, M1. The presence of a considerable amount of silica has been thought to make it more resistant to marine organisms than other Australian species but other factors, such as the nature of its extractives, are involved. **7** S3, SD3. Some mechanical properties are listed on page 428. **8** Marine piling (the bark is often left on for some extra protection against *Teredo* borers but it is difficult to ensure long-term retention of the bark so the merit of the practice may be questionable), poles, sleepers, shipbuilding, wharf and bridge decking, bearings, flooring, panelling, building framework. **9** A common species in New South Wales and southern Queensland.

Turpentine, scrub *Canarium australianum* F. Muell.
Canarium muelleri F. M. Bail.

1 A medium-sized hardwood of the north Queensland and Northern Territory rainforests. The bark exudes a creamy resin with a strong odour of turpentine. **2** Heartwood pale brown to grey-brown. Sapwood white. Moderately fine and even texture. Grain straight. *C. muelleri* can have a high sheen. **3** ADD about 680 kg/m^3. **4** Easy to dry. **5** Easy to work. Glues well. **6** Lyctids S; durability IG4. **7** Provisionally S5, SD6. **8** Plywood, joinery. **9** Not a commercial timber.

Utile *Entandrophragma utile* C. DC.

1 A large hardwood of wide distribution in west and central Africa. **2** Heartwood reddish brown, somewhat similar to sapele but virtually lacking that species' cedar-like odour. Sapwood, to 50 mm wide, pale brown and readily distinguishable from the heartwood. Texture medium and even, a little coarser than sapele. Grain sometimes interlocked, producing an irregular stripe on the quarter-cut surface. **3** ADD about 650 kg/m^3. **4** Variable in seasoning behaviour. Back-cut boards inclined to warp considerably. Shrinkage about 3 per cent radial, 5.5 per cent tangential. **5** Relatively easy to work but sometimes has a considerable blunting effect on saws. Nails and glues satisfactorily. Peels and slices well. Unsuitable for steam bending. The damp wood is corrosive to metals. **6** Lyctids S; durability IG3. **7** Probably S4 or S5. Not quite as strong as sapele. **8** Furniture, decorative veneer. **9** Seldom seen in Australia.

Vitex, New Guinea *Vitex cofassus* Reinw. ex Bl.

1 A hardwood of common occurrence in Papua New Guinea and the Solomon Islands. The species does extend westward through Indonesia to Malaysia. **2** Heartwood pale yellowish brown with a greyish tinge. Sapwood pale yellow. Texture fine and even. Grain can be very interlocked. **3** ADD about 700 kg/m^3. **4** Shrinkage about 2 per cent radial, 4 per cent tangential. **5** Material with interlocked grain can be difficult to work. Its greasy nature may dictate some extra care with adhesives. **6** Lyctids NS; termites NR; durability IG2. **7** SD4 and provisionally S3. Some mechanical properties are listed on page 428.   **8** Building framework, bridge decking, flooring, plywood, piles, poles, sills.   **9** Small quantities occasionally imported.

Walnut, African *Lovoa trichilioides* Harms
Synonym: *Lovoa klaineana* Pierre ex Sprague
Other common names: Benin walnut, Gold Coast walnut

1 A large hardwood of west Africa. Not a true walnut.   **2** Heartwood golden brown, sometimes with narrow streaks of dark brown wood. Texture moderately coarse and even. Grain often interlocked, giving a stripe figure. The radially cut material bears a close resemblance to African mahogany if one ignores the difference in colour, but the tangentially cut wood resembles walnut.   **3** ADD about 550 kg/m³.   **4** Easy to dry. Shrinkage about 2.5 per cent radial, 5 per cent tangential.   **5** Easy to work except for the dressing of the interlocked grain on the radial surface. Nails, screws and glues satisfactorily.   **6** Lyctids S; durability IG3.   **8** Furniture, joinery.   **9** Not seen in Australia.

Walnut, black *Juglans nigra* L.

1 A medium-to-large hardwood mainly of the eastern United States but it also grows to a limited extent in south-eastern Canada.   **2** Heartwood pale to dark brown, often with a purplish tint, and with occasional darker streaks. Sapwood cream. Texture fine and even. Grain usually straight. Fancy figured veneer is obtained from gnarled stumps, branch junctions, etc. The wood resembles European walnut in texture but is usually darker in colour.   **3** ADD about 600 kg/m³.   **4** Slow to dry but little degrade. Shrinkage about 3 per cent radial, 4.5 per cent tangential.   **5** Relatively easy to work. Excellent for carving and turning. Suitable for steam bending. Glues satisfactorily if conditions are carefully controlled.   **6** Lyctids S; durability IG2.   **8** Decorative veneer, furniture, panelling, carving. Because of its good resistance to sudden blows it is favoured for gunstocks.   **9** Only as veneers in Australia.

Walnut, blush *Beilschmiedia obtusifolia* (F. Muell. ex Meissn.) F. Muell.
Other common name: hard bollygum

1 A large hardwood of the coastal rainforests between the Clarence River in New South Wales and the Cairns district of north Queensland.   **2** Heartwood yellow brown, sometimes with a pink tinge. Sapwood whitish. Texture medium and even. Grain straight.   **3** GD about 950 kg/m³; ADD about 750 kg/m³.   **4** Care needed in drying to inhibit checking. Collapse is slight. Shrinkage about 3 per cent radial, 6 per cent tangential.   **5** Hard to work because of its abrasive action on cutting edges.   **6** Lyctids S; durability IG4.   **7** Provisionally S5, SD5. Some mechanical properties are listed on page 428.   **8** Plywood, flooring, panelling, building framework.   **9** Limited to districts of occurrence.

356

Walnut, Brazilian *Phoebe porosa* Mez
Other common names: imbuya, embuia, South American walnut

1 A large hardwood of southern Brazil. **2** Heartwood variable in colour, yellow-brown to chocolate brown, sometimes streaked. May have a greenish tinge. Texture relatively fine and even. Grain variable. Growth rings often prominent. **3** ADD about 640 kg/m³. **4** Easy to dry. **5** Easy to work to a fine finish. **6** Durability IG2. **8** Decorative veneer, furniture, joinery. **9** Small quantities occasionally imported.

Walnut, European *Juglans regia* L.

1 A medium-sized hardwood widely cultivated in Europe and parts of Asia because of its edible nuts as well as its decorative wood. **2** Heartwood greyish brown with irregular dark streaks. Sapwood pale straw. The heartwood colour tends to fade considerably if exposed to strong sunlight. Texture fine and even. Grain often wavy. The gnarled stumps and roots are commonly used as a source of highly figured veneer. **3** ADD about 650 kg/m³. **4** Dries very slowly with little degrade. Shrinkage probably about 2 per cent radial, 4 per cent tangential. **5** Relatively easy to work. Gives a smooth surface. Good resistance to splitting and sudden blows. Suitable for steam bending. Glues satisfactorily. Liable to incur black stains if the damp wood comes in contact with iron. **6** Lyctids S; durability IG3; heartwood some susceptibility to *Anobium* borer attack. **7** S4, SD4. **8** Decorative veneer, furniture, carving, turnery, musical instruments, gunstocks. **9** Seldom imported except as a veneer.

Walnut, New Guinea *Dracontomelum mangiferum* Bl.
Dracontomelum dao Merr. et Rolfe

1 A large hardwood growing in association with taun in lowland forests in Papua New Guinea but of limited availability. Also found in Indonesia, Malaysia and the Philippines in small quantity. **2** Heartwood grey-brown with streaks of darker brown. Sapwood creamy, to 100 mm wide. Texture moderately coarse but even. Grain often interlocked. **3** ADD about 540 kg/m³. **4** Slow to dry but little degrade. Shrinkage about 2 per cent radial, 4.5 per cent tangential. **5** Needs careful working because of the interlocked grain and the wood's dulling effect on cutting edges. **6** Lyctids S; durability IG4. **7** S5, SD6. Some mechanical properties are listed on page 428. **8** Furniture, decorative veneer, panelling, turnery, carving. **9** Small quantities occasionally imported.

Walnut, New South Wales *Endiandra* spp., especially *Endiandra introrsa* C. T. White
Other common names: plumwood, red plum

1 A small-to-medium hardwood of the coastal rainforests of northern New South Wales. **2** Heartwood pinkish brown or pale brown. Moderately fine and even texture. Grain straight. Little figure but rays are prominent on the radial surface. **3** ADD about 830 kg/m³. **4** Slow in drying and inclined to check and split. Shrinkage about 4 per cent radial, 8 per cent tangential. **6** Lyctids NS; durability IG4, M4. **7** Provisionally S4, SD3. **8** Plywood, flooring, panelling. **9** Scarce.

Walnut, Queensland *Endiandra palmerstonii* (F. M. Bail.) C. T. White et W. D. Francis

1 A large hardwood of the north Queensland rainforests. **2** Heartwood variable in colour, basically greyish brown with streaks of chocolate brown, black and pink. Sapwood pale yellow and to 100 mm wide. Texture moderately fine and even. Grain often wavy, producing in conjunction with the range of wood colours a wide variety of figure effects. Unpleasant odour when freshly cut. **3** ADD about 690 kg/m³. **4** Slow to dry, with some risk of checking and end splits. Collapse slight. Shrinkage about 2 per cent radial, 4.5 per cent tangential. **5** Because of its high silica content the dry wood is very abrasive and rapidly dulls cutting edges. It is best reserved for decorative veneer when it can be peeled or sliced in the softer green condition. Moderately good for steam bending. Glues well. Has more than normal resistance to the passage of electric current. In turning it is inclined to bruise on the end-grain. **6** Lyctids S; durability IG4, M4. **7** Provisionally S4, SD5. **8** Decorative veneer, furniture, turnery. **9** Usually only available as a veneer.

Walnut, rose *Endiandra cowleyana* F. M. Bail.
Endiandra muelleri Meissn.
Synonym: *Endiandra discolor* Benth.

1 A hardwood of the Queensland rainforests. **2** Heartwood brown. Texture moderately fine and even. Grain straight. **3** ADD about 770 kg/m³. **6** Durability IG4. **7** Provisionally S5, SD5. **8** Joinery. **9** Limited to districts of occurrence.

Walnut, yellow *Beilschmiedia bancroftii* (F. M. Bail.) C. T. White

1 A medium-to-large hardwood of the north Queensland rainforests. **2** Heartwood pale to lemon yellow. Sapwood not always distinctively defined. Texture coarse but even. Grain usually straight. **3** ADD about 640 kg/m³. **4** Easy to dry. Negligible collapse. Shrinkage about 2 per cent radial, 4 per cent tangential. **5** Has abrasive effect on cutting tools. Glues and nails well. Unsuitable for steam bending. **6** Lyctids S; termites NR; durability IG4, M4. **7** S4, SD5. **8** Plywood, panelling, flooring, building framework. **9** Relatively common in Queensland.

Wandoo *Eucalyptus wandoo* Blakely
Synonym: *Eucalyptus redunca* Schau. var. *elata* Benth.
Powderback wandoo (*Eucalyptus accedens* W. V. Fitzg.) is a very
   similar species that often grows in a mixed stand with wandoo.

1 A medium-to-large hardwood of the 380–500 mm rainfall zone of south-west Western Australia. **2** Heartwood pale yellow-brown to red-brown. Texture fine and even. Grain sometimes interlocked. **3** GD about 1280 kg/m³; ADD about 1100 kg/m³. **4** Careful drying needed to avoid checks and end splits. Shrinkage about 2.5 per cent radial, 4 per cent tangential. **5** Hard to work because of its density but machines to a very smooth surface. **6** Lyctids NS; termites R; durability IG1, AG1, M3. The most durable Western Australian species of eucalypt. **7** S2, SD3. Some mechanical properties are listed on page 428. Powderbark wandoo has been provisionally classified as S3, SD3. **8** Heavy engineering construction, poles, flooring. The wood contains about 10 per cent of tannin and the bark 20 per cent (useful for the leather industry), yet the wood does not cause much corrosion when in contact with steel fixings. Thus, it holds dog spikes well and does not corrode them in its use as a sleeper timber. **9** Only in Western Australia.

Wattle *Acacia* spp.

There are many wattles that produce a very attractive red-brown heartwood resembling that of blackwood (*Acacia melanoxylon*) but because of their usually short life span their size is usually insufficient to be of commercial interest. However, they could have appeal to the wood artisan, carver and turner. Many have excellent shock resistance and make good handles for striking tools. The wide white or pale yellow sapwood is usually susceptible to lyctid borer attack and would require preservative treatment. Some of the larger acacias are described elsewhere (e.g. blackwood, brigalow, brown salwood, gidgee, mulga, raspberry jam); a brief description of minor acacias follows.

Wattle, black *Acacia mearnsii* de Wild.
Synonym: *Acacia decurrens* (J. Wendl.) Willd. var. *mollis* Lindl.,
        formerly *Acacia mollissima* auctt. austral.

1 Common in the eastern states, including Tasmania. Bark has high tannin content. **3** GD about 1000 kg/m³; ADD varies considerably from about 550 to 750 kg/m³. **4** Shrinkage about 4 per cent radial, 6 per cent tangential. **7** S4, SD4. Some mechanical properties are listed on page 428.

Wattle, cedar *Acacia elata* A. Cunn. ex Benth.

1 Mainly a NSW species, where it grows to a medium-sized tree because it has a longer life than most wattles. **9** Common in the Sydney area on the shale soils.

Wattle, ferny *Acacia o'shanesii* F. Muell. et Maiden

1 Native to the east coast and coastal ranges. **3** ADD 800–900 kg/m. **7** Provisionally S4, SD5.

Wattle, golden *Acacia pycnantha* Benth.

1 Native to the southern areas of New South Wales; also found in Victoria and South Australia. **7** Provisionally S5, SD5.

Wattle, golden, Sydney *Acacia longifolia* (Andr.) Willd.

1 A small tree of the coast and tablelands in the eastern states. **3** ADD about 660 kg/m³. **7** S4, SD4.

Wattle, green *Acacia decurrens* (J. Wendl.) Willd.
Acacia irrorata Sieb. ex Spreng.

1 Common in coastal New South Wales and southern Queensland. **3** GD about 1150 kg/m³ (*A. irrorata*); ADD about 720 kg/m³ (*A. decurrens*), about 830 kg/m³ (*A. irrorata*). **4** Shrinkage about 2 per cent radial, 5 per cent tangential (*A. irrorata*). **7** S3 and provisionally SD3. Some mechanical properties are listed on page 429.

Wattle, hickory *Acacia penninervis* Sieb. ex DC.

1 In New South Wales it occurs on the coast, the southern tablelands and the western slopes. Also found in Victoria. **3** ADD 720–820 kg/m³. **4** Shrinkage 1.5 per cent radial, 4 per cent tangential. **7** S4 and provisionally SD4. Some mechanical properties are listed on page 429.

Wattle, ironwood *Acacia excelsa* Benth.

1 Widely distributed in inland eastern Australia. It can grow to 20 m in height. **2** Often has a very attractive figure because of the very interlocked grain. **3** GD about 1350 kg/m³; ADD about 1150 kg/m³. **4** Shrinkage about 2.5 per cent radial, 3.5 per cent tangential. **6** Lyctids NS; durability IG2. **7** Provisionally S2, SD3.

Wattle, silver *Acacia dealbata* Link

1 Found in all the eastern states. **3** GD about 800 kg/m³; ADD ranges from 540 to 720 kg/m³. **4** Shrinkage about 2 per cent radial, 5 per cent tangential. **7** S4 and provisionally SD5. Some mechanical properties are listed on page 429. **9** A closely related species is Bodalla silver wattle, *Acacia silvestris*, and native to the south coast of New South Wales. The wood is very suitable for handles but the tree is small.

Wattle, spear *Acacia rhodoxylon* Maiden

1 Native to central and southern areas of inland Queensland. **2** Very hard and dense. **3** ADD about 1280 kg/m³. **7** Provisionally S1, SD1.

Wattle, white *Acacia bakeri* Maiden

1 A rainforest wattle of southern Queensland with pale yellow heartwood and marble-like figuring on the tangential face. Texture coarse but even. **3** ADD about 900 kg/m³. **5** Easy to work. **7** Provisionally S3, SD4.

Willow *Salix* spp.

1 Willows are hardwoods of common occurrence in Europe and western Asia. Great Britain has several of commercial importance. The cricket bat willow *Salix alba* L. var. *calva* G. Meyer (synonym: *Salix alba* L. var. *coerula* (Sm.) W. Koch) is used for the best quality cricket bats and the white willow *Salix alba* L. and crack willow *Salix fragilis* L. for lesser quality bats. The wood of the various species is similar in general appearance, the main difference being in rate of growth. **2** Heartwood pale reddish brown. Sapwood almost white and very wide in fast-grown wood. Texture fine and relatively even. Grain usually straight. Growth rings are distinct except near the centre of the tree. **3** ADD varies from about 350 to 450 kg/m^3. The cricket bat willow is less dense than the others. **4** Seasons rapidly with little degrade but precautions are necessary against bluestain. Shrinkage about 3 per cent radial, 6 per cent tangential. **5** Easy to work if tools are kept sharp to counteract the woolliness of the wood. **6** Lyctids S; durability IG4. **7** Probably SD8 and below S7. Some mechanical properties are listed on page 429. **8** Artificial limbs, cricket bats, brake blocks, clogs, toys, basket manufacture. In the manufacture of cricket bats, those of best quality have blades entirely of sapwood, with four or five growth rings showing across the face. The blanks are dipped in wax before seasoning to restrict checking. After they are dry the face and edges are pressed by roller to improve resistance to the impact of the ball. Handles are made from layers of Sarawak cane bonded together. Rubber inserts are provided to aid flexibility and sometimes even a piece of spring steel may be fitted in the centre. **9** Very little local production. Material for sporting goods is imported by the manufacturers.

Woollybutt *Eucalyptus longifolia* Link et Otto

1 A large hardwood of the south coast of New South Wales. **2** Heartwood red, rather like that of Sydney blue gum. Texture medium and even. Grain usually interlocked. The dressed surface often has a waxy sheen. **3** GD about 1120 kg/m^3; ADD about 1050 kg/m^3. **4** Slight collapse occurs in drying. Shrinkage about 6 per cent radial, 10 per cent tangential. **6** Lyctids S; termites R; durability IG1, AG1. **7** S2, SD3. Some mechanical properties are listed on page 429. **8** Building framework, sleepers, poles, posts. **9** Common on the south coast of New South Wales.

Woollybutt, northern *Eucalyptus miniata* A. Cunn. ex Schau.
Other common name: Darwin woollybutt

1 A small-to-medium hardwood of scattered occurrence in the Northern Territory north of 15°S latitude and in Queensland on Cape York Peninsula. One of the few northern eucalypts yielding logs of millable size. **2** Heartwood reddish brown or chocolate brown. Texture medium and even. Grain interlocked; often a lot of spiral grain. Very hard. **3** ADD about 1000 kg/m^3. **6** Lyctids S, termites

NR; durability IG2. **7** Provisionally S2, SD3. **8** Fencing, charcoal manufacture. **9** Only in areas of occurrence.

Yarran *Acacia homalophylla* A. Cunn. ex Benth.

1 A hardwood native to the inland plains of New South Wales and Queensland. **2** Very rich dark brown colour. Texture very fine. Sapwood narrow. **3** ADD 1230–1340 kg/m³. **6** Lyctids NS. **7** Provisionally S1, SD1. **8** Could be suitable for musical instruments.

Yasiyasi *Syzygium nidie* Guill.
Syzygium fijiense (Gill). Merr. et Perry
Syzygium curvistylum (Gill). Merr. et Perry
Syzygium brackenridgei C. Muell.

1 Large hardwoods of Fiji and other parts of Oceania. **2** Heartwood brown to red-brown. Sapwood not always clearly distinguishable. Texture medium and even. Grain usually interlocked. **3** ADD about 900 kg/m³. **4** Shrinkage about 4.5 per cent radial, 8 per cent tangential. Prone to surface checking on tangential face. Partial air drying needed before kiln drying. Quarter sawing may be advisable. **5** Not easy to work when dry. Predrilling may be needed when nailing near extremities. **6** Durability IG3. **7** Possibly S3, SD3. **8** General building construction, flooring. **9** Seldom seen in Australia.

Yellowwood *Flindersia xanthoxyla* (A. Cunn. ex Hook.) Domin
Synonym: *Flindersia oxleyana* F. Muell.

1 A large hardwood of the coastal rainforests between the Richmond River in northern New South Wales and the Gympie district in Queensland. **2** Heartwood pale yellow. Sapwood to 20 mm wide and not always clearly distinguishable. Texture medium and even. Grain sometimes interlocked. **3** GD about 900 kg/m³; ADD about 680 kg/m³. **4** Easy to dry. Collapse slight. Shrinkage about 3 per cent radial, 6 per cent tangential. **5** Relatively easy to work. Turns and carves well. Good for steam bending. **6** Lyctids S; durability IG3. **7** S4, SD3. Some mechanical properties are listed on page 429. **8** Furniture, decorative veneer, boat building, handles, carving, turnery, oars, skis. **9** Only in districts of occurrence.

Yertchuk *Eucalyptus consideniana* Maiden

1 A medium-sized hardwood of limited occurrence in the higher country in south-eastern New South Wales and north-eastern Victoria. **2** Heartwood pale brown. Sapwood paler but not always sharply distinguished. Texture moderately coarse but even. Grain slightly interlocked. Gum veins common. The wood has rather similar properties to mountain ash but the log quality is much inferior. **3** ADD about 930 kg/m³. **4** Needs careful drying. Collapse is significant. Shrinkage about 6 per cent radial, 9 per cent tangential; after reconditioning about 4 per cent radial, 6 per cent tangential. **6** Lyctids NS; termites

R; durability IG2, AG1.   **7** S3, SD3. Some mechanical properties are listed on page 429.   **8** Building framework, flooring.   **9** Limited quantities in eastern Victoria.

Yew *Taxus baccata* L.

1 A medium-sized softwood of Europe, western Asia and north Africa.   **2** Heartwood red when freshly cut but it changes to a dark golden brown on exposure. Sapwood white and usually narrow. Texture fine and even. Grain often wavy.   **3** ADD about 650 kg/m³.   **4** Slow in drying. Low shrinkage.   **5** Moderately easy to work. Excellent for turning. Veneers well.   **6** Lyctids NS; durability IG2.   **8** Furniture, decorative veneer, turnery. In ancient times it was much favoured for archery bows.   **9** Seen only in imported articles.

Zebrano *Microberlinia brazzavillensis* A. Chev.
Synonym: *Brachystegia fleuryana* A. Chev.
Other common name: zingana

1 A west African hardwood.   **2** Heartwood pale brown, abundantly striped with irregularly spaced bands of much darker brown and of widely varied width. Texture reminiscent of Brazilian rosewood because of the occasional large pores in an otherwise very smooth surface. Grain variable.   **3** ADD variable, from 650 to 800 kg/m³.   **4** Difficult to season; quarter sawing is advisable.   **5** Easy to work to a smooth lustrous surface. Peels well on the radial surface.   **8** Decorative veneer, fancy turnery.   **9** Seldom seen in Australia.

FURTHER READING

Anderson, R. H. (1956). *The trees of New South Wales.* Sydney: NSW Govt Printer.

Australian/New Zealand Standard. (2001). AS/NZS 1148 *Timber—Nomenclature—Australian, New Zealand and Imported Species.*

Australian Standard. (2005). AS 5604 *Timber—Natural Durability Ratings.*

Berni, C. A., Bolza, E., Christensen, F. J. (1979). South American timbers: the characteristics, properties and uses of 190 species. Melbourne: CSIRO Division of Building Research.

Bolza, E. (1975). Properties and uses of 175 timber species from Papua New Guinea and West Irian. Report 34. Melbourne: CSIRO Division of Building Research.

Bolza, E. and Keating, W. G. (1972). African timbers: the properties, uses and characteristics of 700 species. Melbourne: CSIRO Division of Building Research.

Bolza, E. and Keating, W. G. (1980). The characteristics, properties and uses of 362 species and species groups from South-East Asia, Northern Australia and the Pacific region. Melbourne: CSIRO Division of Building Research.

Bolza, E. and Kloot, N. H. (1963). The mechanical properties of 174 Australian timbers. Technology paper 25. Melbourne: CSIRO Division of Forest Production.

Bolza, E. and Kloot, N. H. (1972). The mechanical properties of 56 Fijian timbers. Technology paper 62. Melbourne: CSIRO Division of Forest Production.

Bolza, E. and Kloot, N. H. (1976). The mechanical properties of 81 New Guinea timbers. Technology paper 11. Melbourne: CSIRO Division of Building Research.

Boomsma, C. D. (1972). *Native trees of South Australia.* Adelaide: SA Woods and Forests Dept.

Bootle, K. R. and Page, L. G. (1982). A comparison of the water absorption characteristics of blackbutt, radiata pine and Douglas fir timber. Internal report. Sydney: Forestry Commission of NSW.

Browne, F. G. (1955). *Forest trees of Sarawak and Brunei.* Sarawak: Govt Printer.

Burgess, P. P. (1966). *Timbers of Sabah.* Sabah: Forest Dept.

Cause, M. L., Weatherhead, T. F., Kynaston, W. T. (1974). The nomenclature, density and lyctus susceptibility of Queensland timbers. Pamphlet 13. Brisbane: Qld Dept of Forestry.

Dept of Forestry, Suva (1969). Fiji timbers and their uses. Pamphlet.

Eddowes, P. J. (1977). *Commercial timbers of Papua-New Guinea.* Port Moresby: Dept Primary Industry.

Fairey, K. D. (1975). Lyctus susceptibility of the commercial timbers used in New South Wales. Tech. pubn 19. Sydney: Forestry Commission of NSW.

Forests Dept of Western Australia (1975). *The forest formations of Western Australia.* Perth: Govt Printer.

Forest Products Laboratory, US Dept of Agriculture (1974). *Wood handbook, agricultural handbook 1972.* Washington: US Govt Print.

Ghali, M. B. (1977). Mechanical and physical properties of New South Wales species of timber. Internal report. Sydney: Forestry Commission of NSW.

Ghali, M. B. (1980). Intrinsic wood properties and utilisation of blue-leaved stringybark. *Aust For Res* 10: 301–9.

Hinds, H. V. and Reid, J. S. (1957). Forest trees and timbers of New Zealand. *NZ For Service Bulletin 12.*

Jane, F. W., Wilson, K., White, D. J. B. (1970). *The structure of wood.* London: A. & C. Black.

Jessome, A. P. (1977). Strength and related properties of woods grown in Canada. Forestry tech. report 21. Ottawa: Eastern For. Prod. Lab.

Kingston, R. S. T. and Risdon, C. J. E. (1961). Shrinkage and density of Australian and other South-West Pacific woods. Technology paper 13. Melbourne: CSIRO Division of Forest Production.

Kloot, N. H. and Bolza, E. (1977). Properties of timbers imported into Australia. Technology paper 17. Melbourne: CSIRO Division of Building Research.

Lavers, G. M. (1969). The strength properties of timbers. *UK For Prod Res Lab Bulletin 50.* 2nd edn. London: HMSO.

Rendle, B. J. (1969). *World timbers.* Vol. 1: Europe and Africa; Vol. 2: North and South America; Vol. 3: Asia, Australia and New Zealand. London: Ernest Benn.

Notes on some uses for wood

Some common uses of wood are described here with a few suggested species for each use mentioned. Such suggestions are given merely as *guidelines and are not to be interpreted as excluding species not mentioned here*. Many of the rainforest species listed are declining very rapidly in availability.

Air dispersers

These are used for producing bubbles (e.g. aquarium use or for making liquid foam).

- Large bubbles: alpine ash, yellow carabeen, rose maple, sassafras, silver silkwood.
- Medium bubbles: white birch.
- Fine bubbles: black apple, ivorywood.

Artificial limbs

Overseas practice: ash, basswood, beech, birch, willow. In Australia, willow and pittosporum have been used, the latter for artificial hands. Plantation poplar is worthy of trial.

Baker's equipment

Wood must be free of taint. Pale colour desirable. Hoop pine, klinki pine, kauri, black pine.

Balconies, sundecks and terraces

The Australian love of the outdoor life is reflected in the popularity of such structures. If they are cantilevered from the main building, and the flooring is of slatted boards that permit water entry to the supporting beams, it is essential that those supports are of durable timber.

There have been many instances of rapid structural failure of balconies supported by the extension of the non-durable softwood floor joists of the upper storey. Decay in such supports may not only endanger the safety of the balcony and its users but may extend along these joists into the main body of the structure, resulting in a substantial repair bill.

The decking boards, too, should be of durable timber since it will be subject to almost nightly dew and thus will often have a relatively high moisture content favourable to decay organisms. The type of board used is generally square dressed (i.e. without tongue and groove) with arrised corners and often with a 'reeded' or 'ribbed' surface. Despite common perception, it does not matter whether the board is fixed with the reeded or ribbed surface uppermost or the flat surface uppermost. The boards are laid with a gap of about 5 mm between the boards to permit rapid shedding of rain.

Hardwoods, cypress and treated softwoods are most commonly used. The extractives leached from hardwoods by rain do stain alkaline surfaces, such as concrete paths and brickwork, so pathways should not be located beneath such decks and the structure should be assembled in such a way that water will not flow from the timber onto the face of the brick wall. Well-maintained exterior stain finishes, if of the more heavily pigmented types, will lessen the risk of such staining but not eliminate it.

The term 'verandah' is applied to the external floored area that receives a large degree of protection from the roof over it but whose boards near the edge do receive a lot of weathering. It is preferable to lay boards parallel to the building's walls so that deterioration is restricted to the few boards on the outside; however, it will be noticed that the majority of verandah floors are laid at right angles to the walls, probably to improve drainage of water from storm rains, but it means that the end of every board is affected by weathering. To avoid having to repair the ends of the boards when most of their length is still in excellent condition, it is worthwhile to maintain a coating on the exposed end-grain plus perhaps the adjacent 200 mm of the face.

Battery separators

The presence of manganese will cut short the life of the separator, hence the need for mineral-free water for topping up.

Quarter-cut veneer (for more uniform swelling) of klinki pine, kauri, Port Orford cedar, redwood, hoop pine.

Bearings

- For machinery: grey box, brush box, forest red gum, river red gum, ironwood, tallowwood, turpentine.
- For instruments: pittosporum, European boxwood.
- For underwater use: lignum-vitae is universally favoured. Crow's ash and forest red gum have been used in lightly stressed situations.

Bee boxes

Wood impregnated with copper–chrome–arsenic (CCA) salts should be avoided as it is likely to cause mortality. Immunisation with boron salts does not seem to have a harmful effect. Since the boxes are often left in ground contact for considerable periods, at least the bottoms should be in durable timber (e.g. heartwood of cypress).

Boat building

Wood has been the traditional material for boat building because of its ease of working and its buoyancy; in more recent times it has been replaced to a considerable extent by aluminium and fibreglass but is still a favoured material for the purpose.

The timber used for such critical parts as planking, stringers, ribs and chines has to be of relatively low shrinkage, virtually free of defects and with straight grain. Unless the boat is to be of glued construction or will be stored out of the water when not in active use, it is not essential to use fully seasoned timber, except for internal fittings. However, its shrinkage does mean that the upper portions and the internal framework should have a moisture content below 20 per cent while the parts below the waterline should not be less than 20 per cent. Because of the considerable period often taken in building a boat, these suggestions are often very difficult to carry out. In order to minimise the effect of shrinkage during construction and while the boat is stored out of the water it is therefore desirable to use only quarter-cut material.

Craft kept on moorings run a very considerable risk of decay. If very durable species are unavailable for the components, preservative-treated timber may be a possibility but since heartwood is very difficult to impregnate satisfactorily it may be necessary to rely on frequent applications of such fungicides as copper naphthenate to the surface of the timbers exposed on the interior of the craft. These surfaces should not be painted as this would tend to prevent evaporation of dampness and hinder the effective application of fungicidal solutions.

Improvements in adhesives have meant that plywood is now sometimes used for the skin of the boat. If the craft is to be kept at moorings it is desirable that such plywood is rot-proofed with non-leachable preservatives. The description of plywood as 'marine grade' only means that it has a highly durable waterproof glue line and is a species of timber that is relatively strong and is capable of providing a smooth surface; it does not infer that the plywood will be resistant to decay.

Because of the wide range of sizes and requirements of marine craft the boat designer will need to consider many factors, such as strength, density, bending and gluing properties, ability to absorb preservatives, and availability, when choosing suitable species.

AS 1738-1975 *Timber for Marine Craft* has been withdrawn by Standards Australia but copies are still available. The Standard gives a list of species that have been found to be satisfactory for the various parts of marine craft and provides grading rules for the quality of material required for the various components. A selection of species, widely differing in the above criteria, are listed in the table below for some of the major parts of a boat. The Standard should be consulted for a more comprehensive listing.

Craft kept at moorings are subject to the dampness and high humidity conditions that favour decay, so it is essential to provide plenty of

Table Uses for marine craft

Species	Approximate air-dry density (kg/m³)	Component
Ash, alpine	620	masts, spars
Ash, silver	670	steam-bent members, stringers, deck frames, masts, spars
Beech, myrtle	700	steam-bent members
Beech, white	500	planking, bulkhead sheathing, decking
Blackbutt	900	planking, bulkhead sheathing, bulkhead frames, engine beds, keels, stern posts, stringers, deck frames
Box, grey	1120	frames, engine beds, keels, stern posts, mooring and towing bits
Brigalow	950	steam-bent members
Cedar, red	420	planking, bulkhead sheathing
Fir, Douglas	530	planking, bulkhead sheathing, bulkhead frames, engine beds, stringers, deck frames, masts, spars
Gum, grey	1080	bulkhead frames, engine beds, keels, stern posts, mooring and towing bits
Gum, red, river	900	keels, stern posts
Gum, spotted	950	planking, bulkhead sheathing, steam-bent members, bulkhead frames, engine beds, keels, stern posts, decking, deck frames, mooring and towing bits, masts, spars
Ironbarks	1120	frames, engine beds, keels, stern posts, mooring and towing bits
Jarrah	820	decking, bulkhead frames, engine beds, keels, stern posts
Karri	900	bulkhead frames, engine beds, keels, stern posts, mooring and towing bits
Kauri	550	planking, bulkhead sheathing, decking
Maple, Queensland	600	planking, bulkhead sheathing, masts, spars
Mahogany, red	950	keels, stern posts
Mahogany, white	1000	keels, stern posts, stringers, deck frames, mooring and towing bits

Table Uses for marine craft (*cont.*)

Species	Approximate air-dry density (kg/m³)	Component
Meranti, red, dark	640–720	planking, bulkhead sheathing
Messmate	780	planking, bulkhead sheathing, bulkhead frames, engine beds
Messmate, Gympie	1000	stringers, deck frames
Oak, tulip	830	steam-bent members
Pine, celery-top	650	planking, bulkhead sheathing, decking, steam-bent members
Pine, hoop	530	planking, bulkhead sheathing, decking, masts, spars
Pine, King William	400	planking, bulkhead sheathing
Quandong, silver	500	steam-bent members, masts, spars
Spruce, Sitka	430	stringers, deck frames, masts, spars
Stringybark, white	850	bulkhead frames, engine beds, keels, stern posts
Stringybark, yellow	870	planking, bulkhead sheathing, decking, stringers, deck frames, masts, spars
Tallowwood	990	planking, bulkhead sheathing, decking, deck frames, engine beds, stringers, mooring and towing bits
Teak	670	planking, bulkhead sheathing, decking
Tuart	1030	steam-bent timbers
Wandoo	1100	decking, decking frames, engine beds, mooring and towing bits

ventilation to the interior to keep the moisture content of the timber components below 20 per cent. If they have not been preservative-treated before use, it is desirable to make regular applications of copper naphthenate to the unpainted internal surfaces to discourage fungal invasion. The other major hazard is possible attack by marine borers, of which the main kinds are described on page 182. Attack is more likely during the warmer months. Small craft that are only intermittently on the water do not need any protective measures but those permanently on moorings need regular slipping and maintenance. Metal sheathing with copper or muntz metal can be used but it is expensive. It should extend about 100 mm above the waterline. Sheathing with fibreglass embedded in synthetic resins is another protective measure but considerable care is needed to ensure satisfactory adhesion to the hull.

Electrochemical corrosion of metal fixings is a common problem because of the dampness of the marine environment. When dissimilar metals are adjacent under such conditions, an electrolytic link is easily provided and the metal closer to the negative end of the following galvanic scale corrodes.

Negative end	Magnesium
	Zinc
	Cadmium
	Aluminium
	Iron and mild steel
	Soft solder
	Lead
	Muntz metal
	Manganese bronze
	Naval brass
	Copper
	Admiralty brass
	Phosphor bronze
	Gunmetal
Positive end	Monel metal

Fully insulated electrical systems are desirable; leakage of current will accelerate the corrosion of fixings. Nails and screws should be of the same metal as the item being attached to the timber. Nails should be punched well below the surface and screws countersunk, with all gaps above them well caulked and painted over to keep salt water away from the metal.

Further reading

Australian Standard. (1975). AS 1738 *Timber for marine craft*.
Baker, A. J. (1974). Degradation of wood by products of metal corrosion. Research Paper FPL 229. USDA Forest Service.
Heath, J. H. and Read, W. J. (1979). Timber in boatbuilding. Tech. Pubn 5 (rev.). Sydney: Forest Commission of NSW.

Bobbins (textile)

Southern sassafras, silver beech, white birch, yellow carabeen.

Boomerangs

The green wood is shaped, twisted and restrained in the desired position until seasoned. Species used by Australian Aboriginals include brigalow, gidgee, mangrove, mulga, myall.

Boot-making

- Lasts: coachwood, broad-leaved tea-tree, sugar maple.
- Heels: coachwood, southern sassafras, brown alder, myrtle beech.
- Wedge heels: bollywood, kauri, camphorwood, hoop pine.

Brush backs and handles

Requirements are fine texture, non-splitting, ability to be bored readily, free of tannins and good appearance. Quarter sawing is advisable for greater stability.

Blackwood, coachwood, miva mahogany, rose sheoak, silver quandong, hoop pine, southern sassafras, Queensland maple, Western Australian sheoak, silver beech.

Buoys

Flame kurrajong, pink poplar, kauri, siris.

Butcher's equipment

- Blocks: tallowwood, forest red gum.
- Tables: hoop pine, Douglas fir.
- Skewers: spotted gum, tulip oak, mountain ash, yellowwood.

Butter churns

Hoop pine, white beech, brown pine, kauri, silver silk wood, King William pine.

Carving

- Soft: blackwood, white beech, bollywood, red cedar, hoop pine, silver quandong, Huon pine, Queensland maple.
- Firm: alpine ash, silver ash, black bean, coachwood, mountain ash, miva mahogany, rose mahogany, silky oak, yellowwood, brown pine.
- Hard: Crow's ash, red almond, river red gum, spotted gum, jarrah, pittosporum, ivorywood.

Chessmen

Black apple, ivorywood, pittosporum.

Cladding

Cladding is normally used either vertically or horizontally; there has been a fashion to apply it at 45° but this is a very questionable practice because of the greater risk of water penetration, particularly at abutting openings. Different profiles are necessary for each method of use in order to provide adequate resistance to water leakage under storm conditions.

Knotty grades of species, such as cypress and radiata pine (the latter requires preservative-treatment with non-leachable preservatives for such exterior use), are often favoured due to their lower cost but can present maintenance problems because of the more rapid failure of coating systems over knots.

Hardboard made from eucalypt chips is a good cladding material and is applied either in sheet form or in strips to simulate traditional cladding.

When using cladding vertically it is important to undercut the bottom to form a drip at the outer edge in order to shed water clear of the material below. Care should be taken to seal the exposed end-grain to prevent moisture absorption.

Clogs

White beech, myrtle beech, radiata pine, southern sassafras.

Clothes pegs

Freedom from staining is essential. Southern sassafras, silver sycamore.

Clutch blocks

Bollywood, pink poplar, coachwood, sassafras, silky oak, yellow carabeen.

Concrete formwork

AS 3610-1995 *Formwork for Concrete* provides rules for the determination of loads likely to occur on formwork. Because of the very considerable weight of wet concrete it is essential that strict structural engineering principles be followed to avoid failure. Timber and plywood are used in large quantities for formwork. Their relatively low density and good insulating properties against temperature change give them an advantage over metals.

If the markings of narrow individual boards on the finished surface are unobjectionable, tongued and grooved solid timber boarding can be used but smooth surfaces require plywood. Manufacturers of plywood have technical publications available on the design and use of their products for concrete formwork.

Formwork in contact with the concrete needs a coating such as is provided by specially formulated 'form oil' to enable it to be removed without damage to either concrete or formwork, thus enabling the latter to be reused many times.

Because of the wet conditions it is necessary to seal the edges of the formwork materials to restrict the swelling arising from moisture uptake. Aluminium- and rubber-based paints are commonly used for the purpose.

The rate of drying out of excess moisture from concrete floors is roughly proportional to the square of the thickness of the floor. Where only one face of the concrete is exposed to drying air, as with a slab-on-ground house foundation, it may take four times as long to dry as a suspended slab of the same thickness.

Further reading

Timber Promotion Council and Monash International University (1997). *Australian Timber Formwork Design Manual.* Victoria.

Cooperage

Acceptability of a particular species will depend on the nature of the contents of the container.

- Heads: miva mahogany, satinay, yellowwood, Western Australian sheoak.
- Staves: Western Australian sheoak, kauri, tulip oak, black wood, yellowwood, messmate.
- Bungs: white beech, southern sassafras, myrtle beech, celery-top pine.
- Shives: white beech, bollywood.

Cross-arms

The Australian Standard pertaining to cross-arms is AS 3818.4-2003 *Timber—Heavy Structural Products—Visually Graded, Part 4: Cross-arms for Overhead Lines.*

AS 3818.1-2003 *Timber—Heavy Structural Products—Visually Graded—General Requirements* gives a comprehensive list of species but does not attempt to segregate them into durability classes. They vary considerably in durability and only a limited number would normally be acceptable to electricity and communication authorities.

Cupboards

Any easily workable species will normally be acceptable.

For the vertical facing material there are numerous alternatives: solid timber, often used with a clear finish; plywood, either of painting grade or with a decorative wood face veneer or synthetic laminate; or particleboard or medium-density fibreboard (MDF) faced with decorative wood veneer or synthetic laminate. Bench tops are usually covered with a decorative laminate but there is increasing use of glued-laminated solid wood panels as a reaction to the sometimes 'clinical' appearance of the synthetic laminate.

MDF is now very commonly used for shelving, having the advantage of availability in wide widths; its front edge is often faced with a strip of solid timber to mask the edge of the MDF.

To ensure that cupboard doors do not distort, it is important that the construction be balanced. For best results the material applied to the outside of the door framing should be matched by material of equivalent behaviour and similar thickness on the inner side of the frame, while the coatings of paint or other covering should be of approximately the same thickness to ensure equal absorption or loss of moisture with changes in environmental conditions.

Diving boards

Spotted gum or laminated boards of Douglas fir.

Drop-hammer boards

Queensland maple, tulip oak, sugar maple.

Dye sticks

Silver sycamore (to avoid staining).

Fencing

Ever since the early days of white settlement timber has been a major fencing material, both for rural and domestic enclosures. In those earlier times, when large areas were cleared for pastoral and agricultural purposes, an abundance of very durable species was available at low cost and fences were often very substantial structures. More recently there has been much greater use of species of lesser natural durability which can be given some form of preservative treatment, or which can be enclosed in soil to which has been added materials such as creosote to deter fungal and termite invasion of the wood.

Farm fencing

Labour now represents a large percentage of fencing costs so the design needs to be simple, involving the minimum of components, and the material as light as possible for easy handling. The traditional heavy fence of closely and evenly spaced posts and large strainers has given way to the use of high-tensile wire with widely spaced supports, which are not necessarily spaced evenly. There is also a trend towards the use of electrically charged wires, where the strength of the supports is of very little importance in providing the desired restraint of animals. Posts that are preservative-treated with creosote or CCA salts are acceptable for use with electric current.

The use of the thinner gauge high-tensile wire has the advantage of greater elasticity without reduction in breaking strain but accurate measurement of wire tension at the time of installation is essential for successful use.

The practice of boring holes through the centre of the post for the purpose of supporting the wire has been replaced by side attachment using staples or wire ties. This change is particularly relevant for preservative-treated round timber in which the boring of holes after preservative treatment would run the risk of exposing untreated wood to fungal and termite invasion.

The use of small-diameter preservative-treated natural rounds of plantation softwoods permits easier hole digging and a lighter burden of transportation, which is of considerable importance in hilly terrain.

The former use of a heavy corner post strainer, fitted with a strut to prevent dislodgement, has been superseded by 'end assemblies' consisting of one or two horizontal stays attached to the last two or three posts, plus a diagonal tension wire.

Gates are now swung from the face of the supporting post, not between the gate posts, so that they can be swung right back against the fence, resulting in less risk of damage to both gate and animal when large numbers of stock are mustered through the gateway.

Any species of timber with a durable heartwood is suitable for split posts. If only small-diameter material with a large percentage of sapwood is available, some form of preservative treatment is necessary and requires the use of the natural round material with its protective ring of preservative sapwood.

AS 1604.1-2005 *Specification for Preservative Treatment—Sawn and Round Timber* sets out the preservative treatments and requirements for penetration and retention.

Domestic fencing

The type of fence to be used around the house depends on whether it is intended mainly as a decorative compliment to the house, a barrier to provide privacy and security, a screen against sun, wind or noise, or a garden subdivider separating the various outdoor activities of the household. Timber provides an aesthetically pleasing and easily constructed enclosure if it is thoughtfully designed and finished.

If a painted fence is required, good-quality seasoned and dressed timbers of good durability, stability and paintability are required but they are expensive. An alternative is to use sawn-surfaced timber in conjunction with a stain-type finish; species prone to checking can be used satisfactorily with such finishes and the state of seasoning of the timber is not as critical to the good performance of the finish.

The biggest domestic market for fencing is in the paling fence, sometimes derided and considered unaesthetic largely because it is usually installed without any thought of giving it a stain finish (relatively cheap and effective finishes are available) or using non-staining nails, or using the basic idea more imaginatively in regard to height, method of attachment of palings and fitting of a capping piece.

The material used in the common paling fence is frequently obtained as a scavenging operation in the forest, or is cut from sawmill off-cuts, so the presence of less durable species or large amounts of sapwood is always a possibility. Despite this, most paling fences give a good service life in relation to their cost, usually lasting at least 15 years, even in high-rainfall coastal areas. The occasional paling of high-percentage sapwood may fail long before this time but it is easily replaced.

Paling fence posts should be of class 1 or class 2 in-ground durability species. Rails should be of class 3 or better out-of-ground durability, while palings may be of relatively low durability provided they are kept clear of the ground. Posts should be free of knots in the vicinity of the mortice, which takes the rails. The amount of wane, want and sapwood should not exceed about 10 per cent of the perimeter of the post or rail, while in palings it should preferably not exceed one-half the thickness by one-third the width. If the sapwood is susceptible to lyctid borer attack, it should be limited to one-third of the perimeter.

If preservative-treated plantation pine is used for the posts, they should be of natural rounds to take full advantage of the wide, treatable sapwood and should be morticed before being preservative-treated. Rails and palings should be free of pith to avoid fractures.

Posts should be buried 600 mm in the ground. The backfilled soil may be puddled with creosote to deter termites. Renewal of this preservative treatment every 5 years is a desirable precaution in termite-prone areas. Posts should not be encased in concrete as it is likely to trap moisture and encourage decay. If posts cannot be embedded in the ground, consider fixing them to a galvanised iron bracket set in concrete.

Posts are usually of nominal cross-section of 100 × 75 mm or 125 × 50 mm, with rails of 75 × 50 mm, and palings of 75 mm or 100 mm width and about 15 mm in thickness. The use of galvanised nails will overcome the risk of nail staining. The nails used are generally 75 × 3.15 mm jolt heads for attaching rails to posts and 40 × 2.8 mm flat heads for connecting paling to rail.

In some states posts are traditionally morticed to house the rails, with the wider face of the post perpendicular to the line of the fence. In other states the wider face of the post is parallel to the line of the fence with the rail bolted to the post.

The advantages of the latter method are that posts are not weakened by morticing and fences are more easily repaired.

Tea-tree fencing

In South Australia very decorative fencing is made from bundles of small-diameter branches of the local broom bush (*Melaleuca uncinata*); this material is also finding a market in the eastern capitals but its high cost is a deterrent. It is usually sold in bundles up to 1.8 m long, with about twenty-five sticks to a bundle, which covers a width of about 650 mm.

In Victoria the stems of other varieties of tea-tree, about 25–30 mm in diameter and well-endowed with pale-coloured corky bark, have been used for many years as a prestige fence.

Fish smoking and curing

Various tea-trees as well as sheoaks, hoop pine, river red gum and spotted gum have been successful. Dry sawdust is used.

Flooring

Over the last 30 years, there has been an increasing use of concrete slab-on-ground as an alternative to the suspended wood floor, mainly on the basis of alleged cost saving. The suspended wood floor has inherent advantages in the correction of any problems that may arise during the life of the building in regard to dampness and termite invasion, as well as enabling repairs and extensions to plumbing, electric wiring and telephone services to be carried out much more easily.

Particleboard and plywood sheeting are often used as a flooring base for non-structural or decorative floor covering, such as carpet, linoleum and timber parquet and timber-overlay flooring.

Australian Standards are available for all types of wood-based flooring. Those for the various timber species are included in the 'Milled products' category indicated in the list of Australian Standards on page 227; there are also standards for flooring made from structural plywood and particleboard, as well as parquetry.

Australian hardwoods have the appearance and wear resistance to make them the equal of any species elsewhere in the world. Except for the very low-density species, most hardwoods are suitable for strip flooring.

There has been an increase in the use of those hardwoods and softwoods that exhibit a lot of feature or character. Modern grading of floorboards is done in such a way that the quality (strength and serviceability) of the boards is the same in each grade, with the differences between each grade being based on the amount of feature or character in the board.

The increasing use of end-matched boards for strip flooring has overcome the perceived need for longer boards as homeowners realise that the length of the board is not related to its quality. A variety of timber-based flooring is now being used, including strip flooring, parquet, overlay, composites and plywood.

The main basis for the choice of which species to use is usually the colour of the finished floor. Colours range from pale straw browns and yellows through to light to pinkish brown and light-to-medium reds to dark reds, dark browns and almost chocolate colours. No matter what species is ordered there will be a range in colour from one board to the next. In some species the range is much greater than in others. Small samples are rarely representative of a whole floor. Some floors are of mixed species—sometimes of similar colours and sometimes dissimilar colours depending on the desired affect.

Here are some example of species in common colours:

- brown colour: white mahogany, yellow stringybark, spotted gum, tallowwood
- yellowish: Crow's ash
- pinkish brown: brush box, turpentine
- light-to-medium red: Sydney blue gum, karri, river red gum
- dark red: jarrah, red mahogany, ironbarks

Flooring, platform

The concept of platform flooring has made considerable headway in domestic construction as a response to the need for more rapid building methods to help counter rapidly rising costs. It involves the laying of the flooring over the whole floor area as soon as the bearers and joists are in position and it extends to the external wall by being located under the wall plate. Double joists are provided under those external walls that run parallel to the joists.

Piers can be set out more evenly over the whole floor area so there is a potential saving in footings, brickwork and termite shields, as well as in the number of bearers and joists required. There is also less waste of the flooring material than when floors are cut in after the internal walls are in position.

Installation of the flooring at this early stage of construction provides a safer working platform, especially in two-storey construction, which should enable work to proceed more rapidly, but the flooring runs the risk of being subject to weathering and expansion before the structure is enclosed against rain and dew.

The exposed flooring material cannot avoid the absorption of a lot of water if exposed for any length of time. The provision of surface sealers is sometimes tried but the amount of wetting that such a flat surface is likely to receive is such that they cannot prevent the ingress of moisture, at least in coastal areas subject to considerable rainfall, so it is most important that builders using the platform-flooring system should organise their operation to ensure rapid enclosure of the structure against the weather. Steps should be taken to drain away any accumulations of water by making a few holes in the floor at locations that will be covered later by skirtings or further internal framing.

Flooring should not be cramped tightly, thus allowing some swelling without serious consequences. A few weeks of weathering will usually only cause some surface checking or opening of joints, which is not of importance when the floor is to be covered with carpet or sheet materials.

Platform flooring cannot be expected to be suitable for a clear-finished feature floor. It can be of plywood, particleboard or timber strip flooring.

Flooring squeaks

The widespread use of carpeting and the consequent reduction in the noise level from foot traffic has resulted in an increased sensitivity to the squeaks that can be emitted by wooden floors. A contributing factor to the squeaking in some instances has been the use of thick underlayments, which in combination with the carpet reduce the ability of the flooring to lose excess moisture derived from the underfloor area; the result is that surfaces that would not have rubbed together previously have now been brought into close contact and when subject to a significant degree of deflection under load may emit a squeak.

There can also be a weather or climatic effect. Flooring systems that provide tight board contact and little deflection may shrink sufficiently in dry weather to create greater deflection under load and just the right amount of board contact to produce a loud squeak. On the other hand, boards that do not squeak under normal circumstances can move sufficiently under highly humid conditions to have the right degree of contact for the production of squeaks.

Summary of causes

The noise is caused by deflection under load and the consequent rubbing together of portions of adjacent boards. Excessive deflection can arise from causes such as the following.

1. The weakness of a section of board due to the presence of a large knot or other defect affecting stiffness.
2. Lack of mutual support for boards due to poor milling or broken tongues and grooves.
3. Too much movement in joists and/or bearers due to excessive spans, inadequate support from piers (packing pieces may become dislodged or piers may sink), or unsuitable quality of timber for the load imposed.
4. Poor nailing: nails may be too short or of too small diameter, or not present in sufficient numbers to hold the floor down firmly. With machine nailing of large areas at a time it is possible that some nails may have completely missed the joist.
5. The flooring may have been cramped too tightly at the time of nailing, giving a domed effect, with the boards not sitting firmly on the joists.
6. The flooring may have been laid at too low a moisture content for the site conditions, resulting in subsequent swelling, which lifts the boards clear of the supporting joists.
7. In old softwood, flooring traffic may have loosened the grip of the nails and all that is needed is re-nailing.
8. The use of narrow boards. If the species or the grade offered has low natural stiffness, the risk of excessive deflection is exacerbated by a narrow width of board.
9. Uneven bearing of the flooring on the supporting joists arising from inaccurate milling or subsequent shrinkage and warping of the joists.

While squeaking can occur at joints in flooring of plywood and particleboard as well as in the normal strip flooring of all species of timber, complaints arise most commonly with cypress because it has a resonant quality that leads to the production of a louder than usual squeak when two surfaces are rubbed together. Because of its relatively low shrinkage, cypress used to be laid in the unseasoned state, when the subsequent shrinkage was usually enough to keep boards from intimate side contact; although the occasional squeak did occur, it was not enough to provoke complaint. In an endeavour to meet the need for a floor of close-fitting appearance for clear finishing the cypress producers were induced to season it before use, leading to the provision of a much more attractively laid floor but one that occasionally suffers from a multitude of squeaks, which are very noticeable when carpet is laid upon it. If carpeting is intended, there is a lot to be said for laying the cypress in a relatively unseasoned state or not cramping it closely, since the appearance of the floor will not be important. When carpeting is proposed for an existing floor, it is important to correct any squeaks before it is laid for they will be much more difficult to attend to later.

Some corrective measures

The first step is to make an inspection of the underfloor area to check on the factors listed above. If the structure is of two storeys, resulting in the underfloor area of the upper floor being inaccessible, correction is obviously more difficult. Where access is readily available, the essential step will be to reduce the deflection in the areas affected, possibly by inserting packing, fitted so that it cannot work loose. Where packing is not possible the screwing of a batten to the underside of the floor to provide mutual support to adjacent boards may be effective.

If appearance is not of importance, skew nailing from one board to another at the point of squeaking may provide the requisite stiffness. Extra nailing into the joists in the vicinity may also be helpful. The use of lubricants, such as French chalk, wax or linseed oil, on the squeaking surfaces may provide a temporary solution but it is unlikely to provide permanent relief. Another approach is to spread the load, and so reduce the amount of deflection, by laying hardboard or other sheet material on top of the floor before fitting the carpet.

In cases where it is impossible to obtain access to the underfloor area, one rather drastic solution is to apply a very liberal coating of a polyurethane floor finish to the surface, working it down the cracks between the individual boards. The finish acts as an adhesive, bonding the boards together and increasing their mutual support. This method should only be undertaken when the moisture content of the boards is at a relatively stable level. Even then, periods of very dry weather are likely to cause sufficient shrinkage to produce some fractures, which may coincide not with the joint between boards but perhaps along the centre of a board, and so affect the appearance of the floor. However, this may be more acceptable to the occupant than continual squeaking.

Garden furniture

Garden furniture is usually exposed to severe weathering and continued dampness. Even where there is an absence of rain, there is the almost nightly dew, while the supporting members are in constant contact with damp soil or masonry. Its design should provide rapid drainage of all contact points between components, ease of access to all parts for regular painting, and a minimum area of contact with damp ground.

Because most people want to be able to move their garden furniture about with ease, the heavy durable hardwoods are generally unsuited for this use so the durable lightweight softwoods such as redwood, western red cedar and the scarce Tasmanian pines (e.g. King William and celery-top) are favoured for the purpose. They need to be free of sapwood, and galvanised fixings should be used to avoid staining. In view of the increasing cost of these favoured species, it may be necessary to revert to a somewhat less durable species, such as Douglas fir, which, if of high ring count and free of sapwood, will give reasonable service. Another possibility would be to consider some of the durable tropical species, such as kwila, which are relatively heavy but not quite as dense as the durable Australian hardwoods. Radiata pine impregnated with preservatives would have the necessary durability and light weight but it is perhaps too prone to surface checking to be widely acceptable for this demanding use.

Glass manufacture

White beech, alpine ash and bollywood have been used satisfactorily for the dies used in making bent safety glass. Poplar is favoured in Europe.

Gun stocks

Queensland maple, coachwood, Queensland walnut, blackwood.

Handles

Hickory and spotted gum are best for striking tools that are subject to severe impact stress. The various acacias and also the tulip oaks usually behave well.

Ash-type eucalypts and the pines are suitable for general utility handles.

- Knife handles: miva mahogany, rose mahogany, Queensland walnut, teak, Brazilian rosewood.
- Chisel handles: Crow's ash, brush box, coachwood, mararie, satinay.
- Saw handles: coachwood, Queensland maple, rose maple.

Hat moulds

White beech, bollywood, flame kurrajong.

Ice-cream spoons and sticks

Hoop pine, klinki pine, radiata pine.

Insulator spindles

Ironbarks, spotted gum, tuart, wandoo, black bean.

Log cabin construction

Nostalgia for the pioneering days often prompts lovers of the bushland to consider the construction of a log cabin from trees on the site, despite the fact that the task is much more difficult than using conventional sawn timber framing and cladding. The large size and uneven shape of the logs, the long period that is required for them to reach equilibrium moisture content and the non-durable nature of the sapwood detract from the practical desirability of the idea.

Selection of logs

To simplify assembly of the walls, logs with a minimum of taper should be sought; the average taper is about 10 mm change in diameter per metre of length. This is a separate issue from that of straightness. Perfectly straight stems will be hard to find so the distance between openings in the walls should be kept small to enable better utilisation of the material available, with unbroken walling limited to a maximum of about 5 metres. Long lengths also present handling difficulties.

All sapwood is liable to decay when continually exposed to wetting by rain. In addition, the sapwood of many hardwoods is susceptible to destruction by lyctid borers within the first few years of service so unless the sapwood of such logs is cut off—a laborious task—it is necessary to select species with a borer-resistant sapwood. While it is possible to have the sapwood impregnated with non-leachable preservatives, this is a quite impractical suggestion to most people interested in making use of the logs on their own property and would only have merit if there was a treatment plant in the district. Prevention of decay of the sapwood that is not susceptible to destruction by borers can be achieved by designing the structure to have wide eaves or overhang or verandah.

While logs might look attractive initially with the bark left on them, it is impossible to keep it intact for more than a few years. Bark beetles will attack the cells at the junction of the wood and bark and loosen it. Removal of bark will be helpful in speeding the drying of the log, particularly with softwoods. Unseasoned logs will undergo a considerable amount of settlement, which will affect the fit and weather tightness of the various components, especially at openings in the wall. Bark will be much easier to remove if this is done as soon as the trees are felled, especially during periods of vigorous growth. The debarked logs need to be stacked, with good air circulation, to dry for at least six months. Because the tangential shrinkage will be about twice the radial shrinkage, it is inevitable that a number of splits will form on the surface of the logs. Severe end splitting is likely to afflict logs from young, fast-growing trees so the application to the end-grain of wax or bituminous paint is desirable to slow down the initial rate of moisture loss and so reduce the development of stresses.

Design of the structure

The mixing of vertically and horizontally oriented logs should be avoided as much as possible, especially if the timber may not be fully seasoned, since shrinkage in the length of the log is very much less than that in its diameter.

A hipped roof makes better use of the protection afforded by roof overhang than does a gable roof.

Termites are likely to be a major hazard in bush areas so it is better to erect the building on piers of impermeable material, such as stone, brick or concrete, rather than on a concrete slab, since it will be easier to control any subsequent termite attack if access to the underfloor area is available.

Fitting of termite caps to the piers will not ensure continuous protection and they should be subject to regular inspection. AS 3660.1-2000 *Termite Management—New Building Work* sets out the requirements for physical and chemical barriers for new buildings (i.e. barriers installed or applied during construction).

The piers should lift the bottom logs at least 400 mm above the ground to provide sufficient space for regular checking for termite activity, indicated by the presence of earth-like tubes, which the termites construct between their nest and food to provide the moisture and darkness necessary for their survival. Special care in providing protection against termites is needed around the base of the chimney, an often neglected spot.

The underfloor area must be kept dry by good site drainage and be well ventilated to keep the humidity relatively low in order to discourage both fungal decay and termite activity. The provision of a layer of polyethylene sheeting over the ground will prevent water vapour rising from the soil (it happens even with dry soil) and help to keep humidity low in the underfloor area. Care should be taken to ensure that water is not ponded on top of the polyethylene sheeting.

In addition to having a considerable width of eaves to keep water well clear of the walls, the roof should have a relatively steep slope to help shed leaves and branches. The roof should be sarked with foil sisalation to protect the interior from leaks from storm rains but its presence requires good ventilation of the roof cavity to prevent condensation, in winter, of water vapour rising through the ceiling from the warmed rooms below. Ventilation under the eaves is easy to provide and can be improved by the provision of additional ventilator space at the roof apex to allow the heated air to escape.

Sealing the gaps between logs

Effective closure of the air gaps between individual logs is a major difficulty. The good insulation achieved by the thickness of the logs will be largely counterbalanced by this gap. It is obvious that unless the logs have been seasoned to moisture equilibrium, gap fillers may be rendered ineffective. Various materials have been used for the purpose (e.g. strips of polyurethane foam and caulking compounds). One method is to brush varnish into the gap between the logs, tamp rock wool insulation into it before the varnish dries and then brush another coating of varnish over the exposed rock wool. Other alternatives, perhaps more effective in making a wall with good insulation value, would be to make a groove in the top and bottom surfaces of the logs and insert a spline to fill both grooves, or provide a hollowed shape in the upper log, which would fit closely over the lower one; this latter solution would probably be too tedious to do on a large scale. If preservative-treated logs are used, their trimming to accommodate such close fitting together could expose untreated wood since it is only the sapwood on the outside of the log that is treatable. Likewise, the notching of logs at corners can expose untreated wood.

Laying the logs

When erecting the walls it is essential to keep all corners as close as possible to the same reference level. If the logs vary a lot in diameter, this will not be easy to achieve; the depth of the notch will have to vary and the butt ends of logs in successive layers will have to be reversed. From the aspect of weatherproofing it is better to remove wood from the underside of the upper log than from the top of the lower log. Either the inside face or outside face of the logs should be made vertical.

The logs may be held together with dowels or steel spikes inserted about 600 mm from corners and at each side of door and window openings. Spiking is done by boring a 20 mm hole halfway through the upper log and a 10 mm hole for the rest of the way through it. A spike 250–300 mm long is then driven through into the lower log. The location of spikes is staggered in alternate layers of logs.

At door and window openings each side jamb is fitted with dowels on each end, which fit into mortices in the sill and head. These side jambs are not nailed to the logs but are held in position by a slot in the ends of the logs, which holds a tongue strip that is fixed to the jamb. This method enables the logs to shrink further without disturbing the frame.

Logs spanning openings should clear the head jamb by perhaps 75 mm (the actual distance will depend on the anticipated shrinkage) to allow further settlement to occur without putting pressure on the head. The gap is packed with compressible insulation material.

Roof framing follows the same principles as in a conventional house; the log at the top of the wall is cut with a flattened surface to provide an even seating for the rafters.

The fireplace is built completely independent of the timber structure and must be cement rendered internally during construction to seal off any small gaps. Insulation must be installed between the brickwork and frame where the chimney pierces the roof.

Lottery marbles

Silver sycamore, ivorywood, yellow boxwood, New Zealand kauri.

Mallets

Brush box, satinay, kanuka box, turpentine, wandoo.

Matches

Splints: hoop pine, cottonwood, poplar. Boxes: hoop pine.

Mauls

Brush box, kanuka box, grey box, tuart, wandoo.

Moth-repelling wood

Port Orford cedar, western red cedar, camphor laurel.

Mushroom boxes

Preservative-treated timber may be used satisfactorily if the treated wood is washed down to remove any chemical sludge and allowed to dry for several weeks before use.

Musical instruments

The acceptability of species for the production of musical instruments is dictated by traditional practice and it is very difficult to obtain acceptance of new ones. The musician expects to hear a certain tone from an instrument and any variant is suspect. Because timber varies considerably in structure and physical properties even within a species, the chances of obtaining musical acceptability with a different species are slim for those parts of the instrument that give it a characteristic tone.

There are many components where decorative value is the most important consideration and in this area the resistance to substitution is less strong.

As many musical instruments were developed in Europe, the favoured species have been those traditionally used by European furniture artisans: timbers such as maple, sycamore, ebony, Brazilian and Indian rosewood, Honduras mahogany, lime and cherry have been widely adopted, with European spruce used for resonant components. The following list gives some species that could be considered by the enthusiastic artisan, without any assurance that the result will be acceptable to the musician. The timber needs to be straight grained, cut on the quarter, free of all defects and adequately seasoned.

Baton

Gidgee, ivorywood.

Castanets

Narrow-leaved red ironbark.

Drum sticks

Ivorywood, silver ash, yellowwood.

Flute

Blackwood, ivorywood, brush box, Crow's ash, brigalow; all lack a sharpness in tone quality.

Guitar

- Belly: King William pine, Sitka spruce.
- Back and ribs: Crow's ash, Queensland maple.
- Arm: silver ash, Queensland maple.
- Fret and bridges: Crow's ash, ironwood, myall, brigalow.
- Fingerboard: ironwood.

Harpsichord

- Soundboard: Traditional species: white Baltic, King William pine, fine-textured Douglas fir, Sitka spruce.
- Keyboard shaft: red cedar, black bean, ivorywood.
- Key facings: black bean, ivorywood.
- Baseboard: brush cypress.
- Casework sides: Crow's ash.
- Bridge: black bean.
- Wrest plank: European beech and sugar maple traditional. Try silver ash.

Lute

Tulip satinwood (*Rhodosphaera rhodanthema* from NSW north coast rainforests).

Mouth organ

Pear is the traditional species. Yellow boxwood could be worth trying.

Piano

- Case: silver quandong, silver silkwood, hoop pine, kauri.
- Keys: hoop pine, kauri, brown pine, black pine.
- Sounding board: hoop pine (must be free of compression wood), King William pine. Kauri in laminations of 3 mm veneer and given a slight curve so that it develops a stress when installed has been tried successfully.
- Bridge: myrtle beech.
- Frame: tulip oak.
- Reed block: coach wood.
- Wrest plank: silver ash, yellowwood, karri plywood.

Violins

- Back: Queensland maple, hoop pine, rose mahogany, rose maple, blackwood.
- Belly: hoop pine, kauri, black pine, brown pine, King William pine.
- Pegs: belah, brush ironbark (*Bridelia exaltata*).
- Bow: grey ironbark, also brush ironbark. The only species widely accepted for violin and cello bows is Pernambuco wood from eastern Brazil, which appears to have just the right degree of springiness. Grey gum has given reasonable performance, as has Western Australian morrell.

Xylophone

- Keys: Crow's ash, kwila.
- Box: rimu, Sitka spruce.

Further reading

Bond, C. W. (1976–77). Wood anatomy in relation to violin tone. *J Inst Wood Sc* 7(5): 30–33 and 7(3): 22–6.

Oars

Alpine ash, silver ash, yellowwood, silver quandong.

Pallets

Pallets, the small platforms of uniform size that enable fork-lift trucks to provide rapid stacking or transfer of goods between warehouse, delivery vehicle and retailer, represent a large market for timber, particularly hardwood, and are a valuable outlet for short lengths. The demand for pallets has increased considerably with the change to containerisation for long-distance transportation and the mechanisation of warehousing. Pallets represent the major form in which solid timber is used in the packaging and transportation of goods.

Pallets consist of one or two decks of boarding held together by bearers, which provide the space for the prongs of the fork-lift truck to enter and pick up the pallet and its load. The components are bound together with machine-driven nails having annular grooved or helically threaded shanks; cement or resin-coated nails are often used with softwoods. The threaded or grooved nails give much better joint strength and withdrawal resistance than is provided by the common smooth shank nail.

The main damage suffered by pallets is to their edge boards, arising from the careless handling of the fork-lift trucks. The fitting of an impact panel to the truck gives a significant reduction in damage.

Individual boards should preferably not be narrower than about 100 mm in order to provide good racking resistance. Timber wider than 200 mm is too inclined to split due to shrinkage stresses. Better impact resistance by the edge boards is obtained by butting two adjacent boards together at such edges.

The tannin staining that eucalypt hardwood pallets may cause as a result of leaching by rain can often be reduced to an acceptable level by giving the pallet material a steaming for several hours before assembly. Such staining is more serious when alkaline goods, such as concrete products, are involved. The alternative is to use the non-staining pine-type softwoods.

The quality of timber required depends on the nature of the load, whether the pallet is to be reused many times, and if it is to be exposed to the weather. Seasoned material would be preferable on the grounds of lower weight, greater stability, and freedom from splitting and nail popping. However, since price is usually a major consideration, most pallets are of unseasoned timber.

The timber should be cut 'square' and to an even thickness and be free of decay, large knots, splits and excessive wane. Sapwood susceptible to lyctid borer attack would be unacceptable in pallets intended for continued use. Surface checks, pin-hole borer holes and stain should be quite acceptable.

Pallet containers are another important form of unitised handling. When the pallet is fitted with slatted sides and ends it is called a 'pallet crate'; if with closed sides and ends, a 'pallet bin'; if a top is added to the latter, a 'pallet box'.

The use of plywood or hardboard provides greater resistance to racking, while their smooth surface can be of importance for pallet bins and pallet boxes.

Paper board

Paper products in the form of corrugated and solid-board containers, folding cartons, rigid boxes and multi-wall sacks represent a major segment of the materials used by the packaging industry. About 50 per cent of the production of the paper manufacturing industry is used in packaging products.

The use of sawn timber for packaging has declined, being replaced for many purposes by these lower density wood-based products, although the increasing use of pallets maintains timber as an important material in the packaging and transportation of goods; it is still essential for the packing of machinery and export goods subject to rough handling and at risk of pilferage.

Some of the most common categories of paper-board product are listed here.

- Packaging papers: bag papers, wrappings, multi-wall sacks.
- Packaging boards: linerboards, folding carton boards, rigid box boards (e.g. shoe boxes).
- Corrugated containers: made from liner boards bonded to each side of a corrugated core.
- Solid-board containers: a number of plies, usually of recycled paper, faced with Kraft liner board.

Pattern-making

White beech, bollywood, white cheesewood, kauri, hoop pine, sugar pine, silver quandong.

Treatment of the timber with a solution containing both borax and boric acid is useful in minimising the scorching of patterns when in use in the foundry. Borax checks flaming but is not a glow retardant, whereas boric acid is just the opposite. The mixture has the added advantage of greater solubility than that pertaining to the individual constituents. Ammonium phosphates are more commonly used as fire retardants but are unsuitable for this particular application because the escape of gases when fired could interfere with the positioning of the foundry sand.

Pencils

Virginian pencil cedar is outstanding.

Polo

Sticks: saffronheart, yellowwood, spotted gum. Heads: broad-leaved tea-tree, kanuka box. Balls: willow.

Saddle trees

Coachwood.

Saunas

Western red cedar, redwood, King William pine.

Scaffold planks

Scaffold planks can be made from one wide piece of timber or from laminations. AS 1577-1993 *Scaffold Planks* gives rules for both visual and mechanical grading of a wide range of acceptable softwood and hardwood species.

Planks purporting to comply with the Standard are required to be at least F11 rating if softwood, and F17 if hardwood; they have to carry a brand, burnt onto the edges, indicating the F rating and the method of grading (visual or mechanical).

Procedures are also given for the proof testing of planks that are the subject of disagreement as to quality.

Softwood planks can be laminated side by side and may be end-joined by finger joints or scarf joints. The same softwoods as are listed in AS 1577 are acceptable. Descriptions are given of the quality of the individual laminate, the preparation of the surfaces, the geometry of the end joins, the types of permissible waterproof adhesive and the method of assembly.

Shingles and shakes

Shingles are produced by sawing but shakes are split by hand along the rays with a wedge-shaped knife, called a 'frow', which is used in conjunction with a maul. Shakes are most frequently used for roofing. Shingles are suitable for this purpose but are also popular for wall cladding.

Shakes are usually thicker and longer (600 mm) than shingles (450 mm). Both may be tapered: in the case of shingles the thickness may vary from about 6 mm at the thinner end to 12 mm at the thicker end, or butt. Both shingles and shakes should be cut radially to avoid cupping when on the roof and the consequent risk of splitting when walked upon.

The number required for a given roof area is dictated by the slope of the roof. Usually there are three thicknesses of timber at any place on the roof; the amount of each piece that is exposed to the weather is determined by its length and the pitch of the roof but it is common for only about a third to be exposed. Extra thickness is often provided at the bottom edge of the roof for extra strength.

A slope of about 15° would be about the minimum that can be used without sarking, but sarking is desirable at all slopes to overcome the problem of the occasional leak, especially in areas subject to cyclonic winds. Such sarking needs to be of a vapour-permeable type in order to prevent condensation occurring in the space between the timber and sarking, for this could lead to decay.

There have been instances where the use of a relatively low roof pitch, in conjunction with an impermeable sarking, has led to some decay within 10 years, even in the durable western red cedar, when the roof was in a damp and shady locality. The decay may be attributable to the retention of moisture under conditions of poor drainage, heavy dew and inadequate opportunities for the drying out of the absorbed moisture. When such a risk is likely, it is suggested that a relatively steep pitch, in excess of 26°, be provided, making sure that the sarking is very permeable or perhaps omitting it.

Shingles and shakes are supported either on closely spaced battens (usually three to each shingle length) or solid boarding. Nails must be of the non-corroding type. Hot-dipped galvanised or aluminium nails are most commonly used.

The main timber used for shingles and shakes is western red cedar, imported from Canada. Rose sheoak is sometimes used for shakes, especially in the restoration of buildings dating from the early days of white settlement, when it was the main species used for this purpose. Because of the small size of the tree the supply is limited.

In the pioneering era the durable eucalypts were used to some extent for the purpose but their often interlocked grain made it difficult to split them.

Further reading

Council of Forest Industries of British Columbia (1979). *Western red cedar shingles and shakes: a handbook of good practice*. Vancouver.

Slats (for blinds)

Red silkwood, redwood, sugar pine, King William pine and western red cedar.

Sleepers

Railway lines have usually been laid on timber sleepers and it is only in recent times that a significant part of the market has been taken by alternatives, mainly prestressed concrete. The alternative has been favoured mainly in areas of very severe termite hazard (especially from the tropical *Mastotermes*) and very high axle loading, as for the iron ore transportation lines of the Pilbara region of Western Australia.

The resistance of the ballast to the sideways buckling of the steel rail is related to the square of the depth of the sleeper so there is a tendency to prefer a deeper section now that rails are being welded into very long lengths. Such lengths result in less mechanical damage to the sleeper but create much more lateral stress in hot weather.

Hardwood sleepers are mostly heartwood but impregnation of the sapwood with preservatives increases the service life of the sapwood and indeed the availability of sleepers. Preservative-treated radiata pine has also found application as sleepers, particularly in New Zealand, when used in conjunction with much larger rail seat plates.

In general, species for sleepers should have high figures for bending, compression parallel to the grain (to give good resistance to spike withdrawal), and compression perpendicular to the grain (to resist wear under the rail seat plate). Care is needed in locating the holes for the attachment of the rail seat plate.

AS 3818.2-2004 *Timber—Heavy Structural Products—Visually Graded—Railway Track Timbers* covers railway track sleepers, railway turnout sleepers, lead and crossing timbers and railway bridge transoms.

AS 3818.1-2003 *Timber—Heavy Structural Products—Visually Graded—General Requirements* lists a number of species suitable for each application. The species are of varying durability so careful selection in relation to particular site conditions and required service life is needed. While decay and termite attack are of importance, shattering of the timber and spike kill (enlargement of the hole in which the rail seat plate spike grips the sleeper) are major factors leading to sleeper replacement.

Further reading

Vaile, R. C. (1979). Upgrading the timber sleeper. *Aust For Ind J* 45(8): 35–9.

Spirit levels

Rose mahogany, Queensland maple, silver quandong.

Turnery

Relatively soft

Brown alder, silver ash, white beech, white birch, bollywood, blackwood, yellow carabeen, red cedar, rose maple, silky oak, sassafras, silver sycamore, silver quandong.

Moderate

Alpine ash, Crow's ash, black bean, silky beech, coachwood, rose gum, miva mahogany, rose mahogany, tulip oak, cypress, messmate.

Hard

Brush box, gidgee, grey gum, river red gum, spotted gum, rose sheoak, tallowwood.

Vats

Essential requirements are straight grain; freedom from sapwood and from defects that could permit leakage or entry of chemicals deeply into the interior of the plank; low shrinkage and swelling; and low permeability. Freedom from coloured extractives may be important in some circumstances. The best timber for vats comes from the outer heartwood.

Softwoods are usually favoured over hardwoods for vat construction involving the intimate contact of wood and chemical. Douglas fir and redwood are the traditionally favoured species but pines with a high resin content may be worthy of trial, provided the material is free of sapwood.

When fitting together the timber components, provision must be made for the swelling that will occur when the vat is filled with aqueous liquids. This will involve some bevelling of the inner edges of the planks, the amount being determined by the shrinkage characteristics of the species used. Wetting of the inside of the plank before assembly will help to ensure that the outside joins do not open when the vat is filled.

Shallow and curved tongues are advisable to lessen the stresses when the vat is filled. The long bolts binding the planks together should not be made very tight until the vat has responded fully to the initial swelling.

If the contents are to be strongly acidic or alkaline, it is better that the vat be lined with an appropriate sheeting or coating resistant to the corrosive effect of the contents. This enables a much wider range of species to be used for the shell of the vat.

Vats can deteriorate if left empty since the timber will dry out and shrink and the vat will leak when first refilled. On the other hand, leaving it full of stagnant water will encourage decay so the contents should be changed regularly or given some relatively neutral fungicidal additive.

It is preferable not to paint the outside surface of the vat. The absence of a coating will allow excess moisture to evaporate and so lessen the risk of decay. If painting is unavoidable, a 'breather' type of paint should be chosen.

Water-cooling towers

- Structure: tallowwood, CCA-treated radiata pine.
- Fill: CCA-treated radiata pine.

Destruction by 'soft rot' fungi is a major problem so radiata pine, adequately loaded with CCA salts, is now most favoured.

Windows

A relatively light weight and dimensional stability under changing atmospheric conditions are required. In recent years western red cedar has been the most commonly used timber but, prior to that, fine-grained Douglas fir and Queensland maple, silky oak, alpine ash and redwood were used. Radiata pine, cut well clear of the tree's core of spiral grain and preservative-treated, may prove adequate if additional steps are taken to inhibit rapid moisture uptake. Meranti and messmate are also used.

Wood flour

Hoop pine, radiata pine, western hemlock.

Recent developments have seen it being used in wood–plastic composites for products such as decking.

Wooden screws

Crow's ash, ivorywood.

Wood wool/cement building boards

Wood wool consists of long shavings, usually cut from a relatively low-density species, and is produced by a special planer fitted with reciprocating spurs and knives. The mechanism holds a short billet of wood and is automatically advanced after each passage of the spurs across the face of the billet. A species with a long fibre length and low in extractives is desirable for good wood wool. The billet needs to be of clear material so as to obtain the maximum length of shavings. Radiata pine is commonly used.

When combining wood wool and cement to form a building board, a species low in extractives content is essential because of the interference by the extractives in the setting and bonding of the cement; pretreatment of the wood wool with small amounts of hydrated lime, calcium chloride, sodium silicate or alum can help to overcome this problem.

The wood wool is mixed with cement in a 1:3 ratio (by weight) in moulds; the mix is pressed to a uniform thickness and set aside for a day to cure before stripping out the boards for several weeks of air drying so that the likely 0.3 per cent shrinkage will occur before marketing.

For ordinary wood wool for use in packaging, extractives are of less consequence and the ash-type eucalypts are commonly used. Poplar is the favoured species for the wood wool pads used in evaporative air coolers.

Wood fibres are used in admixture in the production of the commonly used fibre-cement sheets used for wall cladding and eaves lining in order to make the sheet more resistant to damage. The wood fibres have the advantage of low density and low cost, while increasing the modulus of rupture and impact strength of the sheet.

The organic nature of the wood fibre has some degree of incompatibility with the calcium silicates, aluminates and ferrites of the cement so it is common to pretreat the wood fibres with calcium chloride.

Common metric terms and conversion factors

Prefixes			
Giga (G)	=	1 000 000 000	10^9
Mega (M)	=	1 000 000	10^6
Kilo (k)	=	1 000	10^3
Hecto (h)	=	100	10^2
Deca (da)	=	10	10^1
Deci (d)	=	0.1	10^{-1}
Centi (c)	=	0.01	10^{-2}
Milli (m)	=	0.001	10^{-3}
Micro (µ)	=	0.000 001	10^{-6}
Nano (n)	=	0.000 000 001	10^{-9}

Units of measurement		Abbreviation
Length		
Metre (basic unit)		m
Millimetre	0.001 m	mm
Centimetre	0.01 m	cm
Kilometre	1000 m	km
Nautical mile	1852 m	n mile
Mass		
Kilogram (basic unit)		kg
Gram	0.001 kg	g
Tonne	1000 kg	t
Area		
Square metre (basic unit)		m^2
Square millimetre	$0.000\ 001\ m^2$	mm^2
Square centimetre	$0.000\ 1\ m^2$	cm^2
Hectare	$10\ 000\ m^2$	ha

Units of measurement		Abbreviation
Volume		
Solids:		
Cubic metre (basic unit)		m³
Cubic millimetre	10^{-9} m³	mm³
Cubic centimetre	0.000 001 m³	cm³
Cubic decimetre	0.001 m³	dm³
Fluids:		
Litre	0.001 m³	L
Millilitre	0.001 L	mL
Kilolitre	1000 L (= 1 m³)	kL

Units of measurement	Abbreviation
Speed (velocity)	
Metre per second (basic unit)	m/s
Kilometre per hour (= 0.27 m/s)	km/h
Knot = 1 n mile/h (= 0.514 m/s)	kn
Acceleration—metre per second per second	m/s²
Force	
Newton (basic unit)	N
1 dyne = 10^{-5} N	
Pressure	
Pascal (= 1 N/m²) (basic unit)	Pa
Bar (100 000 Pa)	b
Millibar (100 Pa)	mb
Density	
Kilogram per cubic metre (basic unit)	kg/m³
Tonne per cubic metre (= 1000 kg/m³)	t/m³
Gram per cubic centimetre (= 1000 kg/m³)	g/m³
For fluids only:	
Kilogram per litre (= 1000 kg/m³)	kg/L
Gram per millilitre (= 1000 kg/m³)	g/mL
Temperature	
Kelvin (basic unit)	K
1 degree Celsius = 1 K	°C
Energy	
Joule (basic unit)	J
1 erg = 10^{-7} J	
1 calorie = 4.1868 J	
1 kilowatt hour = 3.6 MJ	

Units of measurement	Abbreviation
Power	
Watt (= J/s) (basic unit)	W
Frequency	
Hertz (basic unit)	Hz
Electric current	
Ampere (basic unit)	A
Electromotive force (electric potential)	
Volt (= W/A) (basic unit)	V
Electric resistance	
Ohm (= V/A) (basic unit)	Ω
Electric conductance	
Siemens (= Ω^{-1}) (basic unit)	S
Electric charge	
Coulomb (basic unit)	C
Electric capacitance	
Farad (= C/V) (basic unit)	F

Conversion factors			
Length			
1 km	= 0.621 371 mile	1 mile	= 1.609 344 km
1 m	= 1.093 61 yd	1 yd	= 0.9144 m
1 m	= 3.280 84 ft	1 ft	= 0.3048 m
1 mm	= 0.039 370 1 in	1 in	= 25.4 mm
Area			
1 km^2	= 0.386 102 mile^2	1 acre	= 0.404 686 ha
1 ha	= 2.471 05 acres		= 4046.86 m^2
1 m^2	= 1.195 99 yd^2	1 yd^2	= 0.836 127 m^2
1 m^2	= 10.7639 ft^2	1 ft^2	= 0.092 903 m^2
1 mm^2	= 0.001 55 in^2	1 in^2	= 645.16 mm^2
Volume			
1 m^3	= 1.307 95 yd^3	1 yd^3	= 0.764 555 m^3
1 m^3	= 35.3147 ft^3	100 super ft	= 0.235 973 m^3
1 m^3	= 423.776 super ft		
1 mm^3	= 6.10237×10^{-5} in^3	1 ft^3	= 0.028 316 8 m^3
1 litre	= 0.035 314 7 ft^3	1 ft^3	= 28.3168 L
1 litre	= 0.219 969 gal	1 gal	= 4.546 09 L
1 litre	= 1.759 76 pint	1 pt	= 568.261 mL
1 mL	= 0.061 023 7 in^3	1 fl oz	= 28.413 mL
1 mL	= 0.035 195 1 fl oz		

Conversion factors *(continued)*

Speed

1 m/s	= 3.280 84 ft/s	1 ft/s	= 0.3048 m/s
1 m/s	= 2.236 94 mile/h	1 mile/h	= 1.609 344 km/h
1 km/h	= 0.621 371 mile/h	1 mile/h	= 0.447 04 m/s

Temperature

1°C	= 1 K = 1.8°F	°C	= 5/9 (°F − 32)
1°F	= 0.555 556°C	°F	= 9/5 °C + 32
1°F	= 5/9°C	1°F	= 5/9 K

Mass

1 tonne	= 0.984 207 ton	1 ton	= 1.016 05 t
1 tonne	= 19.6841 cwt	1 cwt	= 50.8023 kg
1 kg	= 2.204 62 lb	1 lb	= 0.453 592 kg
1 g	= 0.035 274 oz	1 oz	= 28.3495 g
1 kg/m	= 0.671 969 lb/ft	1 lb/ft	= 1.488 16 kg/m
1 kg/m^2	= 0.204 816 lb/ft^2	1 lb/ft^2	= 4.882 43 kg/m^2
1 kg/m^3	= 0.624 28 lb/ft^3	1 lb/ft^3	= 16.0185 kg/m^3

Force

1 MN	= 100.361 ton f	1 ton f	= 9.964 02 kN
1 kN	= 0.100 361 ton f	1 lb f	= 4.448 22 N
1 kN	= 244.809 lb f	(for Janka hardness conversion)	
1 N	= 0.224 809 lb f		
1 N.m	= 0.737 562 lb f ft	1 lb f ft	= 1.355 82 N.m
1 N.m	= 8.850 75 lb f in	1 lb f in	= 0.112 985 N.m
1 N.m		1 ton f ft	= 3.037 03 kN.m
1 N/m	= 0.068 521 8 lb f/ft	1 lb f/ft	= 14.5939 N/m
1 kN/m	= 0.030 590 1 ton f/ft	1 ton f/ft	= 32.6903 kN/m

Pressure

1 MPa	= 0.064 749 ton f/in^2	1 lb f/in^2	= 6.894 76 kPa
1 MPa	= 9.323 85 ton f/ft^2	(for M. of R., M. of E., etc., conversion)	
1 MPa	= 145.038 lb f/in^2	1 lb f/ft^2	= 47.8803 Pa
1 kPa	= 20.8854 lb f/ft^2		

Energy

1 W	= 3.412 14 BTU/h	1 BTU	= 3.931×10^{-4} hph
1 W	= 0.737 562 ft lb f/s	1 BTU	= 0.252 kg cal
1 kWh	= 3413 BTU	1 BTU	= 778.3 ft lb
1 kWh	= 1.341 hph	1 BTU	= 1055 J
1 kWh	= 860 kg cal	1 BTU	= 1.055×10^{10} erg

Conversion factors *(continued)*

Energy *(continued)*

1 kWh	= 2.656 ft lb	1 BTU/h	= 0.2931 W
1 kWh	= 3.601×10^6 J	1 ft lb f	= 1.356 J
1 kWh	= 3.601×10^{13} erg	(for Izod impact conversion)	
1 J	= 9.478×10^{-4} BTU	1 ft lb f	= 1.285×10^{-3} BTU
1 J	= 2.778×10^{-7} kWh	1 ft lb f	= 3.765×10^{-7} kWh
1 J	= 2.388×10^{-4} kg cal	1 ft lb f	= 5.05×10^{-7} hph
1 J	= 0.7376 ft lb f	1 ft lb f	= 3.238×10^{-4} kg cal
1 J	= 1×10^7 erg	1 ft lb f/S	= 1.3558 W

Appendix 2

Moisture meter correction figures

Note: See the comment on page 88 concerning the correction figures and the reason for excluding some common species from this list.

Meter reading (% moisture content)	6	7	8	9	10	11	12	13	14	15	16	17	18	19	20	21	22	23	24
Species								Correct moisture content											
Alder, brown	8	9	10	10	11	12	13	13	14	15	15	16	17	18	18	19	20	20	21
Amberoi	6	7	7	8	9	9	10	11	12	12	13	14	14	15	16	17	17	18	19
Amoora (PNG source)	5	6	7	9	10	11	12	13	14	15	16	17	18	19	20	21	22	23	24
Antiaris (PNG source)	7	8	9	10	11	12	12	13	14	15	16	17	18	19	20	21	22	22	23
Ash, alpine	8	9	10	11	12	13	14	15	16	17	18	18	19	20	21	22	23	24	25
Ash, Crow's	8	9	10	11	12	12	12	13	14	15	16	17	18	19	20	20	21

Meter reading	6	7	8	9	10	11	12	13	14	15	16	17	18	19	20	21	22	23	24
Species	Correct moisture content																		
Ash, European	8	8	9	10	11	12	12	13	14	14	15	16	17	18	18	19	20	21	21
Ash, mountain	8	9	10	11	12	13	14	15	16	17	18	18	19	20	21	22	23	24	25
Ash, silvertop	4	5	6	7	8	9	10	11	12	13	14	15	16	17	18	19	20	21	22
Balsa	–	7	8	9	10	11	12	13	14	15	16	17	18	19	20	21	22	23	24
Baltic, red	–	9	10	11	12	13	14	15	15	16	17	18	18	19	20	21	22	23	24
Baltic, white	–	9	10	11	12	13	14	15	16	17	18	19	20	22	23	24	25	26	27
Bauvudi	7	7	8	9	9	10	11	11	12	13	13	14	15	15	16	17	17	18	18
Bean, black	8	9	10	11	12	13	14	15	16	16	17	18	19	20	21	22	23	24	25
Beech, myrtle	7	8	9	10	11	11	12	13	14	14	15	16	17	18	18	19	20	21	22
Beech, silver	9	9	10	10	11	12	12	13	13	14	14	15	16	16	17	17	18	19	19
Beech, Wau	8	9	11	12	13	14	15	16	17	18	19	20	21	22	23	24	25	26	27
Beech, white (Qld source)	7	8	9	10	11	12	13	14	14	15	16	17	18	19	19	20	21	22	23
Birch, white	8	9	10	11	12	12	13	14	15	15	16	17	18	18	19	20	21	22	22
Blackbutt	7	8	9	10	11	12	13	14	15	16	17	18	19	20	21	22	23	24	25
Blackbutt, WA	8	9	10	11	12	12	13	14	15	16	17	18	19	20	21	22	23	24	25
Blackwood	8	9	9	10	11	12	12	13	14	15	16	16	17	18	19	20	20	21	22
Bloodwood, red	9	10	10	11	12	13	14	15	15	16	17	18	19	19	20	21	22	23	23
Bollywood	7	7	8	9	10	11	12	12	13	14	15	16	16	17	18	19	20	21	22
Box, brush	6	7	7	8	8	9	9	10	10	11	11	12	13	13	14	14	15	15	16

Meter reading	6	7	8	9	10	11	12	13	14	15	16	17	18	19	20	21	22	23	24
Species								Correct moisture content											
Box, grey	9	10	11	12	12	13	14	14	15	16	17	17	18	19	20	20	21	22	23
Box, grey, coast	8	9	10	11	11	12	13	14	14	15	16	17	18	18	19	20	21	22	22
Box, kanuka	8	8	9	10	11	12	12	13	14	15	16	16	17	18	19	20	20	21	22
Brownbarrel	6	7	8	9	10	11	12	12	13	14	15	16	17	18	18	19	20	21	22
Buchanania	5	6	7	8	9	10	10	11	12	13	14	14	15	16	17	18	19	19	20
Butternut, rose	6	7	8	8	9	10	10	11	12	13	13	14	15	16	16	17	18	19	19
Candlenut	–	5	8	10	12	14	16	18	21	23	25	27	29	31	34	36	38	40	42
Carabeen, yellow	7	8	9	9	10	11	12	12	13	14	14	15	16	16	17	18	18	19	20
Cedar, red	8	9	10	11	12	13	14	16	17	18	19	20	21	22	23	25	26	27	27
Cedar, red, western	–	–	8	9	9	10	11	12	13	14	15	16	17	17	18	19	20	21	22
Cedar, South American	–	9	10	11	12	13	14	15	16	16	17	17	18	19	20	21	22	22	23
Coachwood	5	6	7	8	9	10	11	12	13	14	14	15	16	17	18	19	20	21	22
Cypress, white	8	9	10	10	11	12	13	14	15	16	17	18	19	20	21	22	22	23	24
Dakua salusalu	8	9	10	11	11	12	13	14	15	16	17	18	19	19	20	21	22	23	24
Erima	7	8	8	9	10	11	12	12	13	14	15	15	16	17	18	19	19	20	21
Fir, amabilis	–	8	9	10	11	12	13	14	15	16	17	18	19	20	21	22	23	24	25
Gum, blue, southern	7	8	9	10	11	12	12	13	14	15	16	17	17	18	19	20	21	22	22
Gum, blue, Sydney	8	9	10	11	12	13	13	14	15	15	16	17	18	19	19	20	21	22	23
Gum, blue Tasmanian	7	8	9	10	11	12	12	13	14	15	16	17	17	18	19	20	21	22	22

Meter reading	6	7	8	9	10	11	12	13	14	15	16	17	18	19	20	21	22	23	24
Species	Correct moisture content																		
Gum, grey	7	8	8	9	10	11	12	13	14	15	16	17	18	19	20	21	22	23	24
Gum, grey, mountain	8	9	9	10	11	12	13	14	14	15	16	17	18	19	19	20	21	22	23
Gum, lemon-scented	6	6	7	8	9	10	10	11	12	13	13	14	15	16	17	17	18	19	20
Gum, Maiden's	9	10	11	11	12	13	14	15	16	16	17	18	19	20	20	21	22	23	24
Gum, manna	6	7	7	8	9	10	11	12	13	14	14	15	16	17	18	19	20	21	21
Gum, mountain	6	6	7	8	9	10	11	12	13	14	15	16	17	18	19	20	21	22	23
Gum, red, forest	9	10	11	12	12	13	14	15	16	17	18	18	19	20	21	22	23	24	24
Gum, red, river	9	10	11	12	13	14	15	16	17	18	19	20	21	22	23	24	25	26	27
Gum, rose	8	9	10	11	12	13	14	14	15	16	17	18	18	19	20	21	22	23	24
Gum, shining	7	8	9	10	11	11	12	13	14	15	16	17	18	19	20	20	21	22	23
Gum, spotted (NSW source)	7	8	8	9	9	10	10	11	12	12	13	13	14	14	15	15	16	17	–
Gum, spotted (Vic. source)	7	8	9	9	10	11	12	12	13	14	15	15	16	17	18	18	19	20	21
Gum, white, Dunn's	5	6	7	8	9	9	10	11	12	13	13	14	15	16	16	17	18	19	19
Gum, yellow	9	9	10	11	12	12	13	14	15	15	16	17	18	18	19	20	21	21	22
Hardwood, Johnstone River	6	6	7	8	9	10	10	11	12	13	13	14	15	16	17	17	18	19	20
Hemlock, western	7	8	9	10	11	12	13	15	16	17	18	19	20	21	22	23	24	26	27
Hickory	–	–	7	9	11	13	14	16	17	18	20	21	22	24	–	–	–	–	–
Iroko	–	7	7	8	9	10	11	12	13	14	15	15	16	17	18	19	19	20	21
Ironbark, grey (Qld source)	9	10	11	11	12	13	14	15	16	17	18	19	20	21	22	23	24	24	25

Meter reading Species	6	7	8	9	10	11	12	13	14	15	16	17	18	19	20	21	22	23	24
								Correct moisture content											
Ironbark, grey (NSW source)	7	8	9	10	11	12	13	14	15	15	16	17	18	19	20	21	22	23	24
Ironbark, red	10	11	12	12	13	14	15	16	16	17	18	19	20	21	22	22	23	24	24
Ironbark, red, broad-leaved	10	11	12	12	13	14	15	16	16	17	18	19	20	21	22	22	23	24	25
Ironbark, red, narrow-leaved	7	8	9	10	11	12	13	14	14	15	16	17	18	19	20	21	22	23	24
Jarrah	7	8	9	10	11	13	13	14	15	16	17	18	19	20	21	22	23	24	25
Jelutong (Malaysian source)	–	–	–	–	7	8	9	10	11	12	13	14	16	17	18	20	21	22	24
Kamarere (PNG source)	–	8	9	10	10	11	12	13	14	15	16	17	18	19	19	20	21	22	23
Kamarere (Fiji source)	6	7	8	8	9	10	11	11	12	13	13	14	15	15	16	17	17	18	19
Kapur (Malaysian source)	–	3	4	5	6	7	7	8	9	10	11	12	13	14	15	16	17	17	18
Karri	7	7	8	9	10	11	12	13	13	14	15	16	17	18	18	19	20	21	22
Kauri, Qld	9	10	11	12	13	14	15	16	16	17	18	19	20	21	22	23	24	24	25
Kauri, NZ	8	9	10	10	11	12	12	13	13	14	14	15	16	16	17	17	18	18	19
Kauri, Vanikoro	10	11	12	13	13	14	14	15	15	15	16	16	17	17	18	18	18	19	19
Kempas	7	8	8	9	10	11	12	13	14	15	16	17	18	19	20	21	22	23	24
Laran	7	8	8	9	10	11	11	12	13	14	14	15	16	17	17	18	18	19	19
Lumbayau	–	–	–	–	11	12	13	14	15	16	17	18	19	20	21	22	23	24	25
Mahogany, African	–	10	11	12	13	14	15	16	17	18	19	20	21	22	23	24	25	26	27
Mahogany, American	–	7	8	9	10	11	12	13	14	15	16	17	18	19	20	21	22	23	24
Mahogany, brush	8	8	9	10	10	11	11	12	12	13	14	14	15	15	16	16	17	18	18

Meter reading	6	7	8	9	10	11	12	13	14	15	16	17	18	19	20	21	22	23	24
Species	Correct moisture content																		
Mahogany, miva	9	10	11	12	12	13	14	15	15	16	17	18	18	19	20	20	21	22	23
Mahogany, red	9	10	11	12	13	14	15	16	17	18	19	20	21	22	23	24	24	25	26
Mahogany, rose	8	9	10	10	11	12	12	13	14	14	15	16	16	17	18	18	19	20	20
Mahogany, southern	7	8	9	10	11	12	12	13	14	15	16	17	18	19	20	20	21	22	23
Mahogany, white	8	9	10	11	12	13	14	15	16	17	18	19	20	21	22	23	24	25	26
Makoré	–	9	10	11	12	13	14	15	15	16	17	18	18	19	20	21	22	23	24
Malas	6	7	8	9	9	10	11	12	12	13	14	15	15	16	17	18	19	19	20
Maple, Qld	7	9	10	12	13	14	16	17	18	20	–	–	–	–	–	–	–	–	–
Maple, rose	7	8	8	9	10	10	11	12	12	13	14	14	15	16	16	17	18	18	19
Maple, sugar	–	–	7	8	10	12	13	14	15	16	17	18	19	20	21	22	23	24	–
Mararie	9	10	11	11	12	13	14	14	15	16	17	18	18	19	20	21	21	22	23
Marri	7	7	8	9	9	10	11	11	12	13	13	14	15	15	16	17	17	18	19
Matai	8	9	9	10	11	12	12	13	14	15	16	16	17	18	18	19	20	21	22
Messmate	9	10	11	12	12	13	14	15	16	16	17	18	18	19	20	21	22	22	23
Nutmeg (Fiji source)	7	7	8	9	10	11	11	12	13	14	14	15	16	17	18	18	19	20	21
Oak, European	–	7	8	9	10	11	12	13	14	15	16	17	18	19	20	21	22	23	24
Oak, New Guinea	7	7	8	9	10	11	12	13	14	15	16	17	18	19	20	21	22	23	24
Oak, silky, northern	7	8	8	9	10	11	12	13	14	15	16	17	17	18	19	20	21	22	23
Oak, silky, red	7	8	9	9	10	11	11	12	13	13	14	15	16	16	17	18	18	19	20

Meter reading	6	7	8	9	10	11	12	13	14	15	16	17	18	19	20	21	22	23	24
Species							Correct moisture content												
Oak, silky, southern	7	7	8	9	9	10	11	11	12	13	13	14	15	15	16	17	17	18	19
Oak, tulip, blush	8	8	9	9	10	11	11	12	12	13	14	14	15	16	16	17	17	18	19
Oak, tulip, brown	10	10	11	12	12	13	13	14	14	15	16	16	17	18	18	19	19	20	20
Oak, tulip, red	10	11	12	13	14	15	16	17	18	18	19	20	21	22	23	24	25	25	26
Obeche	–	7	8	9	10	10	11	12	13	14	15	15	16	16	17	18	18	19	20
Padauk, African	–	7	7	8	9	10	11	12	13	14	15	15	16	17	18	19	19	20	21
Peppermint, broad-leaved	8	9	10	11	12	13	14	15	16	17	18	19	20	21	22	23	24	25	26
Peppermint, narrow-leaved	9	10	11	11	12	13	14	14	15	16	17	18	18	19	20	21	22	22	23
Persimmon (US source)	–	7	8	9	10	10	11	12	13	14	15	15	16	16	17	18	18	19	20
Pine, black	6	7	8	9	10	11	12	12	13	14	15	16	16	17	18	19	19	20	21
Pine, bunya	9	10	11	12	12	13	14	14	15	16	16	17	18	18	19	20	21	21	22
Pine, celery-top	8	9	10	10	11	12	13	13	14	15	16	16	17	18	19	19	20	21	21
Pine, Corsican (NZ source)	–	–	10	11	12	13	14	15	16	18	19	20	21	22	24	25	26	27	28
Pine, hoop	9	10	11	12	12	13	14	15	16	16	17	18	19	20	21	22	22	23	24
Pine, Huon	9	10	10	11	12	13	13	14	15	16	16	17	18	18	19	20	20	21	22
Pine, King William	9	9	10	11	12	12	13	14	14	15	16	16	17	18	18	19	20	20	21
Pine, klinki	6	7	8	9	10	11	12	13	14	15	16	17	18	19	20	21	22	23	24
Pine, loblolly (Qld source)	8	8	9	10	11	12	13	14	15	16	17	18	19	20	21	22	23	24	25
Pine, longleaf	–	9	10	11	12	13	14	15	16	17	18	19	20	21	22	23	24	25	27

Meter reading	6	7	8	9	10	11	12	13	14	15	16	17	18	19	20	21	22	23	24
Species	Correct moisture content																		
Pine, maritime	9	10	11	12	12	13	14	15	15	16	17	18	18	19	20	21	21	22	23
Pine, white, NZ	–	–	–	–	11	12	12	13	14	15	16	16	17	18	19	19	20	21	22
Pine, Parana	6	7	8	9	10	11	12	13	14	15	16	16	17	18	19	20	21	22	23
Pine, ponderosa	–	7	9	10	11	13	14	15	16	17	18	19	20	21	22	22	23	24	25
Pine, radiata (SA source)	9	10	11	11	12	13	14	15	16	17	18	19	20	21	22	24	25	26	27
Pine, slash (Qld source)	7	8	9	10	11	12	13	14	15	16	17	17	18	19	20	21	22	23	24
Pine, sugar	7	8	9	10	11	12	13	14	15	16	17	18	20	21	22	23	24	25	26
Pine, white, western	–	–	8	9	10	11	11	12	13	14	15	16	17	17	18	19	20	21	22
Quandong, silver	7	7	8	9	10	10	11	12	12	13	14	14	15	16	16	17	18	18	19
Raintree	6	6	7	7	8	8	9	9	10	10	11	11	12	–	–	–	–	–	–
Redwood	8	9	10	10	11	12	13	14	15	16	16	17	18	19	20	20	21	22	23
Rosarosa	8	8	9	10	10	11	12	13	13	14	15	15	16	17	18	18	19	–	–
Sapele	–	9	10	11	12	13	14	15	16	17	18	19	20	22	23	24	25	26	27
Sassafras	8	8	9	10	10	11	12	13	13	14	15	16	16	17	18	18	19	20	21
Sassafras, southern	9	9	10	11	11	12	13	13	14	15	15	16	17	17	18	19	19	20	21
Satinash, grey	7	8	9	9	10	11	12	13	14	15	16	16	17	18	19	20	21	22	23
Satinash, New Guinea	6	7	8	8	9	10	11	11	12	13	13	14	15	16	16	17	18	19	19
Satinash, rose	6	7	7	8	8	9	10	10	11	12	12	13	13	14	15	15	16	–	–
Satinay	6	7	8	9	10	11	12	13	14	15	16	17	18	19	20	21	22	23	24

Meter reading	6	7	8	9	10	11	12	13	14	15	16	17	18	19	20	21	22	23	24
Species							Correct moisture content												
Satinheart, green	9	9	10	10	11	11	12	12	13	13	14	14	15	15	16	16	17	–	–
Sepetir (Malaysian source)	3	4	5	6	7	8	9	10	11	12	13	14	15	16	17	18	19	20	21
Sheoak, river	8	8	9	10	10	11	11	12	12	13	13	14	15	16	16	17	17	18	19
Sheoak, rose	9	9	10	11	11	12	13	13	14	14	14	15	16	16	17	18	18	19	19
Sheoak, WA	9	9	10	11	11	12	12	13	14	14	15	16	16	17	18	18	19	20	20
Silkwood, bolly	9	9	10	11	11	12	12	13	13	14	15	15	15	16	16	17	17	18	18
Silkwood, red	5	6	7	8	8	9	10	10	11	12	12	13	14	14	15	16	17	17	18
Silkwood, silver	9	9	10	11	12	12	13	14	15	15	16	17	18	18	19	20	20	21	22
Spruce, Sitka	–	7	8	9	10	11	12	13	15	16	17	18	19	20	21	22	23	24	25
Stringybark, brown	8	9	10	11	11	12	13	14	15	16	17	18	19	19	20	21	22	23	24
Stringybark, Darwin	7	8	8	10	10	11	12	13	14	15	15	16	17	18	19	20	21	22	22
Stringybark, yellow	10	11	12	13	14	14	15	16	17	18	18	19	20	21	21	22	23	24	24
Sycamore	–	7	7	8	9	10	11	12	13	14	15	15	16	17	18	19	19	20	21
Sycamore, satin	8	9	9	10	11	11	12	12	13	14	14	15	16	16	17	18	18	19	20
Sycamore, silver	9	9	10	10	11	12	12	13	13	14	14	15	16	16	17	17	18	19	19
Tallowwood	6	7	8	10	10	11	12	13	14	15	16	17	18	19	20	21	22	23	24
Tawa	9	9	10	11	11	12	12	12	13	13	14	14	15	15	16	16	17	17	18
Teak	–	7	8	8	9	10	11	12	13	14	15	15	16	17	18	19	19	20	21
Tingle, red	7	9	11	11	12	13	15	16	17	18	19	21	22	23	24	25	27	28	29

Meter reading	6	7	8	9	10	11	12	13	14	15	16	17	18	19	20	21	22	23	24
Species								Correct moisture content											
Tingle, yellow	7	9	10	11	12	13	14	15	17	18	19	20	21	22	23	25	26	27	28
Totara	8	8	9	10	10	11	12	12	13	14	14	15	16	16	17	18	18	19	19
Touriga, red	10	11	11	12	13	14	14	15	16	17	17	18	19	20	20	21	22	23	23
Tuart	9	9	10	11	12	12	13	14	15	15	16	17	17	18	19	20	20	21	22
Turpentine	7	8	9	10	11	12	13	14	15	15	16	17	18	19	20	21	22	23	24
Vitex, New Guinea	7	8	8	9	10	11	12	13	13	14	15	16	17	18	18	19	20	21	22
Walnut, African	–	10	11	12	13	14	15	16	17	18	19	20	21	22	23	24	25	26	27
Walnut, blush	9	10	11	11	12	12	13	14	14	15	16	16	17	18	18	19	19	20	21
Walnut, European	–	9	10	11	12	13	14	15	16	17	18	19	20	22	23	24	25	26	27
Walnut, New Guinea	6	7	8	9	10	11	12	13	14	15	16	17	17	18	19	20	–	–	–
Walnut, Qld	7	9	10	11	12	13	14	15	16	17	18	19	20	22	23	24	25	26	27
Walnut, yellow	6	7	8	8	9	10	10	11	12	12	13	14	14	15	16	17	17	18	19
Wandoo	9	10	11	12	13	14	15	16	16	17	18	19	20	21	22	23	24	25	25
Wattle, hickory	8	8	9	10	11	11	12	13	13	14	14	15	16	16	17	18	18	19	20
Wattle, silver	8	9	10	10	11	12	13	13	14	15	16	16	17	18	19	20	20	21	22
Woollybutt	9	10	10	11	12	13	14	15	15	16	17	18	19	20	20	21	22	23	24
Yertchuk	9	10	11	12	13	14	15	16	17	18	19	20	20	21	22	23	24	25	26

Some mechanical properties

Notes

1. Modulus of rupture, modulus of elasticity and maximum crushing strength are used to decide strength grouping. Impact figures are an indicator of resistance to sudden shock loads. Hardness figures are a measure of resistance to denting. The figures quoted should be used only as broad guidelines.

2. The basic density figures for a number of species have been given. Although of little interest to those concerned with the use of timber for construction purposes, basic density is commonly referred to in the literature associated with the pulp and paper industry. Basic density is a measure of the amount of actual wood substance present and is calculated as the oven-dry mass of a specimen divided by its green volume. If one knows the basic density, it is possible to calculate the approximate mass at any moisture content above the fibre saturation point.

$$\text{Mass at } x \text{ per cent moisture content} = \frac{\text{Basic density} \times (100 + x)}{100} \text{ kg/m}^3$$

Species	Source of test material	Density (see note 2) (kg/m³)			Modulus of rupture (MPa)		Modulus of elasticity (GPa)		Maximum crushing strength (MPa)		Impact (Izod value) (J)		Hardness (Janka) (kN)	
		Basic	Green	Dry	Green	Dry	Green	Dry	Green	Dry	Green	Dry	Green	Dry
Afrormosia	Ghana	–	–	700	108	134	11	13	54	71	–	–	7.1	6.9
Alder, blush	NSW	500	900	600	58	83	10	12	27	44	6.9	6.5	3.2	4.5
Alder, brown	NSW	480	900	600	52	97	10	13	23	42	7.6	8.8	3.0	3.9
Alder, hard	Qld	640	–	780	–	127	–	16	29	59	7.2	11.4	4.6	7.3
Amberoi	Papua New Guinea	310	–	370	36	46	7.6	8.4	17	30	5.9	8.0	1.3	1.6
Amoora	Papua New Guinea	460	–	540	49	85	9.7	12	25	46	8.8	11	2.7	3.8
Antiaris	West Africa	–	–	430	–	59	–	7.2	–	37	–	–	–	2.3
Antiaris	Papua New Guinea	350	–	400	35	51	6.2	7.4	18	32	5.3	11	1.4	1.7
Apple, black	NSW	680	1130	880	85	145	15	17	37	64	15	15	6.7	8.8
Apple, rough-barked	Qld/NSW	680	1180	850	–	110	–	11	–	62	–	18	–	8.6
Apple, smooth-barked	NSW	770	1240	990	83	132	14	16	34	62	15	24	7.3	10
Ash, alpine	Tas., Vic., NSW	490	1050	620	63	110	11	15	33	60	13	18	4.0	4.9
Ash, Blue Mountains	NSW	550	1080	700	67	93	11	13	25	48	14	14	4.5	5.2
Ash, Crow's	NSW	800	1050	950	105	135	14	17	54	70	23	17	8.5	11
Ash, European	Great Britain	–	–	700	66	116	9.5	12	27	53	–	–	4.3	6.1
Ash, mountain	Tas., Vic.	520	1030	680	63	110	13	16	30	63	13	20	3.4	4.9
Ash, red	NSW	610	1100	740	83	134	13	19	38	70	9.0	18	6.2	8.4

Species	Source of test material	Density (see note 2) (kg/m³)			Modulus of rupture (MPa)		Modulus of elasticity (GPa)		Maximum crushing strength (MPa)		Impact (Izod value) (J)		Hardness (Janka) (kN)	
		Basic	Green	Dry	Green	Dry	Green	Dry	Green	Dry	Green	Dry	Green	Dry
Ash, silver, northern	Qld	560	–	680	70	103	10	13	32	56	14	16	4.4	5.3
Ash, silver, Queensland	Qld	520	–	620	62	92	11	13	29	52	14	14	3.5	5.0
Ash, silver, southern	NSW	570	–	700	61	122	12	17	26	65	9.3	9.4	3.1	6.5
Ash, silvertop	NSW, Vic.	670	1200	820	69	136	10	17	38	70	12	20	7.2	9.5
Ash, white	NSW	550	950	700	65	139	11	23	35	78	14	–	4.6	5.6
Balsa	Ecuador	–	–	170	–	19	–	3.8	–	12	–	–	–	0.4
Baltic, red	Europe	–	–	480	44	83	7.7	10	21	45	–	–	2.0	2.6
Baltic, red	Great Britain	–	–	510	46	89	7.3	10	22	47	–	–	2.2	3.0
Baltic, white	Europe	–	–	420	39	72	7.4	10	18	37	–	–	1.5	2.1
Baltic, white	Great Britain	–	–	400	36	66	6.3	8.5	17	35	–	–	1.4	2.0
Banksia, wallum	Qld	–	–	650	–	56	–	–	–	33	–	–	–	4.2
Basswood, New Guinea	Papua New Guinea	330	–	390	40	61	8.7	9.6	18	36	6.9	7.6	1.2	1.7
Bean, black	NSW	570	1100	770	64	115	14	15	34	65	4.8	11	7.4	7.5
Beech, canary	Qld	–	–	610	–	97	–	–	–	52	–	6.0	–	4.0
Beech, European	Great Britain	–	–	690	65	118	9.8	13	28	56	9.3	14	4.3	6.4
Beech, European	Italy	–	–	675	–	108	–	10	–	52	–	–	–	5.7
Beech, myrtle	Tas.	580	–	700	71	108	12	14	33	56	12	13	4.4	5.9

Species	Source of test material	Density (see note 2) (kg/m³)			Modulus of rupture (MPa)		Modulus of elasticity (GPa)		Maximum crushing strength (MPa)		Impact (Izod value) (J)		Hardness (Janka) (kN)	
		Basic	Green	Dry	Green	Dry	Green	Dry	Green	Dry	Green	Dry	Green	Dry
Beech, negrohead	NSW	610	1050	770	69	125	12	16	33	63	17	14	5.4	7.6
Beech, New Guinea	Papua New Guinea	640	–	830	74	128	15	16	37	69	18	18	5.2	6.2
Beech, red	New Zealand	–	980	720	63	79	12	13	27	52	16	6.2	3.4	5.6
Beech, silky	NSW	580	1030	720	70	110	11	15	33	59	12	9.5	4.6	7.2
Beech, silver	New Zealand	510	900	550	52	84	8.8	12	24	42	11	12	2.7	3.2
Beech, Wau	Papua New Guinea	390	–	480	47	79	8.3	9.8	26	45	12	7.9	3.4	3.0
Beech, white	NSW	430	950	500	50	74	8.3	11	25	40	6.4	5.4	2.9	2.9
Beech, white	Papua New Guinea	400	–	470	47	61	8.7	8.8	26	36	8.7	6.3	2.1	2.0
Belah	NSW	950	1250	1150	121	121	15	16	51	48	18	13	8.1	20
Belian	Sabah	–	–	1000	143	178	18	18	80	94	–	–	13	13
Birch, white	NSW	500	980	640	65	95	12	14	29	53	9.2	9.5	3.8	4.5
Blackbutt	NSW, Qld	710	1100	900	100	144	17	19	48	77	21	22	7.3	9.1
Blackbutt, New England	NSW	700	1150	930	81	140	12	14	41	68	17	19	6.8	9.5
Blackbutt, Western Australian	WA	680	1120	850	66	99	12	13	37	65	13	11	5.5	6.9
Blackwood	Tas.	570	870	640	70	99	13	13	33	48	15	13	4.6	5.9
Bloodwood, brown	NSW	870	1250	1050	95	89	12	13	51	65	13	6.9	8.5	13
Bloodwood, red	NSW	750	1150	900	93	115	13	15	50	70	15	11	8.5	8.8

Species	Source of test material	Density (see note 2) (kg/m³)			Modulus of rupture (MPa)		Modulus of elasticity (GPa)		Maximum crushing strength (MPa)		Impact (Izod value) (J)		Hardness (Janka) (kN)	
		Basic	Green	Dry	Green	Dry	Green	Dry	Green	Dry	Green	Dry	Green	Dry
Bollywood	NSW	410	760	500	53	74	10	11	24	40	8.9	8.0	2.3	2.7
Bonewood	NSW	680	1100	860	81	164	16	23	36	67	13	16	7.0	10
Box, brush	NSW, Qld	710	1160	900	85	123	12	15	38	68	17	15	7.9	9.5
Box, grey	NSW, Vic.	900	1170	1120	105	163	15	20	52	80	19	18	11	15
Box, grey, coast	NSW, Vic.	880	1180	1100	103	163	17	21	50	73	23	26	10	13
Box, kanuka	NSW	640	1160	840	81	145	17	19	36	64	17	20	4.1	8.0
Box, steel	NSW	–	1290	1130	90	136	14	19	43	82	21	–	9.2	17
Box, swamp	Qld, NSW	600	1040	900	62	82	7.0	9.4	30	54	11	8.7	6.0	9.0
Box, white-topped	NSW	800	1230	1030	98	163	17	18	47	71	20	13	8.2	14
Box, yellow	Vic.	900	1300	1100	85	122	11	14	46	68	18	12	11	13
Brigalow	NSW	780	1100	900	112	127	14	18	48	58	16	16	8.4	10
Brownbarrel	Vic., NSW	570	1140	750	80	107	14	14	36	65	18	13	5.7	6.4
Calophyllum	Papua New Guinea	500	–	590	59	102	11	14	34	58	9.9	12	3.6	4.6
Camphorwood	NSW	460	840	560	56	93	10	14	24	43	8.4	13	3.2	4.1
Candlebark	Vic.	550	–	740	61	95	10	13	30	55	13	11	5.0	5.9
Carabeen, yellow	NSW	520	880	620	64	107	11	15	28	55	9.0	7.8	3.2	4.9
Carbeen	NSW	770	1160	1000	81	–	15	–	38	–	13	–	5.3	–

Species	Source of test material	Density (see note 2) [kg/m³] Basic	Green	Dry	Modulus of rupture (MPa) Green	Dry	Modulus of elasticity (GPa) Green	Dry	Maximum crushing strength (MPa) Green	Dry	Impact (Izod value) (J) Green	Dry	Hardness (Janka) (kN) Green	Dry
Cedar, Alaska	North America	–	–	500	45	78	8.5	11	21	45	–	–	2.0	2.6
Cedar, pencil, Virginian	USA	–	–	520	48	61	4.5	6.1	25	42	–	–	2.9	4.0
Cedar, Port Orford	Great Britain	–	–	415	34	68	3.9	5.5	14	29	–	–	1.7	2.6
Cedar, Port Orford	USA	–	–	–	43	78	9.8	12	22	45	–	–	1.8	2.5
Cedar, red	NSW	350	640	420	47	65	9.0	9.4	25	36	5.0	5.5	2.1	2.3
Cedar, red	Papua New Guinea	310	–	375	35	59	6.3	7.9	20	32	5.0	3.9	1.6	1.7
Cedar, red, western	Canada	–	–	380	37	54	7.2	8.3	19	34	–	–	1.2	1.5
Cedar, red, western	Great Britain	–	–	370	38	65	5.4	7.0	18	35	–	–	1.6	2.0
Cedar, red, western	USA	–	–	–	35	53	6.3	7.7	19	35	–	–	1.2	1.6
Cedar, South American	Brazil	–	–	–	44	78	8.1	9.8	21	41	–	–	2.0	2.5
Cedar, South American	Nicaragua	–	–	360	36	54	6.0	7.0	19	31	–	–	1.6	2.2
Cedar, white	Qld	390	640	450	–	71	–	–	–	35	–	6.6	–	2.5
Cheesewood, white	Papua New Guinea	310	–	385	36	60	7.8	9.1	20	29	7.5	4.2	1.9	1.7
Coachwood	NSW	490	850	620	59	100	12	14	28	48	11	12	3.4	4.6
Cottonwood, eastern	USA	–	–	400	35	55	6.5	8.6	15	28	–	–	1.7	1.9
Cypress, black	NSW	590	780	710	63	74	8.0	9.0	32	45	7.7	3.6	5.2	6.6
Cypress, coast	NSW	490	880	550	69	61	9.0	8.2	33	45	–	3.1	4.4	–

Species	Source of test material	Density (see note 2) (kg/m³)			Modulus of rupture (MPa)		Modulus of elasticity (GPa)		Maximum crushing strength (MPa)		Impact (Izod value) (J)		Hardness (Janka) (kN)	
		Basic	Green	Dry	Green	Dry	Green	Dry	Green	Dry	Green	Dry	Green	Dry
Cypress, white	Qld, Vic.	580	770	680	71	79	7.7	9.0	40	53	7.8	4.6	5.6	6.5
Doughwood	NSW	430	770	530	48	75	8	11	22	38	5.8	5.8	2.4	3.6
Ebony	Nigeria	–	1010	–	–	189	–	18	–	92	–	–	–	14
Ebony	West Africa	–	–	820	–	117	–	11	–	59	6.0	4.8	–	9.5
Erima	Papua New Guinea	310	–	370	36	53	6.5	8.2	23	36	–	–	1.5	1.6
Erima	Sabah	–	–	350	37	52	5.3	6.3	22	33	–	–	1.4	1.7
Fir, alpine	USA	–	–	360	34	59	7.2	8.9	16	34	–	–	1.2	1.6
Fir, alpine	Canada	–	–	390	36	55	8.7	10	17	35	–	–	1.2	1.6
Fir, amabilis	Canada	–	–	440	38	69	9.3	11	19	41	–	–	1.4	2.0
Fir, amabilis	USA	–	–	460	39	73	8.7	12	18	45	–	–	1.4	1.9
Fir, balsam	Canada	–	–	390	37	58	7.8	9.7	17	34	–	–	1.3	1.8
Fir, balsam	USA	–	–	400	34	52	6.6	8.5	17	31	–	–	1.3	1.8
Fir, Douglas	NSW	410	730	510	56	90	12	13	26	55	–	–	2.1	3.1
Fir, Douglas	Canada	–	–	540	52	89	11	13	25	50	–	–	2.1	3.0
Fir, Douglas	Canada (coast type)	–	–	560	56	97	11	13	27	55	–	–	2.3	3.2
Fir, Douglas	Great Britain	–	–	500	53	91	8.3	11	25	48	–	–	2.4	3.4
Fir, Douglas	New Zealand	–	750	480	56	98	11	13	28	54	–	–	2.5	3.3

Species	Source of test material	Density (see note 2) (kg/m³)			Modulus of rupture (MPa)		Modulus of elasticity (GPa)		Maximum crushing strength (MPa)		Impact (Izod value) (J)		Hardness (Janka) (kN)	
		Basic	Green	Dry	Green	Dry	Green	Dry	Green	Dry	Green	Dry	Green	Dry
Fir, Douglas	USA (coast type)	–	–	540	52	84	11	13	27	51	–	–	2.2	3.2
Fir, Douglas	USA (mountain type)	–	–	–	50	86	9.3	12	24	47	–	–	1.9	2.6
Fir, grand	USA	–	–	420	40	61	8.6	11	20	37	–	–	1.6	2.2
Fir, noble	USA	–	–	430	43	74	9.5	12	21	42	–	–	1.3	1.8
Fir, red, Californian	USA	–	–	430	40	72	8.1	10	19	38	–	–	1.6	2.2
Giam	Papua New Guinea	–	–	1000	119	169	22	24	70	94	18	22	9.2	10
Gidgee	Qld	1100	1330	1250	–	159	–	18	–	101	–	16	–	19
Greenheart	Guyana	–	–	970	140	180	16	21	67	90	–	–	8.4	11
Guarea	West Africa	–	–	550	74	103	8.9	9.4	35	53	–	–	3.9	4.0
Gum, blue, southern	Vic.	700	1100	900	78	146	11	20	40	83	16	23	7.3	12
Gum, blue, Sydney	NSW	650	1070	850	91	140	16	18	44	68	16	18	6.4	9.0
Gum, grey	NSW	850	1240	1080	110	140	16	18	51	72	19	21	10	14
Gum, grey, mountain	Vic., NSW	690	1100	880	97	142	15	18	41	77	17	20	7.0	10
Gum, Maiden's	Vic., NSW	740	1100	950	83	147	14	19	43	84	21	22	7.5	11
Gum, manna	Tas., Vic., NSW	550	1100	750	74	108	13	14	34	61	18	12	5.4	6.0
Gum, mountain	Vic., NSW	560	1100	700	67	117	11	13	32	50	15	8.2	5.1	5.7
Gum, red, forest	Qld, NSW, Vic.	900	1200	1050	85	120	12	14	44	70	19	16	12	12

Species	Source of test material	Density (see note 2) (kg/m³)			Modulus of rupture (MPa)		Modulus of elasticity (GPa)		Maximum crushing strength (MPa)		Impact (Izod value) (J)		Hardness (Janka) (kN)	
		Basic	Green	Dry	Green	Dry	Green	Dry	Green	Dry	Green	Dry	Green	Dry
Gum, red, river	Qld, Vic.	710	1130	900	64	101	8	11	33	55	14	8.1	7.7	10
Gum, rose	NSW, Qld	510	950	620	79	122	13	17	36	66	15	16	5.3	7.5
Gum, round-leaved	NSW	690	1220	960	81	140	14	23	38	54	10	11	–	12
Gum, scribbly	NSW, Qld	600	1150	930	60	95	10	13	30	60	9.5	10	5.5	7.5
Gum, shining	Vic.	530	1050	700	62	99	10	13	31	58	15	16	4.8	5.8
Gum, spotted	NSW	740	1150	950	99	150	18	23	50	75	20	24	8.0	11
Gum, white, Dunn's	NSW	610	1100	800	74	135	17	22	34	69	12	21	5.5	7.2
Gum, yellow	Vic.	870	1200	1010	87	111	11	12	44	67	17	8.5	9.1	11
Hemlock, western	Canada	–	–	510	50	88	9.5	12	25	52	–	–	2.2	3.0
Hemlock, western	Canada	–	–	480	48	81	10	12	25	47	–	–	2.1	2.7
Hemlock, western	Great Britain	–	–	430	41	76	6.8	8.0	20	41	–	–	2.0	2.6
Hemlock, western	USA	–	–	–	42	70	8.4	10	21	43	–	–	1.9	2.6
Hickory	Canada	–	–	–	71	132	11	16	30	58	–	–	6.0	9.5
Hickory	USA	–	–	–	76	139	11	15	32	64	–	–	–	–
Iroko	West Africa	–	–	660	74	90	8.3	9.4	35	55	–	–	4.8	5.6
Ironbark, grey	NSW	890	1210	1120	120	181	20	24	60	95	24	27	11	14
Ironbark, red	NSW, Vic.	920	1220	1130	108	135	16	17	54	75	17	14	11	13

Species	Source of test material	Density (see note 2) (kg/m³)			Modulus of rupture (MPa)		Modulus of elasticity (GPa)		Maximum crushing strength (MPa)		Impact (Izod value) (J)		Hardness (Janka) (kN)	
		Basic	Green	Dry	Green	Dry	Green	Dry	Green	Dry	Green	Dry	Green	Dry
Ironbark, red, broad-leaved	NSW	910	1210	1140	110	167	18	24	60	79	17	18	12	14
Ironbark, red, narrow-leaved	NSW	910	1160	1090	116	118	15	16	59	70	18	13	12	14
Ironwood	NSW	810	1100	1020	105	185	20	20	43	84	20	24	9.5	9.7
Ironwood, Cooktown	NT	1030	–	1220	140	–	–	–	85	–	22	–	13	–
Ivorywood	NSW	660	1110	860	69	148	12	20	28	66	12	19	5.6	10
Jarrah	WA	670	1170	820	68	112	10	13	36	61	13	10	5.7	8.5
Jelutong	South-East Asia	–	–	400	39	50	8.0	8.1	21	27	–	–	1.5	1.7
Kamarere	Papua New Guinea	540	–	690	71	105	12	14	48	70	18	19	4.4	5.3
Kapur	Sabah	750	–	–	82	119	11	14	41	66	–	–	4.0	5.4
Karri	WA	690	1200	900	73	132	14	19	36	72	21	24	6.0	9.0
Kauri, East Indian	Papua New Guinea	–	–	490	41	67	7.6	9.3	21	43	8.1	4.3	2.6	2.7
Kauri, New Zealand	New Zealand	–	820	560	54	90	11	13	23	39	14	11	2.1	3.3
Kauri, North Queensland	Qld	400	720	480	46	64	6.8	7.8	24	38	5.4	2.3	2.3	2.3
Keruing	Philippines	–	–	590	64	112	12	16	30	59	–	–	3.6	5.3
Keruing	Sabah	–	–	770	82	137	12	14	39	72	–	–	4.7	5.7
Keruing	Sabah	–	–	640	70	110	13	14	35	60	–	–	3.2	4.6
Kurrajong, flame	NSW	320	800	420	31	34	9.4	7.0	16	20	4.5	6.2	1.1	1.3

Species	Source of test material	Density (see note 2) (kg/m³) Basic	Green	Dry	Modulus of rupture (MPa) Green	Dry	Modulus of elasticity (GPa) Green	Dry	Maximum crushing strength (MPa) Green	Dry	Impact (Izod value) (J) Green	Dry	Hardness (Janka) (kN) Green	Dry
Kwila	Papua New Guinea	650	–	830	103	147	15	18	55	81	18	14	7.6	8.6
Kwila	Qld	–	–	770	–	130	–	12	–	63	–	7.7	–	7.2
Larch, European	Great Britain	–	–	545	53	92	7.9	9.9	24	47	–	–	2.4	3.6
Larch, European	New Zealand	–	750	560	51	68	9.1	12	22	49	–	–	2.0	4.3
Larch, western	Canada	–	–	640	60	107	11	14	31	61	–	–	2.6	4.2
Larch, western	USA	–	–	560	53	90	10	13	26	53	–	–	2.3	3.7
Lignum-vitae	Central America	–	–	–	–	–	–	–	–	79	–	–	–	20
Mahogany, African	Ghana	–	–	530	60	83	7.7	9.2	28	46	–	–	3.2	4.1
Mahogany, African	West Africa	–	–	–	52	76	8.1	9.6	25	44	–	–	3.0	3.8
Mahogany, American	British Honduras	–	–	500	–	83	–	8.8	–	44	–	–	–	3.1
Mahogany, American	Central & South America	–	–	–	64	80	11	10	31	46	–	–	3.1	3.6
Mahogany, brush	NSW	550	900	650	64	108	12	14	28	56	15	12	4.0	5.8
Mahogany, miva	NSW	540	1120	670	65	92	12	11	31	54	12	7.2	5.1	5.3
Mahogany, Philippine, dark red	Philippines	–	–	–	55	83	10	12	26	43	–	–	2.6	3.2
Mahogany, Philippine, light red	Philippines	–	–	440	51	78	9.8	11	25	40	–	–	2.1	2.6
Mahogany, red	NSW, Qld	790	1150	950	78	140	16	18	50	76	14	15	9.0	12
Mahogany, rose	NSW	590	1120	720	70	116	10	12	39	68	11	–	5.3	8.3

Species	Source of test material	Density (see note 2) [kg/m³]			Modulus of rupture (MPa)		Modulus of elasticity (GPa)		Maximum crushing strength (MPa)		Impact (Izod value) (J)		Hardness (Janka) (kN)	
		Basic	Green	Dry	Green	Dry	Green	Dry	Green	Dry	Green	Dry	Green	Dry
Mahogany, southern	NSW, Vic.	720	1180	920	84	130	15	18	46	77	18	18	7.0	9.0
Mahogany, white	NSW	780	1200	1000	101	130	16	17	49	76	17	14	8.5	10
Makoré	Ghana	–	–	610	75	101	8.2	10	37	53	–	–	4.1	4.9
Malas	Papua New Guinea	680	–	800	105	152	16	19	55	84	20	21	7.2	9.5
Mallet, brown	WA	810	1120	980	113	179	15	19	53	94	–	–	9.9	15
Mangrove, grey	NSW	690	1150	850	62	76	9	9	36	45	–	6.9	5.9	8.4
Mangrove, red	Papua New Guinea	–	–	980	108	157	19	23	59	85	20	20	11	11
Maple, Queensland	Papua New Guinea	–	–	560	50	85	9.2	11	25	50	8.9	11	2.8	3.2
Maple, Queensland	Qld	440	–	580	–	77	–	10	–	44	–	11	–	4.7
Maple, rose	NSW	570	980	720	73	130	14	19	33	61	11	13	4.2	6.9
Maple, sugar	Canada	–	–	740	71	115	12	14	31	56	–	–	5.2	7.3
Maple, sugar	USA	–	–	–	69	109	11	13	28	54	–	–	4.3	6.4
Mararie	NSW	700	1040	840	75	173	11	21	32	64	15	13	5.8	10
Marfim, Pau	Brazil	–	–	–	99	130	–	–	42	57	–	–	6.8	–
Marri	WA	650	–	850	78	125	14	17	41	66	20	23	6.6	7.1
Matai	New Zealand	550	1100	610	62	74	8.5	9.1	28	47	5.2	19	3.0	3.4
Meranti, red, dark	Sabah	–	–	–	68	92	9.7	11	34	53	–	–	3.1	3.5

Species	Source of test material	Density (see note 2) (kg/m³)			Modulus of rupture (MPa)		Modulus of elasticity (GPa)		Maximum crushing strength (MPa)		Impact (Izod value) (J)		Hardness (Janka) (kN)	
		Basic	Green	Dry	Green	Dry	Green	Dry	Green	Dry	Green	Dry	Green	Dry
Meranti, red, light	Malaysia	–	–	–	63	88	9.7	11	32	50	–	–	2.5	2.8
Meranti, red, light	Sabah	–	–	450	50	74	7.2	9.1	25	45	–	–	2.0	2.4
Meranti, white	Sabah	–	–	–	61	81	9.1	9.7	32	48	–	–	2.9	3.2
Meranti, yellow	Sabah	–	–	–	67	91	9.0	11	32	48	–	–	3.2	3.7
Merawan	Papua New Guinea	–	–	700	97	110	15	16	44	64	10	16	4.7	4.5
Messmate	Vic., NSW	630	1080	780	75	118	14	15	35	61	16	15	5.3	7.1
Messmate, Gympie	Qld	810	–	1000	94	137	14	17	49	73	21	13	7.7	12
Myall	NSW	940	1280	1100	123	189	17	19	64	60	16	23	13	–
Oak, European	Great Britain	–	–	690	59	97	8.3	10	28	52	–	–	4.7	5.5
Oak, New Guinea	Papua New Guinea	550	–	670	57	95	12	15	28	57	14	18	4.8	4.1
Oak, silky, southern	Qld	520	1100	620	–	92	–	–	–	40	–	–	–	3.7
Oak, silky, red	NSW	670	1100	830	81	139	15	17	42	63	13	17	7.0	10
Oak, tulip, blush	NSW	630	1050	810	68	124	15	21	33	66	11	19	6.3	8.8
Oak, tulip, brown	NSW	700	1050	860	90	118	16	18	40	69	12	15	5.6	7.3
Oak, tulip, red	Qld	630	–	800	79	126	12	15	37	61	–	–	6.4	9.0
Oak, white, American	USA	–	–	750	57	105	8.6	12	25	51	–	–	4.7	6.0
Obeche	Nigeria	–	–	370	37	54	4.6	5.5	19	28	–	–	1.9	1.9

Species	Source of test material	Density (see note 2) [kg/m³]			Modulus of rupture (MPa)		Modulus of elasticity (GPa)		Maximum crushing strength (MPa)		Impact (Izod value) (J)		Hardness (Janka) (kN)	
		Basic	Green	Dry	Green	Dry	Green	Dry	Green	Dry	Green	Dry	Green	Dry
Osage-orange	Vic.	–	–	950	–	177	–	13	–	85	–	–	–	–
Peppermint, broad-leaved	Vic.	640	1100	820	73	110	11	14	38	66	13	12	6.3	8.4
Peppermint, narrow-leaved	Vic.	590	1100	800	68	117	11	14	35	62	12	12	5.0	7.1
Pine, black	Papua New Guinea	–	–	430	44	65	8.4	9.5	21	40	5.6	3.3	2.0	2.0
Pine, bunya	Qld	390	–	460	42	71	12	13	22	45	6.2	6.9	1.7	2.3
Pine, Caribbean	Central America	–	–	770	67	106	11	13	33	56	–	–	3.4	5.0
Pine, Caribbean	NSW	410	990	480	46	67	5.3	5.4	20	35	3.4	2.2	2.7	–
Pine, celery-top	Tas.	530	1050	650	69	98	9.4	12	36	56	7.6	6.5	3.9	4.5
Pine, Corsican	Corsica	–	–	–	63	–	10	–	26	–	–	–	2.8	–
Pine, Corsican	Great Britain	–	–	480	42	84	7.3	9.2	20	44	–	–	2.0	2.9
Pine, Corsican	New Zealand	–	990	530	46	77	9.5	11	23	50	–	–	2.2	3.1
Pine, hoop	Qld, NSW	450	680	530	48	90	10	13	28	53	9.1	5.6	3.0	3.4
Pine, jack	Canada	–	640	500	44	78	8.0	10	20	41	–	–	1.8	2.6
Pine, jack	USA	–	–	480	41	68	7.4	9.3	20	39	–	–	1.8	2.5
Pine, King William	Tas.	340	–	400	41	69	5.3	6.8	21	37	5.7	4.9	1.8	2.0
Pine, klinki	Papua New Guinea	380	–	450	42	77	10	12	22	44	8.4	6.5	2.0	2.4
Pine, loblolly	NSW, Qld	470	970	550	38	77	5.9	7.7	20	40	11	6.6	2.0	3.1

Species	Source of test material	Density (see note 2) (kg/m³)			Modulus of rupture (MPa)		Modulus of elasticity (GPa)		Maximum crushing strength (MPa)		Impact (Izod value) (J)		Hardness (Janka) (kN)	
		Basic	Green	Dry	Green	Dry	Green	Dry	Green	Dry	Green	Dry	Green	Dry
Pine, loblolly	USA	–	–	–	50	88	9.7	12	24	49	–	–	2.0	3.1
Pine, lodgepole	Canada	–	640	460	39	76	8.8	11	20	43	–	–	1.6	2.2
Pine, lodgepole	USA	–	–	460	38	65	7.4	9.2	18	37	–	–	1.5	2.1
Pine, longleaf	USA	–	–	660	60	101	11	14	30	58	–	–	2.6	3.9
Pine, maritime	Great Britain	–	–	480	36	77	6.6	8.9	17	40	–	–	1.7	2.7
Pine, Parana	South America	–	–	530	50	95	9.0	11	28	54	–	–	2.5	3.5
Pine, radiata	Kenya	–	–	510	41	80	7.7	9.0	19	43	–	–	2.2	3.6
Pine, radiata	New Zealand	–	930	480	41	76	7.3	9.1	18	41	–	–	2.2	2.8
Pine, radiata	SA, Vic.	400	800	500	42	81	8.1	10	19	42	12	6.9	2.1	3.3
Pine, slash	NSW, Qld	450	1000	530	42	85	7.0	9.7	22	41	8.0	5.6	2.1	3.4
Pine, slash	USA	–	–	690	61	110	11	14	30	63	–	–	2.8	4.5
Pine, sugar	USA	–	–	410	35	55	6.5	8.3	17	33	–	–	1.4	1.7
Pine, white, New Zealand	New Zealand	–	820	450	43	66	6.6	7.9	17	35,	6.5	–	2.0	3.0
Pine, white, western	Canada	–	580	410	33	64	8.2	10	17	36	–	–	1.2	1.7
Pine, white, western	USA	–	–	440	36	66	8.1	10	18	39	–	–	1.4	1.6
Pine, yellow, western	Canada	–	750	510	39	73	7.8	9.5	20	42	–	–	1.9	2.6
Pine, yellow, western	USA	–	–	450	34	63	6.7	8.7	17	36	–	–	1.4	2.0

Species	Source of test material	Density (see note 2) [kg/m³]			Modulus of rupture (MPa)		Modulus of elasticity (GPa)		Maximum crushing strength (MPa)		Impact (Izod value) (J)		Hardness (Janka) (kN)	
		Basic	Green	Dry	Green	Dry	Green	Dry	Green	Dry	Green	Dry	Green	Dry
Pine, yellow, western	NSW	310	960	370	24	57	8.0	5.2	12	33	15	6.1	1.9	–
Planchonella, red	Papua New Guinea	460	–	595	60	88	11	12	29	52	11	14	3.1	3.9
Poplar, hybrid	NSW	–	740	440	59	87	7.2	12	22	42	11	18	2.9	3.9
Poplar, pink	NSW	380	800	450	33	66	8.0	11	14	32	3.4	5.1	1.5	2.3
Purpleheart	Guyana	–	–	865	105	147	14	17	57	79	–	–	9.2	11
Quandong, silver	Qld, NSW	430	750	500	51	72	10	11	26	53	12	8.2	2.5	2.8
Ramin	Sarawak	–	–	660	71	134	10	14	39	72	–	–	2.9	5.8
Rauli	Chile	–	–	580	–	92	–	9.2	–	50	–	–	–	3.6
Redwood	USA	–	–	450	52	69	8.1	9.2	29	42	–	–	1.8	2.1
Rimu	New Zealand	520	960	600	51	77	8.4	9.0	23	37	7.1	5.6	2.8	3.5
Rosewood, Indian	South-East Asia	530	–	600	63	117	8.2	12	31	64	–	–	5.6	12
Rosewood, New Guinea	Papua New Guinea	500	–	615	74	95	10	12	38	58	13	10	4.2	4.7
Rosewood, scentless	NSW	540	–	650	64	122	11	15	26	43	8.5	7.5	5.0	7.1
Saffronheart	NSW	770	1130	950	118	198	18	21	54	96	16	16	9.0	13
Salwood, brown	Qld	–	–	700	–	128	–	–	–	60	–	–	–	5.9
Sapele	West Africa	–	–	670	74	110	10	12	36	59	–	–	4.5	6.7
Sassafras	NSW	480	950	600	60	99	11	14	30	52	8.9	8.0	3.1	4.1

Species	Source of test material	Density (see note 2) (kg/m³)			Modulus of rupture (MPa)		Modulus of elasticity (GPa)		Maximum crushing strength (MPa)		Impact (Izod value) (J)		Hardness (Janka) (kN)	
		Basic	Green	Dry	Green	Dry	Green	Dry	Green	Dry	Green	Dry	Green	Dry
Sassafras, socket	NSW	530	1020	650	70	112	13	17	33	57	11	10	4.1	6.0
Sassafras, southern	Tas.	420	–	630	–	99	–	–	–	50	–	13	–	4.7
Satinash, grey	Qld	–	–	700	61	103	9	11	33	50	15	11	4.8	5.6
Satinash, New Guinea	Papua New Guinea	610	–	770	66	110	12	16	39	68	16	14	4.2	7.7
Satinash, rose	NSW	530	900	700	60	89	9.0	11	26	51	12	12	3.2	5.2
Satinay	Qld	640	–	840	77	129	11	16	38	70	9.9	7.1	5.2	8.3
Sepetir	Sarawak	–	–	660	81	125	10	13	39	64	–	–	4.2	6.3
Sheoak, river	NSW	580	970	770	72	112	11	12	33	53	17	22	8.0	–
Sheoak, rose	NSW	770	1160	920	113	145	17	20	58	72	18	17	12	14
Spruce, black	Canada	–	590	490	41	78	9.1	10	–	42	–	–	1.7	2.4
Spruce, black	USA	–	–	450	37	72	7.3	11	18	37	–	–	1.6	2.3
Spruce, Engelmann	Canada	–	–	440	39	70	8.6	11	19	42	–	–	1.5	2.0
Spruce, Engelmann	USA	–	–	390	32	64	7.1	8.9	15	31	–	–	1.2	1.8
Spruce, red	Canada	–	560	450	41	72	9.1	11	19	39	–	–	1.6	2.3
Spruce, red	USA	–	–	460	40	70	8.2	11	18	41	–	–	1.6	2.2
Spruce, Sitka	Canada	–	500	430	38	75	9.1	11	18	40	–	–	1.5	2.3
Spruce, Sitka	Canada	–	–	440	37	70	9.5	11	18	38	–	–	1.5	2.2

Species	Source of test material	Density (see note 2) (kg/m³)			Modulus of rupture (MPa)		Modulus of elasticity (GPa)		Maximum crushing strength (MPa)		Impact (Izod value) (J)		Hardness (Janka) (kN)	
		Basic	Green	Dry	Green	Dry	Green	Dry	Green	Dry	Green	Dry	Green	Dry
Spruce, Sitka	Great Britain	–	–	385	34	67	5.9	8.1	16	36	–	–	1.6	2.1
Spruce, Sitka	USA	–	–	–	39	70	8.5	11	18	39	–	–	1.6	2.3
Spruce, white	Canada	–	610	420	35	63	7.9	9.9	17	37	–	–	1.2	1.9
Spruce, white	USA	–	–	450	39	68	7.4	9.2	18	38	–	–	1.4	2.1
Stringybark, blue-leaved	NSW	690	1070	880	96	135	14	17	40	63	12	14	5.0	7.5
Stringybark, brown	Vic., NSW	650	–	900	87	130	13	16	43	70	19	15	5.4	7.5
Stringybark, Darwin	NT	880	–	1050	145	–	–	–	74	–	28	–	9.6	–
Stringybark, diehard	NSW	610	1000	770	98	–	14	–	–	–	15	–	–	–
Stringybark, red	Vic., NSW	690	1060	900	89	123	11	16	43	63	13	16	6.6	8.7
Stringybark, silvertop	NSW	530	1030	860	87	143	15	18	38	73	17	18	5.5	8.8
Stringybark, white	NSW, Qld, Vic.	680	1100	880	92	133	14	17	43	68	15	15	6.8	8.8
Stringybark, yellow	NSW, Vic.	690	1100	870	90	132	14	17	44	72	20	14	6.3	8.5
Sycamore	Great Britain	–	–	560	66	99	8.4	9.4	28	48	–	–	3.9	4.9
Sycamore, pink	Qld	590	–	710	86	130	13	16	40	64	23	14	5.9	6.8
Sycamore, satin	Qld	510	–	620	–	107	–	13	33	55	8.4	9.1	3.4	3.9
Sycamore, silver	NSW	480	920	630	–	95	12	15	28	50	11	7.7	3.1	5.7
Tallowwood	NSW, Qld	800	1230	990	106	134	18	18	51	73	20	17	7.6	8.6

Species	Source of test material	Density (see note 2) (kg/m³)			Modulus of rupture (MPa)		Modulus of elasticity (GPa)		Maximum crushing strength (MPa)		Impact (Izod value) (J)		Hardness (Janka) (kN)	
		Basic	Green	Dry	Green	Dry	Green	Dry	Green	Dry	Green	Dry	Green	Dry
Taun	Papua New Guinea	580	–	695	67	106	11	14	31	60	14	14	4.2	6.5
Tawa	New Zealand	560	1070	720	67	108	11	14	30	58	11	11	4.6	7.1
Teak	Myanmar	–	–	640	84	106	8.8	10	43	60	–	–	4.1	4.5
Teak	India	–	–	630	76	88	10	11	38	49	–	–	4.8	4.6
Tea-tree, broad-leaved	NSW, NT	610	1070	750	76	97	9.2	13	35	53	14	11	6.6	7.3
Terminalia, brown	Papua New Guinea	390	–	465	44	68	8.3	9.9	21	37	8.9	8.3	2.5	2.8
Totara	New Zealand	410	950	480	45	53	6.3	7.4	21	38	3.7	2.3	2.3	2.4
Touriga, red	Qld	600	–	730	58	94	8.5	10	28	60	16	12	4.6	6.5
Tuart	WA	840	1250	1030	81	125	12	16	46	72	18	16	9.4	11
Turpentine	NSW, Qld	680	1130	930	83	142	14	16	42	76	14	9.5	6.5	12
Vitex, New Guinea	Papua New Guinea	610	–	705	80	113	12	14	42	64	15	7.3	5.1	5.6
Walnut, black	Canada	–	–	670	62	103	11	13	29	54	–	–	4.1	5.9
Walnut, black	USA	–	–	600	66	101	9.8	12	30	52	–	–	4.0	4.5
Walnut, blush	NSW	610	950	750	81	118	21	18	35	58	9.7	7.7	–	6.2
Walnut, New Guinea	Papua New Guinea	470	–	540	59	81	9.7	11	30	46	11	10	3.3	3.7
Wandoo	WA	920	–	1110	101	142	14	17	55	82	20	16	9.9	15
Wattle, black	NSW	630	900	740	89	124	10	18	46	41	27	39	9.9	9.2

Species	Source of test material	Density (see note 2) [kg/m³]			Modulus of rupture (MPa)		Modulus of elasticity (GPa)		Maximum crushing strength (MPa)		Impact (Izod value) (J)		Hardness (Janka) (kN)	
		Basic	Green	Dry	Green	Dry	Green	Dry	Green	Dry	Green	Dry	Green	Dry
Wattle, green	NSW	680	1150	830	82	106	16	17	42	63	15	30	7.7	11
Wattle, hickory	NSW	680	–	800	106	135	12	15	47	70	29	39	7.0	8.3
Wattle, silver	Vic.	420	800	680	60	87	10	12	30	52	14	19	4.0	5.1
Willow, cricket bat	Great Britain	–	–	420	31	62	5.6	6.6	14	27	–	–	1.8	2
Woollybutt	NSW	840	1120	1070	87	128	13	16	48	77	16	13	8.8	11
Yellowwood	NSW	560	900	680	70	135	12	19	31	71	16	16	3.5	8.2
Yertchuk	Vic., NSW	730	–	930	81	129	13	16	45	75	15	16	7.2	10

Index